RELIGION AND AIDS TREATMENT IN AFRICA

This book critically interrogates emerging interconnections between religion and biomedicine in Africa in the era of antiretroviral treatment for AIDS. Highlighting the complex relationships between religious ideologies, practices and organizations on the one hand, and biomedical treatment programmes and the scientific languages and public health institutions that sustain them on the other, this anthology charts largely uncovered terrain in the social science study of the Aids epidemic.

Religion and AIDS Treatment in Africa

Saving Souls, Prolonging Lives

Edited by

RIJK VAN DIJK
African Studies Centre, Holland

HANSJÖRG DILGER
Freie Universität Berlin, Germany

MARIAN BURCHARDT
Max Planck Institute for the Study of Religious and Ethnic Diversity, Göttingen

THERA RASING
University of Lusaka (UNILUS), Zambia

ASHGATE

Published by
Ashgate Publishing Limited
Wey Court East
Union Road
Farnham
Surrey, GU9 7PT
England

Ashgate Publishing Company
110 Cherry Street
Suite 3-1
Burlington, VT 05401-3818
USA

www.ashgate.com

British Library Cataloguing in Publication Data
A catalogue record for this book is available from the British Library

The Library of Congress has cataloged the printed edition as follows:
Religion and AIDS treatment in Africa : saving souls, prolonging lives / edited by Rijk van Dijk, Hansjörg Dilger, Marian Burchardt and Thera Rasing.
pages cm
Includes index.
ISBN 978-1-4094-5669-8 (hardcover : alk. paper) — ISBN 978-1-4724-2840-0 (ebook) — ISBN 978-1-4724-2841-7 (epub) 1. AIDS (Disease)—Treatment—Africa. 2. AIDS (Disease)—Treatment—Religious aspects—Christianity. I. Dijk, Rijk van, 1959- editor of compilation. II. Dilger, Hansjörg, editor of compilation. III. Burchardt, Marian, editor of compilation. IV. Rasing, Thera, editor of compilation.
RA643.86.A35R45 2014
362.19697'920096--dc 3

2014000528

ISBN 9781409456698 (hbk)
ISBN 9781472428400 (ebk – PDF)
ISBN 9781472428417 (ebk – ePUB)

MIX
Paper from responsible sources
FSC® C013985
www.fsc.org

Printed in the United Kingdom by Henry Ling Limited, at the Dorset Press, Dorchester, DT1 1HD

Contents

List of Figures

Notes on Contributors

Felicitas Becker obtained her PhD in African History from the University of Cambridge. She has taught at School of Oriental and African Studies, London, and Simon Fraser University, Vancouver, and now holds the post of University Lecturer in African History at Cambridge University. Her research interests focus on social history and Islam in modern East Africa. She is the author of *Becoming Muslim in Mainland Tanzania, 1890–2000* (OUP, 2008) and of articles in *Journal of African History*, *Journal of Religion in Africa*, *African Affairs and Africa*.

Marian Burchardt is a Researcher at the Max Planck Institute for the Study of Religious and Ethnic Diversity. His PhD, which he received from the University of Leipzig's Cultural Studies Department, explores the entanglements of religion, biomedicine and sexuality in South Africa's fight against HIV/AIDS from a transnational perspective. His research interests include the sociology and anthropology of religion, modern social thought, medical anthropology, the sociology of the body, transnationalism and globalization. His articles appeared in, amongst others, *Oxford Development Studies* and *Culture, Health and Sexuality*. One of his recent publications is 'Subjects of Counselling: Religion, HIV/AIDS and the Management of Everyday Life in South Africa', in *AIDS and Religious Practices in Africa*, edited by Becker and Geissler (Brill, 2009).

Hansjörg Dilger is a Professor of Social and Cultural Anthropology at Freie Universität Berlin. He has conducted long-term fieldwork on HIV/AIDS and social relations in Tanzania, focusing on the dynamics of kinship and Neo-Pentecostalism in the context of rural–urban migration, as well as on the identity politics and the limitations of collective action in urban NGOs. Dilger is author of the book *Living with AIDS: Illness, Death and Social Relationships in Africa* (Frankfurt, 2005, in German). He is also co-editor of the volume *Morality, Hope and Grief: Anthropologies of AIDS in Africa* (Oxford, 2010, with Ute Luig). His articles were published in *Anthropological Quarterly*, *African Journal of Aids Research*, *Journal of Religion in Africa*, *Medical Anthropology* and *Africa Today*. Dilger's current book project is about Christian and Muslim Schools in Dar es Salaam. He is a member of the steering committee of the Research Network Religion and AIDS in Africa.

Benjamin Kobina Kwansa studied Social and Medical Anthropology for his postgraduate programmes in the University of Ghana and the University of Amsterdam, where he successfully defended his PhD dissertation titled 'Safety in the midst of Stigma: Experiencing HIV/AIDS in two Ghanaian Communities.' His research interests are in the areas of constructions of masculinities, gender and health, HIV/AIDS, sexual and reproductive health, religion and health, and family, population and development. Between 2002 and 2006 he worked in various capacities at the Family, Population and Development Unit, and the NUFU-sponsored Care and Globalisation Project, at the Institute of African Studies, University of Ghana, where he is currently a Research Fellow. He is currently finalizing his PhD dissertation titled 'Safety in the midst of stigma: Experiencing HIV/AIDS in two Ghanaian communities'.

Alexander Leusenkamp studied cultural anthropology/culture, organization and management at the Free University of Amsterdam. Currently he is both a Lecturer in Public Health at Windesheim Honours College and a PhD candidate at the Amsterdam Institute of Social Science Research. His PhD research focuses on the implementation of HIV/AIDS antiretroviral treatment (ART) programmes in Uganda, aiming at meso-level health care management and cooperative networks involving NGOs, donors and government institutions. In addition he has conducted research on indigenous healers' perceptions regarding HIV/AIDS in Botswana, and on trade-related intellectual property rights in relation to the import of HIV/AIDS medication in Kenya.

Dominik Mattes is a Research Associate at the Institute of Social and Cultural Anthropology, Freie Universität Berlin. His doctoral research is focusing on social dynamics within the public HIV/AIDS treatment programme in Tanzania as well as the treatment's impact on patients' and their families' life worlds, conceptualizations of 'healing', and the more general discourse of HIV/AIDS. Besides HIV/AIDS, his research interests include anthropology of pharmaceuticals, global health policy, and anthropology of biomedicine.

Caroline Meier zu Biesen received her PhD degree at the Institute of Social and Cultural Anthropology, Freie Universität Berlin. Her thesis explores transformations of medical knowledge and practices entailed by the global transfer of the Chinese medicinal plant *Artemisia annua*. Her research interests include (critical) medical anthropology, anthropology of pharmaceuticals, social inequality and health, traditional medicine, bioprospecting, malaria and HIV/AIDS. She is currently working at the Center for Area Studies (CAS) at the Freie Universität Berlin with a postdoctoral research project which is applying the area of traditional medicine, modern science and antimalarial phytomedicine on Zanzibar.

Louise Mubanda Rasmussen has a background in development studies. Between 2006 and 2010 she researched various HIV/AIDS interventions in Uganda with an emphasis on Catholic organizations. She obtained her PhD degree in African Studies from the University of Copenhagen in 2011 on the basis of a thesis entitled 'From dying with dignity to living with rules: AIDS treatment and holistic care in Catholic organisations in Uganda'. She is currently working at the Department of Society and Globalization at Roskilde University with a postdoctoral research project on the local experiences with celebrity-driven development projects in Malawi.

Bjarke Oxlund is an Associate Professor at the Department of Anthropology, Faculty of Social Sciences at University of Copenhagen. In his PhD thesis from 2009, 'Love in Limpopo: Becoming a man in a South African university campus', he focused on the social development of young men in the rural province of Limpopo in a context of HIV and AIDS. His most recent publications include articles on research ethics, soldiers and HIV/AIDS in Rwanda, university reform, masculinities, and situational analysis as a research method.

Amy Patterson is Professor in the Department of Politics at University of the South, Sewanee, Tennessee, USA. She is editor of *The African State and the AIDS Crisis* (Ashgate, 2005) and author of *The Politics of AIDS in Africa* (Lynne Rienner Publishers, 2006) and *The Church and AIDS in Africa: The Politics of Ambiguity* (FirstForum Press, 2011). She has published articles on HIV and AIDS, civil society, and gender in Africa in *Africa Today*, *Journal of Modern African Studies*, *Canadian Journal of African Studies*, *African Journal of AIDS Research*, *Contemporary Politics*, and *African Studies Review*. She has conducted fieldwork in Senegal, Ghana and Zambia. As a Fulbright Scholar in 2011, she conducted research on political empowerment and social capital development among members of secular and religious support groups for people living with HIV and AIDS in Zambia. She teaches courses on international relations, global health and development, and African politics.

Thera Rasing (PhD 2001, Erasmus University, Rotterdam) studied Anthropology (specialized in Religious Anthropology) and Women and Development, both at the Free University, Amsterdam. Since 1992 she has conducted extensive research on female initiation rites and wedding ceremonies, gender relations, sexuality, traditional and Christian religion, urbanization, globalization and HIV/AIDS in Zambia. From 1995 to 2001 she was affiliated to the African Studies Centre, Leiden, the Netherlands. She worked as Lecturer at the University of Amsterdam and as Senior Lecturer at the Catholic University Malawi, both at the Department of Anthropology. From 2005 to 2010 she was Senior Lecturer at the Gender Studies Department at the

University of Zambia, and was the Head of the Gender Studies Department for two years. She is currently working as researcher at the Ministry of Community Development Mother and Child Health in Zambia. Her main publications are: *The Bush Burnt, the Stones Remain: Female Initiation Rites in Urban Zambia* (LIT Verlag, 2001) and 'The Persistence of Female Initiation Rites: Reflexivity and Resilience of Women in Zambia', in *Situating Globality: African Agency in the Appropriation of Global Culture*, edited by W. van Binsbergen and R. van Dijk (Brill, 2004).

Anthony Simpson teaches social anthropology at the University of Manchester. From 1974 to 1997 he taught English in a Catholic mission boarding school for boys in Zambia where he developed an interest in anthropology and psychology. He is the author of *'Half-London' in Zambia: Contested Identities in a Catholic Mission School* (Edinburgh University Press, 2003), an ethnography of the school that he calls St Antony's. His recent book, *Boys to Men in the Shadow of AIDS: Masculinities and HIV Risk in Zambia* (Palgrave Macmillan, 2009), is an intimate, longitudinal study which analyses the lives of a cohort of former students of St Antony's and explores how the risk of HIV infection has shaped constructions of masculinity and sexual practices.

Jack Ume Tocco is a postdoctoral researcher at the HIV Center for Clinical and Behavioral Studies at the New York State Psychiatric Institute and Columbia University in New York City. He received a PhD in Anthropology and an MPH from the University of Michigan, and an MA is Social Anthropology from the School of Oriental and African Studies, University of London. His dissertation examines the Islamic response to AIDS in northern Nigeria. He was a U.S. Peace Corps Volunteer in Niger from 2001 to 2003 and has worked as a consultant for the World Bank and Population Council in Nigeria. He has published in journals including the *African Journal of AIDS Research* and *Culture, Health, and Sexuality*.

Rijk van Dijk is an anthropologist working at the African Studies Centre, Leiden and a Professor in the study of Religion and Sexuality in Africa at the University of Amsterdam. He is an expert on Pentecostalism, globalization and transnationalism, migration, youth and healing. He has done extensive research and published on the rise of Pentecostal movements in urban areas of Malawi, Ghana and Botswana. He is the author of *Young Malawian Puritans* (ISOR Press, 1993) and has co-edited eight books. With Ria Reis and Marja Spierenburg he co-edited *The Quest for Fruition through Ngoma* (James Currey, 2000) and with Wim van Binsbergen *Situating Globality: African Agency in the Appropriation of Global Culture* (Brill, 2004). His current research deals with the religious, in particular Pentecostal, engagements with the domains of sexuality and HIV/AIDS in Botswana. Recently published articles, entitled 'Gloves in Times of AIDS: Pentecostalism, Hair and Social Distancing in Botswana', in *AIDS and Religious Practices in Africa*, edited by Becker and Geissler (Brill, 2009) and 'Marriage, Commodification and the Romantic Ethic in Botswana', in *Markets of Well-Being: Navigating Health and Healing in Africa*, edited by Marleen Dekker and Rijk van Dijk (Brill, 2010), deal with insights gained from this ongoing research. He is also the chair of the International Research Network on Religion and AIDS in Africa. In addition, he is the editor-in-chief of the journal *African Diaspora: A Journal of Transnational Africa in a Global World*, which is published by Brill, Leiden.

Acknowledgements

Some of the chapters in this book were first presented at the international symposium on 'Prolonging Life, Challenging Religion? ARVs, New Moralities and the Politics of Social Justice' held in Lusaka, Zambia, 15–17 April 2009. The symposium was organized by the International Research Network Religion and AIDS in Africa. Josien de Klerk's support was crucial for the organizing process. Importantly, the editors of this book wish to express their gratitude to the Volkswagen Foundation in Germany for sponsoring the symposium, as well as Justo Mwale College in Lusaka for hosting the event. We also thank the other participants of the symposium, as well as the anonymous reviewers whose thoughts and input provided an important source for revising the chapters. Ann Reeves from the African Studies Centre in Leiden kindly took over the language editing, and Linn Leißner (Freie Universität Berlin) did a marvellous job with preparing the final manuscript for print. Gratitude is also expressed towards the *African Journal of AIDS Research*, where earlier versions of some of the chapters in this book have been previously published.

Introduction

Religion and AIDS Treatment in Africa: The Redemptive Moment[1]

Hansjörg Dilger, Marian Burchardt and Rijk van Dijk

Introduction

This edited volume critically interrogates emerging intertwinements between religion and biomedicine in Africa in the context of AIDS treatment. In the complex relationships between religious ideologies, practices and organizations on the one hand, and biomedical treatment for AIDS (antiretroviral treatment: ART; antiretrovirals: ARVs) on the other, new dynamics are evolving in the fields of healing, care and provision of services.

Within the last 10 years, social science scholarship on religion in Africa has increasingly turned towards investigating the role of religion in the struggle against HIV/AIDS (Prince, Denis and Van Dijk 2009; Burchardt 2009a; Patterson 2011). In the initial years of the epidemic, and in the absence of treatment, the disease was seen primarily as a behavioural matter. This allowed religious groups to play a role in attempting to change behaviour along dogmatic moral lines of conduct. This moral agenda – which was complemented by the provision of care and support for those getting sick and dying from HIV/AIDS – came under pressure with the growing availability of ART at the turn of the twenty-first century. Religious groups subsequently became involved in the provision of ART, once again by incorporating antiretroviral treatment into specific moral agendas which were in turn changed by, and adjusted to, the language and requirements of biomedical interventions.

Simultaneously, medical anthropologists began to conceptualize the significance of religious imaginaries and communities, within medical traditions and practices, as they bear on the ways in which HIV/AIDS is experienced and dealt with (Becker and Geissler 2007; Dilger 2001). This volume seeks to engage *both* fields of investigation – medical anthropology and the study of religion in Africa – in relation to HIV/AIDS, by combining their theoretical

[1] An earlier version of this chapter appeared in the *African Journal of AIDS Research* (AJAR) 9/4 (2010), in a special section on religion and antiretroviral therapy. Permission to reprint – in part or in whole – from that publication was kindly granted by AJAR.

and methodological insights and applying them to empirical case studies on emerging 'religious spaces' in the context of ART in Africa.

Two questions stand out: first, how can we create a better understanding of these emerging religious spaces in relation to HIV/AIDS? Second, is it possible to ensure use of a language that allows agnostic sciences such as anthropology and history to talk about matters of life and death in the context of HIV/AIDS in a way which accounts for the fact that in many African societies, people and institutions – and also theologians – often express these issues in terms of faith? This volume demonstrates that HIV/AIDS-related issues can be better understood if the relevance of religion is acknowledged, and vice versa if the study of religion incorporates the challenges arising from HIV/AIDS. This is visible with regard to (theological) discussions about the meanings of life and death, of healing and health, and of sexuality, intimacy, and the body (see Chitando 2007; Balogun 2010; Togarasei 2010; Haddad 2011). There is no question of being celebratory about the religious responses to HIV/AIDS (as some of the theological literature quoted here also acknowledges); but we argue that these responses do need to be studied and problematized not only from a theological point of view, but also from a social science perspective.

The emergence of HIV has been co-productive in the emergence of new religiosities (that is, devotional life) that inform individual and social identities, and which consequently bear on policies and political and economic realities. The chapters in this edited volume address this comparatively, with Christian, Islamic and African ritual and 'traditional' practices all approached through ethnographically grounded reflections that draw attention to the specific social, cultural and political configurations emerging at the intersection of religion and HIV/AIDS. With this approach, we follow up on previous studies that have explored the cultural, moral and political responses that various (religious) actors in society have developed in relation to the disease and which give the HIV epidemic particular shape and meaning (Schoepf 2001; Poku and Whiteside 2004; Campbell 2003; Patterson 2006; Rödlach 2006; Dilger and Luig 2010).

Why Study Religion in Relation to ART?

Why are biomedical mass treatment programmes for HIV/AIDS important for the study of religion? On the one hand, biomedical mass treatment initially seemed to undermine the focus on HIV prevention, which had hitherto been quite enthusiastically adopted by many religious groups. At this very moment, religious reservations amongst conservative groups about biomedical HIV/AIDS treatment are surfacing (see, e.g., Horn 2012), especially in the context of public health pilot programmes in which treatment is directly used for prevention in terms of a 'population approach'.[2] On the other hand, we see that religious communities and organizations continue to be engaged with HIV/AIDS, in treatment and otherwise.

In the context of their engagement with and in HIV treatment programmes, religious groups have been confronted once again by a range of existential concerns over divine healing, the provision of medicines, health resources and ethics. Ideological contestations have emerged in some cases, whereby religious ideologies have questioned or contested the moral acceptability of ART rollout (as being opposed to God's perceived omnipotence as the ultimate source of a cure). Hence, there is a need for a multidisciplinary approach to mass treatment programmes. Conversely, by studying religion, we realize how studies of ART can be enhanced by including religious processes of meaning making, legitimacy, morality and identity formation, and how these become crucial to understanding the efficacy of HIV treatment and care.

From the perspective of the social scientific study of religion, three conceptual concerns are central here. First, religious engagements with and discourses around HIV/AIDS have produced shifts in the location of religious traditions in the public and civil spheres, and reconfigured their place in structures of governance (Burchardt 2013). Exploring these shifts offers insights into the complex entanglements of religion, state policies and the transnational assemblages of institutions, values and technologies. Second, there is a need to explore how the inherited but rapidly changing patterns of religious diversity are mapped onto the domains of therapeutic and medical pluralism, and vice versa. Different religions feed in specific ways into the shaping, cultural value and attractiveness of therapeutic styles or regimes. Third, we need to investigate how engagements with biomedicine engender shifts in the meaning of specific religious practices and ideas (for example 'salvation') and how such shifts are variously negotiated, incorporated and also rejected (Dilger 2007).

The following section gives a brief overview of the larger field of HIV/AIDS research and how it relates to recent studies on religion and ART in Africa. Next, we describe how insights from these studies can be fruitful in formulating a notion of what happens when religion meets ART and brings about a new stage in the interaction between religion and the disease: what we refer to as 'the redemptive moment'. Medically, anthropologically and theologically engaging with concepts of 'prolonging life' and the 'afterlife' has created a unique dynamic, variously explored by the authors in this edited volume.

---

[2] These views were reported from pilot projects in Swaziland during an expert meeting on 'Treatment as Prevention' at the University of Amsterdam in February 2012.

Overview of the Study of Religion and HIV/AIDS

Just as religious communities and organizations in sub-Saharan Africa were latecomers in responding to HIV/AIDS, researchers were initially reluctant to acknowledge the multiple ways in which religious faith and practices are involved with the disease. When religion was adopted as a subject in HIV/AIDS research in Africa, it was first described with regard to its perceived negative impact on the interventions of HIV/AIDS programmes and the life situations of people living with HIV (for exceptions see Garner 2000; Dilger 2001). In fact, during much of the 1990s the public representation of religious responses to HIV and AIDS was dominated by (Christian) discourses on infection as divine retribution for individual or collective failures to adhere to sanctioned (and strongly gendered) models of conduct. Likewise, in Islamic contexts HIV infection has mostly been considered as indicating illicit sexual contact and deviance from divine instruction. As a corollary, some Christian churches and Islamic communities began to promote strict adherence to religious sexual teachings on premarital abstinence and fidelity in marriage as a form of HIV prevention.

Social science researchers, theologians and HIV/AIDS activists have criticized these religious responses to HIV because they contribute to stigma in many cases (Burchardt 2010a; Haddad 2011). The volume by Haddad (2011) also demonstrates the extent to which an internal critical debate of these views emerged within religious circles in Africa, a critical debate which nevertheless seemed to resonate little in more fundamentalist religious orientations (Horn 2012).

Importantly, religious constructions of HIV and AIDS as a problem of sexuality and sexual relationships have illuminated the manifold ways in which religious beliefs and cosmologies are entangled with the forging of sexual ties, with some religious leaders making renewed claims to authority over sexual practices in the name of the 'sacredness of sex'. Much of this research ties in with broader questions about the ways in which expressions of sexuality and gender – as well as relationships of healing and care – are given particular spiritual significance within the moralistic agendas of Pentecostal and evangelical Christianity (and partially concerning mainline churches) that are flourishing across sub-Saharan Africa. A few discrete dimensions of this are distinguished below.

Sexuality, Sin and Healing: Christian Responses to HIV/AIDS

Firstly, in the wake of envisioning and imagining Christian discourse as HIV prevention, responses to the HIV epidemic have come to produce new forms of speaking about sexuality and gender relations (Leclerc-Madlala 2005; Christiansen 2009). This has entailed reliance on inherited (if hitherto less emphatically promoted) Christian ideals as well as the partial adoption of public health discourses championing notions of responsible sexuality and its discursive cognates (Burchardt 2010b). Both developments seem to coalesce in what Becker and Geissler (2009) have termed 'the prescriptive turn in religious life'; in other words, the notion that one of the prime preserves of religion is to enjoin upon followers and thereafter monitor behavioural change.

Secondly, there are specific ways in which HIV and AIDS have been incorporated into Pentecostal discourses and moral constructions. If not always explicitly, the evangelical notion of 'being saved' has increasingly taken to include AIDS in the list of evils from which twice-born Christians are delivered (Dilger 2007; Christiansen 2009; Gusman 2009). Here, acquiring membership of a Pentecostal community through conversion is conceived of as saving individuals from the threat of AIDS illness, sometimes replacing the biomedical notion of sexual HIV transmission with the idea of 'immunity by faith' (Burchardt 2010a). The most controversial issue in faith-based HIV prevention is invariably condom promotion, which many churches equate with promulgating sexual promiscuity (Parsitau 2009). In various African countries, the emergence of a conservative public discourse on sexual morality and abstinence has been facilitated and reinforced by the building of international evangelical alliances, not least through the establishment of the United States President's Fund for AIDS Relief (PEPFAR) (Dilger 2009; Gusman 2009).

Thirdly, we are faced with questions about the processes whereby people take up religious injunctions on sexual life and then collectively negotiate them in the context of often competing cultural orientations, or else reject them. Some studies (e.g. Garner 2000; Agadjanian 2005) have compared mainline and Pentecostal churches regarding the influence of church teachings on HIV prevention and sexual practices, with contradictory results. Although religious discourses on sexual self-restraint may address both women and men alike, they may also meet with a social reality in which sexual practices (just as the experience of HIV) are inserted into arrangements of domination that are profoundly gendered (Sadgrove 2007; Burchardt 2010b).

Fourthly, religious thoughts and practices can be analysed in relation to practices of healing and mourning, as well as the building of (gender specific) networks and communities of support. Klaits (2010) has described how an Apostolic church in urban Botswana shaped experiences and practices of grief and mourning among its followers, and how the church contributed essentially to its members' efforts to turn the experience of dying from the stigmatized disease into a morally acceptable death. The neo-Pentecostal church in urban Tanzania described by Dilger (2007) has become an informal network of care and support for its mostly female followers in the context of urbanization and modernization processes. In a similar vein, Burchardt (2010b) argues that churches and faith-based organizations in urban South Africa have become social arenas in which gender constructions are renegotiated and reconfigured in relation to HIV.

Moral Decay and Politicized HIV: Muslim Experiences of HIV/AIDS

To some extent, the above-mentioned prescriptive turn in religious life has also become manifest in Islamic contexts, not only as a scholarly category or perspective but as a way in which people have (re)constructed the significance of religion. Among Muslim youths in the Kenyan town of Kisumu, Svensson (2009) found a pervasive sense in which Islamic forms of facing HIV were constructed through the notion of 'following instructions'. He also highlighted the fundamental importance of religious scriptures to Muslim interpretations. The chapters by Tocco (this volume) and Balogun (2010) show us that the role of the scriptures in grappling with HIV disease has gained renewed salience with the arrival of ART.

Drawing on research among Muslims in mainland Tanzania, however, Becker (2009, this volume) argues that Muslims' attitudes may also be influenced by the wider political context. This context has been shaped by longer processes of economic decline, resulting in mistrust of the state and its ability to generate progress, as well as perceptions of being sidelined in government politics. Muslims' ideas of their own marginalization in the Tanzanian state have led to distrust or even the rejection of government messages, including those about HIV prevention and control.

From a conceptual perspective, this implies that the influence of Islam on constructions of HIV and AIDS may have less to do with Islamic beliefs than with interpretations of the structural location of Muslims in society. Where Muslims' beliefs matter, they do so in ways quite different from those found in Christian contexts. Again, on the basis of reference to the scriptures, as the virus has been seen as being God's will (cf. Tocco this volume; Balogun 2010), Muslims have tended to accept HIV rather than demonize it. As a result, stigma and silence appear less a product of shame than they are associated with the fact that there was no hope for people with AIDS-related illnesses before the arrival of ART (Becker 2009).

In various Islamic contexts, HIV has been taken as a symbol for moral decay, epitomized by the loosening of gender segregation and as one in a series of concerns with sexuality, such as prostitution and the influence of tourism on sexual mores, as in the case of Zanzibar (Beckmann 2009). Much of the condemnatory discourse on HIV in Islamic reformist movements seems to have constructed this moral decay as a result of outside influences, somehow echoing discourses of moral superiority which Van Dijk (2009) also found to have been reactivated in Pentecostal responses to HIV in Botswana. Interestingly, in Zanzibar Muslim discourses of decay have been inscribed into narratives of intergenerational conflict, in which the older generation accuses the younger (Beckmann 2009), while in Uganda Pentecostalism has seen the rise of a born-again 'Joseph generation' that holds the older generation responsible for the spread of HIV (Gusman 2009). All this research demonstrates the need to explore the ways in which religion ties in with larger social and political contexts and cultural sensibilities, on the basis of which meanings of HIV are collectively constructed.

Challenges for Future Research

While the relationship between religion and HIV/AIDS has been discussed in a number of recent publications and conferences (see Becker and Geissler 2007, 2009; Prince, Denis and Van Dijk 2009), a more holistic and comparative approach is required. In particular, existing research has been characterized by a bias with regard to the work of Christian churches and organizations, with an emphasis on (neo-)Pentecostal churches. The responses of former Christian mission churches as well as Muslim communities and organizations have been discussed to a lesser extent (but see Christiansen 2010).

In addition, substantial research has been done on African 'traditional' religions *before* the introduction of ART. Anthropologists have analysed the healing claims of witch finders in the context of local power relations (Yamba 1997) and how HIV/AIDS has been incorporated into local disease categories that associate the illness with the non-observance of ritual prescriptions (Mogensen 1995; Wolf 2001; Heald 2002; Green 2003). Furthermore, they have shown how notions of purity and impurity have become contested with regard to mourning rituals and ritual cleansing practices for widows (e.g. Offe 2010; Prince 2007). They have also shown how these debates on purity and ritual have become implicated in local discussions pertaining to burials and the social and moral belonging of (deceased) persons with HIV (Dilger 2005, 2008). However, there is still a need to understand how the field has been (re)shaped by the growing presence of ARV medications and biomedical programmes in the context of transnational development/collaboration, especially in sub-Saharan Africa.

Against this backdrop, a crucial question is: how does the growing interest of international HIV/AIDS organizations and donors in the involvement of different faith-based organizations in HIV/AIDS responses affect these religious traditions? The recent developments in HIV treatment also pose new questions about religious perceptions and practices surrounding life, death and healing, and the shifting nature of religious involvement in governance and international development policies. We suggest that the answers to these questions are intimately tied to the growing availability of ART in wide parts of sub-Saharan Africa, and that the terms on which this treatment has been grafted onto wider therapeutic landscapes have engendered the production of new religious spaces. It is within these spaces that notions of life and its moralities are being negotiated and configured.

ART in Africa[3]

While an estimated 2.1 million people with HIV had access to ART in sub-Saharan Africa as of the end of 2009 (WHO, UNAIDS and UNICEF 2010), social science research on the new medications has remained scarce. Initial concerns that cultural factors were presenting a major obstacle to the successful introduction of ART in African countries were eventually modified in light of the multiple structural obstacles that have hindered access to ART on the subcontinent. These obstacles include a lack of confidentiality at HIV treatment centres as well as the long waiting times and costs arising for patients making regular visits (Hardon et al. 2007). Furthermore, recent studies have highlighted how the massive impact of ART funds has challenged and transformed institutional setups in East Africa (Hardon and Dilger 2011), thereby leading to new inequalities and frictions within clinical settings and among health staff (Sullivan 2011).

Apart from focusing on issues of access, adherence (see Ware et al. 2009) and the implications of global treatment programmes for local health systems, few publications have dealt with the way in which ART has become embedded in patients' social and family networks, and how the treatment affects understandings of health, illness and healing. A study on the introduction of ART in Senegal (Desclaux et al. 2004) provided initial insights into the social effects of this treatment on patients and their families. The authors interpret ART as a catalyst for social and familial change due to a growing individualization of ART patients and increasing dissociation from their families. Other studies have focused on the way in which societal discussions about ART – and the treatment programmes that have been built around ART – have led to new forms and understandings of political activism and citizenship in different African countries (e.g. Robins 2004; Nguyen 2005). In a seminal article, Nguyen (2005) subsumed the various practices, values and ideas that have emerged in the context of a globalized health response to HIV under the concept of therapeutic citizenship – a transnationalized form of biological citizenship that makes claims on the global economic and social order based on a 'shared therapeutic predicament'. According to Nguyen (2005: 125f.), the social and cultural practices that have evolved in this context over the last 10 to 15 years have been organized around a complex set of 'confessional technologies' and processes of self-fashioning that are closely interwoven with internationally acclaimed forms of HIV/AIDS activism and essentially draw their legitimacy from the economic, political and biological inequalities that exist in a globalizing world. This kind of citizenship may explain 'exemplary adherence' among some ART patients in West Africa (Nguyen et al. 2007).

[3] The authors want to thank Dominik Mattes for providing information about some of the literature discussed in this section.

Similarly, Burchardt (2009b) explores how efforts in South Africa concerning treatment adherence tie into negotiations of subjectivity in the context of counselling and have engendered new sites of governmentality. Whyte, Whyte and Kyaddondo (2010) demonstrate that the medical personnel of governmental and non-governmental institutions play a crucial and often difficult role as mediators between individual patients and their families, national health policies and transnational donor organizations. Finally, in Uganda Kyakuwa (2009) describes how the translation of ethical guidelines into professional relationships within an ART programme had to be negotiated in relation to the moral commitments and obligations that the 'entangled' health workers (HIV-positive nurses) experienced with their patients and clients, who were often members of the same community.

While interesting and innovative work has been done on the introduction of ART in recent years, few studies have addressed the way in which the availability of these life-prolonging drugs has affected individual and communal understandings of life, death, healing and stigma in the context of HIV. In a study in Uganda, Mogensen (2010) focuses on the dynamics of disclosure in the context of ART and analyses how the decision to speak to third parties about one's HIV infection is embedded in varying levels of sociality and moral commitment. Her research points to the need for in-depth ethnographic research that can highlight the variety and negotiability of people's positions and practices in the context of family relations over the life course of individuals. Mattes' (2011, this volume) study on ART patients and their families in coastal Tanzania highlights that the 'biopower' that is exerted on individual ARV users only partly contributes to producing a self-responsible patient in the sense of 'therapeutic citizens.' He shows how frictions implicated in the therapeutic process and the production of adherent patients are strongly influenced by perceived gender roles and economic constraints, as well as by the logics of traditional healing and people's struggle to maintain mostly kinship-based networks of support (Mattes 2011).

Incorporating the Perspective of Religion

Building on earlier studies on ART, as well as the existing literature on religion and HIV, we argue in this volume that the introduction of ART in sub-Saharan Africa has created a specific historical momentum that has challenged religious practices, ideas and thinking in unique ways, and has triggered the formation of new religious spaces. At the same time, religious practices and institutions – with their multiple local manifestations and transnational links – have shaped the implementation and appropriation of ARV medications by national authorities, health institutions and the recipients of ART, as well as their respective social and family networks.

Our argument is that these mutually intertwined dynamics can be designated as the 'redemptive moment' in the larger history of the HIV epidemic in Africa. The use of the term 'redemptive' fulfils the above-mentioned need to create a working language for the complex analytical challenges that the field of religion and ART presents. The term redemptive appeals to social scientists for whom the transitory nature of the excitement and hope connected to the introduction of ART seems obvious. It may also appeal to theologians and religious practitioners since redemption indicates particular discursive regimes of soul-saving practices. Christianity has become particularly influential in supplying such dominant themes, tropes and manners of speech, suggesting the redemption of the individual as the granting of a 'new life' by divine intervention. Furthermore, by highlighting the transitoriness of the 'redemptive *moment*', the term does not only shed critical light on the way in which ART has become the magic bullet of global development, informed by increasingly medical perspectives; additionally, it also reveals the anxieties and insecurities that the global economic crisis and declining funds, as well as the continued challenge to make people comply with the requirements and side effects of long-term treatment, entail for the field of HIV/AIDS. We argue that this term will provide workers in both anthropology and theology with an analytical tool to speak conceptually to one another about changes and continuities. The next section explores in more detail how new faith, hope, and expectations meet the predicaments of everyday life in African societies.

'The redemptive moment'

The introduction of ART in Africa has, since the beginning, been closely linked to religious thinking and practice, and more specifically to redemptory language and images.[4] While in the late 1990s the HIV epidemic in Africa was seen as a development and security crisis, since the early 2000s the introduction of ART has marked a new era in its history. This new era has triggered hopes and expectations among local, national and international organizations and governments, and most of all among patients and their families, that the immeasurable experiences of loss and suffering of the 1980s and 1990s might soon become relics of the past. While for many years Africa had been caught up in a 'state of abjection' due to the globalizing world order, with the HIV epidemic being the most explicit marker of the continent's marginalized position in the globalized political economy (Comaroff 2007), the introduction of ART seemed to indicate a reversal of this trend.

[4] However, religious organizations were strikingly absent when it came to challenging global and national power relations with regard to the introduction of ART in Africa.

The anxieties and hopes that surrounded the introduction of ART in Africa were driven by treatment activist groups like the Treatment Action Campaign in South Africa, which claimed the treatment of people with HIV or AIDS as a human right, thus challenging the status quo of the political, legal and moral world order. Through the pressure of local activist groups, the foundation of new international bodies and initiatives like the Global Fund and PEPFAR set up the institutional framework for this new era. Funds began to pour into African healthcare budgets to almost excessive degrees; new structures and frameworks were established to implement HIV treatment regimes at a breath-taking pace enabling people with AIDS to return to their normal social lives. 'From despair to hope' was the phrase used by Doctors without Borders in 2001[5] to summarize the sentiment that characterized the situation in many African countries, and which was sustained by activist organizations as well as by policy shifts in the HIV/AIDS response (on 'the Lazarus effect' see Richey and Ponte 2011: 77ff.; Simpson, this volume).

The almost miraculous nature of the arrival of ART in Africa was closely linked to the interventions of the United States government and its involvement in the religious field in Africa and beyond. Even the sternest critics of former President George W. Bush, who was closely linked to the evangelical field, acknowledge that the Bush administration's PEPFAR initiative saved millions of lives in Africa. Bono, the lead singer in the rock band U2 and one of the most outspoken HIV activists on the global scene, made this connection very clear in 2005: 'I think [Bush has] done an incredible job, his administration, on AIDS ... 250,000 Africans are on anti-viral drugs. They literally owe their lives to America. In one year that's been done.'[6] Awareness of the special bond between the United States and Africa was increasingly instilled in the minds of ordinary people in Africa, as is exemplified in a quote by an American nurse who described her encounter in Uganda with a patient on ARV drugs in 2010: 'Just today, a patient came up to me in the parking lot and said, "Thank you, American." I said, "For what?" He said, "For my medicine. You care if I live or die."'[7]

In Africa, local processes of carving out religious spaces for dealing with and negotiating the consequences of HIV and AIDS are increasingly mediated through interconnections with globally operating regimes of development aid and humanitarian assistance (Prince, Denis and Van Dijk 2009). As religious communities presented themselves as being mobilized and proactive, and were perceived as reliable and, most importantly, socially and morally embedded

[5] See: http://www.doctorswithoutborders.org/publications/alert/article.cfm?id=3319&cat=alert-article.

[6] Thus quoted on America.gov, a website produced by the US Department of State's Bureau of International Information Programs (see: http://www.america.gov/st/washfile english/2005/June/20050627175254sssillE0.3220789.html).

[7] See: http://www.nytimes.com/2010/05/10/world/africa/10aids.html?pagewanted=2.

institutions in transnational policy domains, their role in donor dominated development networks was enhanced. The PEPFAR programme in particular (but also other donor initiatives) contributed to the generating of new opportunity structures for religious actors and new horizons for reasserting their positions in the public spheres of African countries. Thus, while the bulk of the available PEPFAR money (initially US$15 billion over a period of five years) was used for the rollout of ARVs and the establishment of infrastructure for providing treatment, religious actors also benefited from (and triggered) shifting priorities in the field of HIV prevention.

In this regard, abstinence promotion became PEPFAR's preferred method for programmes addressing youth populations, whereas 'be faithful' programmes were designed primarily for married couples or older people in monogamous sexual relationships. Condoms, in turn, were to be offered only to the 'most-at-risk populations', including 'prostitutes' and their clients, migrant workers, people in discordant relationships, drug users, and men who have sex with men. Consequently, the plan did not support intervention efforts that promoted condoms or reduction in sexual partners for young people, especially those under the age of 14 (Dilger 2009: 95; Burchardt 2013). Emerging social science discourses on 'religion and development' have explored the effects of and local engagements with these shifts in global agendas and politics of funding, and have criticized the alleged secularist assumptions of earlier development paradigms (Bornstein 2005; Deneulin and Bano 2009).

Religion and the Global Development Framework: Challenges and Opportunities

Much of the financial support provided for the implementation of ART in Africa has been channelled through the religious field. The decision to involve religious organizations in healthcare provision should not come as a surprise, as religious organizations – especially the former (Christian) mission organizations but also actors from the Islamic field – have played a central role in healthcare provision on the continent over the last 100 years (Vaughan 1991). However, the funds that have become available for the introduction of ART since the early 2000s have not only been allocated to established religious organizations, such as in Zambia where mainline Christian churches have been operating successfully in the ART field for many years (see Patterson this volume). The promises and hopes raised by the growing availability of HIV treatment funds also challenged the less-established religious organizations (such as the Pentecostal churches) and in some cases Islamic organizations, to develop their own policies on HIV/AIDS and ART.

In this regard, the globalized HIV/AIDS response has created opportunities for a wide range of religious organizations to adopt responsibility in responding to the epidemic, and has helped them to adjust their language, practices and institutional arrangements to the expectations and standards of (mostly Western driven and predominantly Christian) development frameworks and accountability structures (Dilger 2009). Most importantly, however, the growing institutional engagement of religious organizations in HIV/AIDS-related activities has seemed to make up for the fact that religion was losing ground in one of its most traditional domains, that is health and healing. The growing availability of biomedical treatment and the expected concurrent medicalization of people's lives in the context of HIV queried the (continued) relevance of religious actors in the field of healing: what role does religious healing play in a world where people's problems are increasingly solved by the rapidly growing (mostly secularly defined) HIV/AIDS industry?

From the start, ART in Africa has never been what it was hoped or expected to be. We therefore conceive of the dynamics described here as 'a moment', highlighting the transitoriness and fragility of global development configurations. The PEPFAR initiative has been criticized for a range of reasons, and not only for its preference for the involvement of religious actors in the HIV/AIDS response and its explicit support of religious groups' often morally conservative agendas (Sadgrove 2007). The comparative abundance of funds for HIV/AIDS-related treatment and infrastructure has also created overwhelming challenges for healthcare systems in Africa regarding absorption of the available funds into existing infrastructure. In some cases, the over-availability of resources for HIV and AIDS in comparison to other health problems has reinforced inequalities and conflicts within some health institutions, where health staff have to compete for better working conditions and career opportunities (Sullivan 2011; Leusenkamp this volume). At the same time, current discourses on policy shifts away from 'vertical' programmes such as HIV/AIDS towards broader health agendas (for example maternal health) reflect the transitoriness of the structures and hopes that were put in place by a particular framework of health governance and agenda setting at the turn of the century.

Moreover, while medicine adherence rates in some healthcare settings in Africa have turned out to be high (Ware et al. 2009), the new era of HIV treatment has not produced the medicalized, disciplined, or responsible patients that a project of this size anticipated. Several chapters in this volume demonstrate that religiously driven healing practices in many African countries continue to flourish, and that bodies and people have not been disciplined by the available biomedical treatment regimes in the ways envisaged (or at least hoped for) by national and international policymakers as well as local healthcare providers (Tocco this volume, Kwansa this volume). Thus, along with the strong stigma that continues to surround an HIV-positive diagnosis and HIV-related illnesses, the biopower that is exercised by rigid treatment regimens and transnationally funded healthcare interventions cannot be viewed independently of the social and moral priorities formulated by communities, families, religious organizations and leaders in relation to the disease (Dilger 2012). Their behaviours and actions are shaped along with or in contestation of the biomedical ideas, material circumstances, and HIV treatment regimes that have come to configure the ART rollout in wide parts of sub-Saharan Africa (ibid.).

It is becoming clear that the introduction of ART in Africa has become a story of hope, success, and opportunities as much as it has been shaped by anxieties, contradictions, and conflict. Most importantly, the hopes and opportunities that were so closely implicated in the introduction of ART over the last few years – in relation to healing, openness about HIV, de-stigmatization – are now being questioned not only by the above-mentioned policy shifts but also by recent reports about decreasing funds and the non-sustainability of treatment programmes in the wake of the global financial crisis,[8] concerns that have been expressed in relation to the 'ART hype' in Africa since the beginning. This in turn sheds critical light on the question of whether the massive ART rollout has actually been able to produce the wide reaching conceptual and cultural shifts, as envisaged for people's everyday lives. Rather, perhaps 'medicalization' in the context of mass treatment will remain the ideological driving force of this particular historical momentum, all the while it continues to be challenged by the ways in which religious and cultural meanings and practices appropriate, transform, and sometimes subvert biomedical truths and practices in their daily, context-specific applications.

Dominant Themes in this Volume

The 11 chapters present a multidisciplinary approach (including political science, sociology, anthropology, religious studies and history), and cover different regions of sub-Saharan Africa, with case studies from South Africa, Ghana, Nigeria, Tanzania, Uganda, Zambia and Zanzibar. The chapters are based on empirical research and take into account the broad diversity and historical contingencies that have shaped religious responses to HIV treatments in recent years. The book is organized according to three thematic concerns.

Part I: Agency, Subjectivity and Authority

The chapters of this section explore biomedical treatment and its consequences as a horizon through which to address sociological and theoretical concerns

8 See: http://www.nytimes.com/2010/05/10/world/africa/10aids.html?pagewanted=2.

regarding agency, subjectivity and authority. They draw attention to how the culturally and academically circulating binary of African culture-cum-tradition versus religion is unsettled (as in the construct of 'African Traditional Religion') through changing co-implications of medical traditions. In this context, the chapters demonstrate how interactions between religion and the rollout of ARVs produce new notions of self-fashioning, identity and cultural styles of healing. The chapters follow individual negotiations, explorations and contestations of emerging trajectories, and place them in the wider cultural and historical contexts of specific societies.

Felicitas Becker discusses how in the context of Tanzania the discourses surrounding ART provision encourage new forms of self-reflection and self-control. The underlying concepts to these discourses are often based on Weberian or Foucauldian notions of subject formation, discipline and the power of ideology, and they impose distinctions between 'modern' and 'pre-modern' selves and therefore tend to relegate Africans to a 'pre-/not-yet-quite-modern' sphere in ways that need to be problematized. Styles of self-fashioning that are developed in the context of ART must be seen as related to the wider personal projects ART users pursue. Such personal projects are typically reflected in aspirations to upward social mobility, which born-again Christianity nurtures. Becker argues that the context-specific 'styles' of comportment and interaction that Tanzanians have developed in managing their extremely changeable and hybrid social environments are transferred to the situation of ART recipients, producing patients who adopt new stances on the care of the self as part of their treatment regime and develop a 'compliant patient' style.

Marian Burchardt's chapter begins with an ethnographic account of the biomedical activism of a Pentecostal group from the South African city of Cape Town. He suggests that there are three crucial theoretical concerns at stake in the study of ART and religion: first, hierarchies and differentiations of knowledge; second, processes of subject formation; and third, the differential logics of therapeutic habitus and practices. He defends the concepts of governmentality and subject formation and suggests that, in order to elucidate the empirical diversity of such processes, they can be fruitfully construed in terms of the different logics of what – drawing on Bourdieu's theory of practice – he calls 'therapeutic habitus'. He defines the therapeutic habitus as the embodied generative principles that mediate the complex relationships between the objective circumstances of patients and their therapeutic ideas, beliefs, orientations and practices. In the last part of the chapter, Burchardt analyses how therapeutic choices are shaped by the therapeutic habitus. Drawing on two autobiographical stories and ethnographic data linked to them, he shows that people's therapeutic choices are far from arbitrary and, in fact, are often not even 'choices' at all.

Bjarke Oxlund explores the manner in which the Zion Christian Church (ZCC) in South Africa – one of the largest African independent denominations –

positions itself in relation to the ways in which HIV-infected members engage with treatment. As a healing oriented African Independent Church that embraces ancestor worship and the belief in witchcraft, the ZCC does not subscribe to a viral aetiology of HIV/AIDS nor does it recommend ART. Meanwhile, the symptoms often associated with HIV and AIDS lend themselves easily to a ZCC interpretation of misfortune brought about by breaches of moral rules and social taboos. Oxlund explores how in concrete cases these ideological and moral interpretations interact with the understandings of HIV/AIDS, especially when it concerns students enrolled at the University of Limpopo who have been exposed to biomedical notions of therapy. The chapter deals with the complexities that ZCC converts face in reconciling their subject positions in their lives as they are caught between worship, kinship and therapeutic citizenship in a highly contradictory environment where divine healing, care and support from the ZCC congregation oppose the pursuit of ART.

Through a long-term study among Catholic men in Zambia, Anthony Simpson discusses the hope and excitement associated with the introduction of ART. He shows that while most of the men had experiences of HIV, either through the loss of relatives or friends, or from being infected themselves, religion played a varying and often contradictory role for them. Especially during the early 2000s (that is before ART), HIV/AIDS was framed largely in a discourse of sin and the need to lead a morally upright life. From 2004 onwards, the men increasingly described religion as a source of hope and support for those with the HIV infection. Continued secrecy around HIV in Zambia, however, shows that for these men, religious education was of little help in cultivating health seeking competencies, particularly those linked to disclosure, which are crucial in mediating access to health facilities, voluntary counselling and testing, and ART. The chapter highlights the multiple and often inconsistent meanings that religion has produced in relation to HIV and the way in which these meanings have shaped men and women's gendered identities and experiences over an extended period of time.

Part II: Contesting Therapeutic Domains and Practices

The second set of chapters deals with how religious communities and practices shape therapeutic ideas and hopes. On the one hand, such processes entail the redrawing of boundaries between and the shaping of distinct therapeutic domains: biomedicine, the Holy Spirit and traditional healing. On the other hand, as religious communities' constructions of disease and cure draw on non-biomedical ideas, there are also contestations and blurring of these boundaries, creating overlaps and contradictory assemblages (for example where pastors promote a 'magic cup' or Holy Water to cure AIDS). The chapters discuss how practices surrounding illness and healing have become embedded in the wider histories of religious diversity in specific localities. They illuminate the manifold struggles of patients, churches, and health personnel to establish meaningful relations in the wake of a primarily biomedical HIV/AIDS response. In addition, they highlight how religious practices shape the manufacturing of heterogeneous therapeutic strategies.

Jack Ume Tocco shows how the introduction of ART in northern Nigeria has been connected to a flourishing of Islamic healing practices and to recent political shifts in the country, which in turn have been associated with the introduction of *sharia* law and a wider reorientation of society in the region. While the introduction of ART has challenged the religious authority of Islam and Islamic leaders, this challenge is negotiated differently by various actors. While the Nigerian Supreme Council for Islamic Affairs fully endorsed the national government's treatment guidelines for HIV/AIDS in its 2009 National Islamic Policy on HIV/AIDS, many Islamic traditional healers 'stake their professional reputations on their ability to cure patients of their ills', including HIV and AIDS. This position is viewed critically by some of Tocco's (male) interviewees, who state that the healers' claims for a cure are false. The contribution hints at the analytical difference to be drawn between 'medicine' and 'cure', as well as the complex contestations of values and practices that shape Islamic perspectives on HIV and ART in Nigeria.

Benjamin Kobina Kwansa also addresses the issue of religious and medical authority in relation to ART and the way it is negotiated and contested by healers, patients, and religious and medical institutions in Ghana. He provides ample evidence that the behaviour of people with HIV or AIDS in Ghana is only partially shaped by religious prescriptions and frameworks, since people with HIV make context dependent use of different spiritual therapies, including those offered by Pentecostal churches, traditional priests, and Islamic healers. The negotiations and compromises people make in this wider context of medical pluralism are best understood through a pragmatic approach that analyses healing practices first and foremost with regard to people's moral and social priorities, as well as the aspired outcome of spiritual healings. This sheds light on social science assumptions about beliefs which cannot be understood within a stable cognitive framework of reference for action, but that are subject to negotiation and (shifting) experience.

Dominik Mattes describes how in 2011 Tanzanian newspapers began featuring reports on an herbal 'miracle cure' for HIV/AIDS and other major chronic diseases. Hundreds of thousands of people flocked to receive the 'magic cup' from a retired Lutheran pastor who claimed to act according to Godly instruction. The close entanglement of religious faith and scientific evidence in the form of the 'magic cup' triggered a heated discussion among governmental and scientific bodies, religious leaders of various denominations, as well as sceptical or approving Tanzanian citizens. Drawing from the discussion that took place on the national scale, Mattes localizes the conceptualization of distinguishable and interconnected healing domains (biomedical, herbal and spiritual/religious) in the experiences of HIV-positive people in urban Tanga. Despite the massive rollout of ART and respective efforts to promote it as the only effective remedy for HIV/AIDS, patients continue to flexibly navigate the diverse therapeutic landscape in the search for a cure. More thorough scrutiny of the articulation between ART and religious promises of healing is just as necessary as a closer examination of traditional healers' endeavours to develop medications against HIV/AIDS in order to fully understand patients' strategies to cope with the disease and their decisions to stop taking their 'hospital medicine'.

Part III: Emergent Organizational Forms in Times of ART

The third set of chapters focuses on organizational dynamics: the ways in which ART rollout provide the context for religious organizations to re-imagine and reconfigure their place in structures of welfare, development and networks of medical humanitarianism. The chapters by Amy Patterson, Alexander Leusenkamp, Louise Rasmussen and Caroline Meier zu Biesen highlight emerging conflicts over eligibility, resource diversion, and authority, and point out the ambivalent perceptions of institutional change among religious leaders and communities. These chapters take an institutional perspective to explain how the reshaping of religious spaces in the era of biomedical treatment for HIV is enabled and constrained by a variety of institutional interactions. These shifts are taking place between religious actors, states and external donors, as well as within the religious field itself. Describing the multiple ways in which access to donor resources reveals and reconfigures the distribution of power between religious and state actors, these chapters also provide a sense of how donor organizations have reinserted themselves into systems of governance in Africa.

Amy Patterson's contribution starts with the observation that church involvement with HIV/AIDS and ART has differed strongly in Ghana and Zambia, in terms of scope and over time. Her chapter explains these differences using a multilevel approach that takes into account how the specific shape of civil society, the state and international relations influence church activities. She shows that the nature of church activities depends on their representation in the national HIV/AIDS policy arena, but also on the place of HIV/AIDS on national policy agendas. Simultaneously, the power of church bodies is massively enhanced if, as in the case of Zambia, their access to funds is not mediated through the state but through direct interaction with donors. A fascinating account is offered of how the highly complex mosaics of church initiatives in both countries are constantly reconfigured as a result of shifting political opportunities, and also how churches strive to shape these opportunities themselves.

Alexander Leusenkamp highlights how the presence of religious organizations in ART rollout programmes in rural Uganda, especially Catholic Relief Services, has come to produce new religious spaces within local governance networks. Here, the arrival of ART has been accompanied by an ever closer alignment of donors and religious service organizations, precipitating the reinforced marginalization of state actors. Emphasizing the fact that religious service organizations operate under a bishop's authority, the chapter reminds us how strongly religious HIV/AIDS activities can be shaped by inherited church hierarchies, even if the official responsibility for biomedical interventions lies with governmental agencies. In this sense, Leusenkamp's study provides a telling example of how official and formal organization works as 'myth and ceremony' (Meyer and Rowan 1977). The chapter serves as an admirable example of the benefits of in-depth ethnographic research for unearthing how governance works at ground level.

Employing a Foucauldian perspective on governmentality, Louise Rasmussen analyses counsellors and community workers' attempts in a Roman Catholic Centre in Kampala (KCCC) to shape the lives of people with HIV and AIDS. Exploring Catholic notions of healing, Rasmussen demonstrates how counsellors and community workers employ these notions as a practice aimed to restore *wholeness*; a moral and spiritual injunction towards 'comprehensive healing'. However, observations of counselling and home visits show that these ideals of holistic care are under pressure, both from the bio-political concerns associated with the expansion of ART in Uganda and from the dominant neoliberal rationalities of international development. These forces are reshaping the organizational form and mission of KCCC such that it is becoming more and more a 'machine' of government meant to ensure good treatment outcomes, through counselling and home visiting comprising techniques to enhance clients' responsible self-government.

Caroline Meier zu Biesen explores how church-related self-help groups for people with HIV in Tanzania have adopted the use of a Chinese medical plant – *Artemisia annua* – in their efforts to delay the point at which they should start taking ARV medicines. This 'revolutionary' acceptance by the church of the Artemisia herbal tea not only caused a protracted fight between the church and biomedical practitioners, who did not think much of this kind of 'herbalism', but its acceptance also changed the organizational mode and placement of these church-based groups. Use of the Artemisia tea now places these groups at the forefront of the effort to create more space for alternatives to biomedicine. It has also profoundly reshaped these groups into social spaces of empowerment; empowerment not only at the level of the individual in need of personal support and care, but also empowerment on a communal level, which contravenes the institutional power that a priori is vested in the biomedical domain. It changes the manner in which this church-based organization – which has created its own rituals around the cultivation of *Artemisia annua* and the consumption of the herbal tea – is meaningful for individual members and their self-help groups in creating new forms of citizenship that so far have hardly been described for the domains of 'traditional' or 'alternative' medicine.

Taken together, the chapters in this volume emphasize the need to explore how religion has become intertwined with the evolving HIV epidemic in sub-Saharan Africa, and how HIV treatment programmes and healthcare interventions are established (or withdrawn) on the continent. There are no single forms of Islam, Christianity or African traditional religions that shape people's practices and experiences in the context of HIV and ART in uniform ways. Instead, the chapters highlight the manifold articulations that internally differentiated and contested religious ideologies and practices offer with regard to disease, treatment, and healing. This edited volume provides a unique perspective on the topical and theoretical challenges that will surely characterize research on ART in the coming years, especially studies focusing on the relationship between religion and the wider field of HIV/AIDS and medicine in sub-Saharan Africa.

References

Agadjanian, V. 2005. Gender, religious involvement, and HIV/AIDS prevention in Mozambique. *Social Science and Medicine*, 61(7), 1529–39.

Balogun, A.S. 2010. Islamic perspectives on HIV/AIDS and antiretroviral treatment: The case of Nigeria. *African Journal of AIDS Research*, 9(4), 459–66.

Becker, F. 2009. Competing explanations and treatment choices: Muslims, AIDS and ARVs in Tanzania, in *AIDS and Religious Practice in Africa*, edited by F. Becker and P.W. Geissler. Leiden: Brill, 155–88.

Becker, F. and Geissler, P.W. 2007. Introduction – Searching for pathways in a landscape of death: Religion and AIDS in East Africa. *Journal of Religion in Africa*, 37(1), 1–15.

Becker, F. and Geissler, P.W. (eds) 2009. *AIDS and Religious Practice in Africa*. Leiden: Brill.

Beckmann, N. 2009. AIDS and the power of God: Narratives of decline and coping strategies in Zanzibar, in *AIDS and Religious Practice in Africa*, edited by F. Becker and P.W. Geissler. Leiden: Brill, 119–54.

Bornstein, E. 2005. *The Spirit of Development: Protestant NGOs, Morality, and Economics in Zimbabwe*. Stanford, CA: Stanford University Press.

Burchardt, M. 2009a. Religion and AIDS in South Africa: A cultural sociology. PhD thesis, Department of Cultural Studies, University of Leipzig.

Burchardt, M. 2009b. Subjects of counselling: HIV/AIDS, religion and the management of everyday life in South Africa, in *AIDS and Religious Practice in Africa*, edited by F. Becker and P.W. Geissler. Leiden: Brill, 333–58.

Burchardt, M. 2010a. 'Life in brackets': Biographical uncertainties of HIV-positive women in South Africa. *Forum Qualitative Sozialforschung/Forum: Qualitative Social Research* 11(1). [Online]. Available at: http://nbn-resolving.de/urn:nbn:de: 0114-fqs100135 [accessed: 6 February 2013].

Burchardt, M. 2010b. Ironies of subordination: Ambivalences of gender in religious AIDS-interventions in South Africa. *Oxford Development Studies*, 38(1), 63–82.

Burchardt, M. 2013. Faith-based humanitarianism: Organizational change and everyday meanings in South Africa. *Sociology of Religion*, 74(1), 30–55.

Campbell, C. 2003. *'Letting Them Die': Why HIV/AIDS Prevention Programmes Fail*. Oxford: James Currey.

Chitando, E. 2007. *Living with Hope: African Churches and HIV/ AIDS*. Geneva: WCC (World Council of Churches) Publications.

Christiansen, C. 2009. When AIDS becomes part of the (Christian) family: Dynamics between kinship and religious networks in Uganda, in *Social Security in Religious Networks*, edited by C. Leuthoff-Grandits, A. Peleikis and T. Thelen. London: Berghahn Books, 23–43.

Christiansen, C. 2010. Development by churches, development of churches: Institutional trajectories in rural Uganda. PhD thesis, Faculty of Social Sciences, University of Copenhagen.

Comaroff, J. 2007. Beyond bare life: AIDS, (bio)politics, and the neoliberal order. *Public Culture*, 19(1), 197–219.

Deneulin, S. and Bano, M. 2009. *Religion in Development: Rewriting the Secular Script*. London and New York: Zed Books.

Desclaux, A., Lanièce, I., Ndoye, I. and Taverne, B. (eds) 2004. *The Senegalese Antiretroviral Drug Access Initiative: An Economic, Social, Behavioural, and Biomedical Analysis*. Paris: Agence Nationale de Recherches sur le SIDA.

Dilger, H. 2001. 'Living PositHIVely in Tanzania': The global dynamics of AIDS and the meaning of religion for international and local AIDS work. *Afrika Spectrum*, 36(1), 73–90.

Dilger, H. 2005. *Leben mit AIDS: Krankheit, Tod und soziale Beziehungen in Afrika. Eine Ethnographie*. Frankfurt a.M.: Campus,

Dilger, H. 2007. Healing the wounds of modernity: Salvation, community and care in a neo-Pentecostal church in Dar Es Salaam, Tanzania. *Journal of Religion in Africa*, 37(1), 59–83.

Dilger, H. 2008. 'We are all going to die': Kinship, belonging and the morality of HIV/AIDS-related illnesses and deaths in rural Tanzania. *Anthropological Quarterly*, 81(1), 207–32.

Dilger, H. 2009. Doing better? Religion, the virtue-ethics of development, and the fragmentation of health politics in Tanzania. *Africa Today*, 56(1), 89–110.

Dilger, H. 2012. Targeting the empowered individual: Transnational policy-making, the global economy of aid, and the limitations of 'biopower' in Tanzania, in *Medicine, Mobility, and Power in Global Africa: Transnational Health and Healing*, edited by H. Dilger, A. Kane and S. Langwick. Bloomington, IN: Indiana University Press, 60–91.

Dilger, H. and Luig U. (eds) 2010. *Morality, Hope and Grief: Anthropologies of AIDS in Africa*. New York and Oxford: Berghahn Books.

Garner, R.C. 2000. Safe sects? Dynamic religion and AIDS in South Africa. *Journal of Modern African Studies*, 38(1), 41–69.

Green, E. 2003. *Rethinking AIDS Prevention: Learning from Successes in Developing Countries*. London: Praeger.

Gusman, A. 2009. HIV/AIDS, Pentecostal churches, and the 'Joseph generation' in Uganda. *Africa Today*, 56(1), 67–86.

Haddad, B. (ed.) 2011. *Religion and HIV and AIDS: Charting the Terrain*. Pietermaritzburg: University of KwaZulu-Natal Press.

Hardon, A., Akurut, D., Comoro, C., Ekezie, C., Irunde, H., Gerrits, T., Kglatwane, J., Kinsman, J., Kwasa, R., Maridadi, J., Moroka, T.M., Moyo, S., Nakiyemba, A., Nsimba, S., Ogenyi, R., Oyabba, T., Temu, F. and Laing, R. 2007. Hunger, waiting time and transport costs: Time to confront challenges to ART adherence in Africa. *AIDS Care*, 19(5), 658–65.

Hardon, A. and Dilger, H. 2011. Global AIDS medicines in East African health institutions: Introduction. *Medical Anthropology*, 30(2), 136–57.

Heald, S. 2002. It's never as easy as ABC: Understandings of AIDS in Botswana. *African Journal of AIDS Research (AJAR)*, 1(1), 1–10.

Horn, J. 2012. *Not as Simple as ABC: Christian Fundamentalisms and HIV and AIDS Responses in Africa*. Toronto, ON: AWID (Association for Women's Rights in Development) Press.

Klaits, F. 2010. *Death in a Church of Life: Moral Passion during Botswana's Time of AIDS*. Berkeley, CA: University of California Press.

Kyakuwa, M. 2009. Ethnographic experiences of HIV-positive nurses in managing stigma at a clinic in rural Uganda. *African Journal of AIDS Research*, 8(3), 367–78.

Leclerc-Madlala, S. 2005. Popular responses to HIV/AIDS and policy. *Journal of Southern African Studies*, 31(4), 845–56.

Mattes, D. 2011. 'We are just supposed to be quiet': The production of adherence to antiretroviral treatment in urban Tanzania. *Medical Anthropology*, 30(2), 158–82.

Meyer, J.W. and Rowan, B. 1977. Institutionalized organizations: Formal structure as myth and ceremony. *American Journal of Sociology*, 83(2), 340–63.

Mogensen, H.O. 1995. *AIDS is a Kind of Kahungo that Kills: The Challenge of Using Local Narratives when Exploring AIDS among the Tonga of Southern Zambia*. Oslo: Scandinavian University Press.

Mogensen, H.O. 2010. New hopes and new dilemmas: disclosure and recognition in the time of antiretroviral treatment, in *Morality, Hope and Grief: Anthropologies of AIDS in Africa*, edited by H. Dilger and U. Luig. Oxford and New York: Berghahn Books, 61–79.

Nguyen, V.-K. 2005. Antiretroviral globalism, biopolitics, and therapeutic citizenship, in *Global Assemblages: Technology, Politics, and Ethics as Anthropological Problems*, edited by A. Ong and S. Collier. Oxford: Blackwell Publishing, 124–44.

Nguyen, V.-K., Ako, C.Y., Niamba, P., Sylla, A. and Tiendrébéogo, I. 2007. Adherence as therapeutic citizenship: Impact of the history of access to antiretroviral drugs on adherence to treatment. *AIDS*, 21(supplement 5), S31–S35.

Offe, J.A. 2010. Diseased and dangerous: images of widows' bodies in the context of the HIV epidemic in northern Zambia, in *Morality, Hope and Grief: Anthropologies of AIDS in Africa*, edited by H. Dilger and U. Luig. Oxford and New York: Berghahn Books, 270–91.

Parsitau, D.S. 2009. 'Keep Holy distance and abstain till He comes': Interrogating a Pentecostal church's engagement with HIV/AIDS and the youth in Kenya. *Africa Today*, 56(1), 45–64.

Patterson, A. 2006. *The Politics of AIDS in Africa*. Boulder, CO: Lynne Rienner.

Patterson, A. 2011. *The Church and AIDS in Africa: The Politics of Ambiguity*. Boulder, CO: Lynne Rienner.

Poku, N.K. and Whiteside, A. (eds) 2004. *Global Health and Governance: HIV/AIDS*. New York: Palgrave Macmillan.

Prince, R. 2007. Salvation and tradition: Configurations of faith in a time of death. *Journal of Religion in Africa*, 37(1), 84–115.

Prince, R., Denis, P. and Van Dijk, R. 2009. Introduction to special issue – Engaging Christianities: Negotiating HIV/AIDS, health, and social relations in East and southern Africa. *Africa Today*, 56(1), v–xviii.

Richey, L.A. and Ponte, S. 2011. *Brand Aid: Shopping Well to Save the World*. Minneapolis, MN: University of Minnesota Press.

Robins, S. 2004. 'Long live Zackie, long live': AIDS activism, science and citizenship after apartheid. *Journal of Southern African Studies*, 30(3), 651–72.

Rödlach, A. 2006. *Witches, Westerners, and HIV: AIDS and Cultures of Blame in Africa*. Walnut Creek, CA: Left Coast Press.

Sadgrove, J. 2007. 'Keeping up appearances': Sex and religion amongst university students in Uganda. *Journal of Religion in Africa*, 37(1), 116–44.

Schoepf, B.G. 2001. International AIDS research in anthropology: Taking a critical perspective on the crisis. *Annual Review of Anthropology*, 30, 335–61.

Sullivan, N. 2011. Mediating abundance and scarcity: Implementing an HIV/AIDS-targeted project within a government hospital in Tanzania. *Medical Anthropology*, 30(2), 202–21.

Svensson, J. 2009. 'Muslims have instructions': HIV/AIDS, modernity, and Islamic religious education in Kisumu, Kenya, in *AIDS and Religious Practice in Africa*, edited by F. Becker and P.W. Geissler. Leiden: Brill, 189–220.

Togarasei, L. 2010. Christian theology of life, death and healing in an era of antiretroviral therapy: Reflections on the responses of some Botswana churches. *African Journal of AIDS Research*, 9(4), 429–35.

Van Dijk, R. 2009. Gloves in times of AIDS: Pentecostalism, hair and social distancing in Botswana, in *AIDS and Religious Practice in Africa*, edited by F. Becker and P.W. Geissler. Leiden: Brill, 283–306.

Vaughan, M. 1991. *Curing their Ills: Colonial Power and African Illness*. Cambridge: Polity Press.

Ware, N.C., Idoko, J., Kaaya, S., Biraro, I.A., Wyatt, M.A., Agbaji, O., Chalamilla, G. and Bangsberg, D.R. 2009. Explaining adherence success in sub-Saharan Africa: an ethnographic study. *PLoS Med*, 6(1), 39–47.

Whyte, S.R., Whyte, M. and Kyaddondo, D. 2010. Health workers entangled: Confidentiality and certification, in *Morality, Hope and Grief: Anthropologies of AIDS in Africa*, edited by H. Dilger and U. Luig. Oxford and New York: Berghahn Books, 80–101.

Wolf, A. 2001. AIDS, morality and indigenous concepts of sexually transmitted diseases in Southern Africa. *Afrika Spectrum*, 36(1), 97–107.

World Health Organization (WHO), UNAIDS and UNICEF 2010. *Towards Universal Access: Scaling-Up Priority HIV/AIDS Interventions in the Health Sector, Progress Report 2010*. Geneva: WHO.

Yamba, B.C. 1997. Cosmologies in turmoil: Witchfinding and AIDS in Chiawa, Zambia. *Africa*, 67(2), 200–23.

PART I
Agency, Subjectivity and Authority

Chapter 1

Fashioning Selves and Fashioning Styles: Negotiating the Personal and the Rhetorical in the Experiences of African Recipients of ARV Treatment

Felicitas Becker

Introduction

The increasing availability of ART in Africa has greatly reduced the terror attendant on an HIV-positive diagnosis. It has also given rise to debates about the effects such treatment, and the specific ways it is administered, has on the patients beyond safeguarding them from full-blown AIDS. Some of this literature suggests that the discourses surrounding ART provision encourage new forms of self-reflection and control, described sometimes as ethical self-fashioning or subject formation. This chapter problematizes these interpretations from several angles. The underlying concepts can be derived variously from Weber or Foucault, but in both cases imply a distinction between 'modern' and 'pre-modern' selves and therefore tend to relegate Africans to a 'pre/not-yet-quite-modern' sphere that is difficult to conceptualize. Moreover, observers need to connect self-fashioning in the context of ART to the wider social projects pursued by ART providers, such as the upwardly mobile social identities that born-again Christianity helps create. Most importantly perhaps, researchers also need to pursue the political and rhetorical dimensions of pronunciations on ART recipients' self-care, whether by recipients or providers. The chapter argues that such strategic speech or 'context-appropriate' rhetoric is not 'mere' rhetoric but an instantiation of a very entrenched and effective kind of practice. It is related to what James Ferguson has described as the context-specific 'styles' of comportment and interaction that Africans have developed in managing their extremely changeable and hybrid social environments. These findings do not negate the possibility of subject formation in the context of ART provision, but situate it as one of several related processes that need to be studied together.

One day in the mid 2000s, Tatu Mohamed, the sister of my long-standing research assistant in the provincial Tanzanian town of Lindi, showed me a kind of scrapbook she had made in preparation for her marriage. Although she knew little English and did not normally speak it, many of the captions were in English. They included the sentence 'I will respect my body' as well as references to cleanliness, purity and self-care. The illustrations were predominantly of modestly yet fashionably dressed women and items of comfortable domesticity, including soaps and skincare products. The English captions were cut from a printed text and read like extracts from an 'abstinence education' manual.

This document reflected currents in the social life of Tatu's home town, Lindi, as well as her particular circumstances. Anxiety about AIDS was then running very high and the disease was commonly attributed to a crisis in sexual morals. At the same time, vocal criticism from young reformists had prompted mainstream Muslims, such as Tatu's family, to emphasize their Islamic credentials, including the maintenance of the proprieties of women's behaviour (Becker 2007, 2009; Beckmann 2009). But at the same time, an ongoing road-building project in the district had brought in English-speaking strangers, encouraged trade in the sort of consumption goods represented in Tatu's scrapbook and created opportunities for transactional sexual encounters.

Personally, Tatu had had to gain acceptance from a distant father and meddling stepmother for a suitor from out of town who was also a convert from Christianity, and had only just reached the stage of setting up her own household. In a sense, Tatu (considered the most diplomatic among their number by her siblings) had won a certain amount of independence after her wedding by first demonstrating the self-restraint required to have the marriage permitted. 'Self-restrained' here denotes a quality her parents and neighbours would have understood partly in terms of an established Islamic discourse on women's modesty. But the scrapbook suggests that it has also taken on overtones of a more recent derivation, related to the sort of self-care advice long given to HIV-positive people and reworked for ART recipients, and perhaps also to a wider 'post-permissive' drift in Western discourses on sexuality, evident for instance in the American 'true love can wait' campaigns. Certainly, her actions in putting together this scrapbook were not purely strategic. If so, she would have had no reason to share this object with a visiting outsider like myself, however friendly.

The existence of this scrapbook and its contents can be seen as indications of the occurrence of a process which, in the context of AIDS, has been described as the construction of new forms of selfhood around the management of HIV, of ethical self-regulation fostered by treatment regimes that are often accompanied by a new or intensified religious orientation. Burchardt (2009: 346–7) uses the terms 'ethical selfhood' and 'ethical subject formation' (see also Nguyen 2009; Van Dijk 2009; Dilger 2012). In this view, ART, delivered in the form of programmes with in-built control mechanisms, not only provides for survival but also inserts Africans into a process whereby medical providers seek to reshape their subjectivities in ways inspired by deracinated religious or technocratic discourses, and shaped by the conditions neoliberal governance imposes on aid provision.

Tatu's scrapbook suggests that such changes can reach beyond those who themselves are subject to ART regimes. ART was available at the time in Lindi but only through a private practice. PEPFAR-funded provision was being prepared but was slowed down by problems of coordination between the different agencies involved. The empirical material in this chapter mainly deals with people party to communal and, as Tatu's example shows, also very personal debates about sexuality and public morality in times of AIDS and ART, rather than with recipients of ART and the attendant counselling. Nevertheless, I argue that the insights obtainable from this material are relevant to the discussion of 'subjects of counselling' more specifically. Put differently, the aim is to place the examination of subject formation in a wider context than that of ART provision and counselling and to trace some of the processes at play here to a longer history of Africans making sense of AIDS.

The above-mentioned observations on subject formation have immediate plausibility. Even with ART, an HIV-positive diagnosis remains a personal crisis and learning to live with it is likely to require a profound reorientation. Patients have to reconsider their relationships, their use of their body and their place in the world. Moreover, the presence of an ethical element in much of the advice given to HIV-positive patients, even before ART, is undeniable: it is indeed about taking care of one's body as well as one's relations, and many patients draw upon their religious allegiances in this process. It is also evident that the language in which advice on the management of AIDS as a survivable condition is couched has specific institutional origins and is bound up with particular visions of personhood (Prince 2012). As Dilger (2012) puts it, it is a language about empowered or to-be-empowered individuals heavily conditioned by international donor organizations that are providing funding for AIDS/ART education and care projects.

The concepts at play are not, however, without problems. The demands for personal reform in the context of ART counselling can be far-reaching, as can be the claims by recipients of counselling. It is difficult even to ask how true these claims are because the question smacks of what Glassman (2011: 50) has called the 'implication of insincerity': the observer appears to either ascribe hypocrisy or a form of 'false consciousness' to the observed. But at the same time, the intellectual authorities who, implicitly or explicitly, validate the concept of the self, from Freud to Foucault, would agree that purely verbal evidence is a poor guide to the processes under discussion. Moreover, a focus on the self is a poor guide to the interactive, interpersonal, sometimes collective nature of processes of subject formation in the context of AIDS/ART counselling.

This chapter explores the possibility of adapting Ferguson's concept of 'style' and the development of context-specific styles by groups of African actors to the description of the changes wrought by AIDS and ART programmes. The attraction of this concept is threefold. Firstly, it recognizes that actors may speak and comport themselves in different registers in different contexts without being insincere in any of them. Following Judith Butler, Ferguson (1999: 99) calls the styles he examined 'strategies of survival under compulsory systems': they are ways of working with the practical necessities and cultural possibilities that actors face and that vary between contexts.

Secondly, Ferguson (1999: 99) calls these styles 'motivated, intentional and performative, but not simply chosen or lightly slipped into'. They are both intuitive and pragmatic, capturing the tentative way in which intellectual, ethical and social positions are developed and adopted in the 'rough and tumble of everyday struggle' (Glassman 1995). This is useful because it cautions against expecting too much cohesion of the resulting stances, and against literal acceptance of verbal claims. Moreover and thirdly, 'style' thus conceived acknowledges the interpersonal nature of this quest for tenable positions in shifting social contexts. It therefore helps to think about the ongoing processes of personal reorientation in the context of ART programmes without opening up a chasm between the individual nature of changes to the self and the interpersonal nature of treatment programmes.

The Theoretical Antecedents of the Concept of 'Self'

Different terms are used to describe the process under discussion, with ethical self-fashioning, ethical subject formation and new forms of care of the self all jostling with each other. This multiplicity reflects the difficulty of defining not only the ongoing process of change but also the thing that is changing. What is a self? The term oscillates between meanings established in developmental psychology, psychoanalysis, the study of ethical religions as inspired by Max Weber, the study of intimate, 'capillary' forms of power as inspired by Foucault, and meanings in literary studies and philosophy that draw on all of the above (Bosma and Gerlsma 2003; Weber 1988; Foucault 2008; Irigaray 1985; Bhabha 1995). In the context of AIDS-related changes, it refers to a phenomenon as impossible to ignore or dismiss as it is to pin down.

The following attempts to identify and disentangle at least some of the overtones of the notion of 'self' that are important in the present context. Three strands of discussion can be identified. Firstly, there is the long-standing proposition of the existence of specifically African forms of the self, typically glossed as less monadic than Western ones. Secondly, there is the proposition, associated with modernization theory, that selves have been changing, or ought to have been changing in Africa due to the social change induced by colonial and post-colonial upheavals. Thirdly, there is the Foucauldian suggestion that the self owes its existence not to advances in personal autonomy but rather to advances in social control; that selves are increasingly being coaxed into being by intimate, to some extent embodied forms of power that are often described as 'biopower'. Evidently, the term 'self' can be called upon to do different kinds of work in a discussion of medically induced social change.

The proposition of a more relational, less individualist form of personhood prevailing on the continent is old and widespread (e.g. Gulliver 1971; Mbiti 1969). It has recently been restated in a sophisticated way by Geissler and Prince (2010: 164), who observe that among the people they observed in western Kenya, 'personhood ... is not centred on an autonomous and bounded self, which then engages with others ... the boundaries between persons, others and things are fluid and permeable' (see also Kresse 2007). The enormous reach and density of personal networks in Africa is indisputable, and Geissler and Prince's assertion that the atomized individual is not taken as a given in their Kenyan research site is convincing.

Nonetheless, the kind of 'networked' personhood they describe is not incompatible with active individualism, as they would also acknowledge (see also Prince 2012). Perceptive studies of social relations in Africa at times emphasize the subtly conflict-focused character of the networks sustaining selves in Africa: they are animated by the self-centred and conflicting designs and desires of their members (e.g. Mitchell 1956; Falk Moore 1996). Such a tense and political personal network possibly makes the contours of the individual self sharp in circumstances where deeply personal interests are at stake. Tatu's quiet and determined campaign to leave her paternal household and enter the marriage she desired comes to mind. Ultimately, therefore, the proposition of the relational self in Africa cannot support a specific account of the way selves are changing because the pre-existing selves are already very open to interpretation. Nevertheless, the prevalence of such networked personhood is quite compatible with the absorption and elaboration of new, including more individualist, ethical stances and social practices. This is part of what the developing literature on AIDS and self-fashioning is about.

Secondly, there is the Weberian proposition of individualization as a part of the ongoing modernization in Africa. In its strong form, this narrative is now largely discredited. In the mid twentieth century, it was widely used to class Africans, with other inhabitants of the 'Third World', as not-yet-modern, in counter-distinction to the modern West.[1] The association of HIV/ART with the operations of a technocratic medical bureaucracy, the manifest need for self-control and self-reflection to minimize risks in one's sexual and personal life, is easily associated with the concept of rationalization, which was central to

---

[1] For a genealogy of such ideas in area studies more generally, see Lockman (2004) and, for Africa, Comaroff and Comaroff (1993).

dividing the world into modern countries and those in need of modernizing, which in this mode of reasoning include all of Africa.

Observers of ART and 'ethical subject formation', to use Burchardt's term, need not therefore be understood to be bringing back modernization theory through the back door. Even where they do not address their relationship with modernization theory explicitly, it is clear that they differ from its classical version in a crucial respect: these theories regularly posited secularization as another core element of modernization, in addition to individualization. This 'secularization hypothesis' has of late become highly controversial, some would say obsolete. Whatever may be salvaged from it, it is clearly orthogonal to the recent work on subject formation among subjects of counselling, where religious elements often mix with medical ones.

The differences between the modern African individuals predicted in the 1960s (Ferguson 1999) and processes of individuation and self-reflection under study today reflect the end of optimism and of the naïve universalism once inherent in notions of progress or modernization among researchers. The 'subjects of counselling' (Burchardt 2009) are kindred to the modern Africans once prophesied by modernization theorists in that their lives are inserted into bureaucratic or bureaucratizing institutional structures. But these structures are no longer seen as emancipatory or rational in a positive sense. They are essential lifelines for people stalked by a slow death, and their behaviour is conditioned by ever-scarce funding as well as religious/ideological orientations that their clients have to take in their stride. Overall, recent accounts of subject formation serve more to counteract modernization-theoretical ideas of individualization as an increase in personal sovereignty than to underpin them.

Concomitantly, the echoes of Michel Foucault are the strongest overtones in the literature on ART and subject formation. His insistence that the development of a self-reflexive sexual self in Europe is at heart an extension of power, of diffuse forms of social control, into the most intimate regions of life, gives a good deal of drama to the processes under discussion. But Foucault gives little thought to the possibility that the configurations of institutions he examined – of psychiatry, schools, prisons and the different partly institutionalized forms of speech he called 'discourse' – could weaken as well as grow. In Africa, by contrast, the transience of institutions dedicated to 'programmes', always started with the fiction that organizations would eventually make themselves superfluous as programmes become self-sustaining, is a hallmark of the institutional contexts of subject formation (Prince 2012). Of course, this transience does not mean that such institutions can have no effect on personhood. But how these effects survive the institutions is a question in itself.

As Stoler (2010), one of the strongest proponents of the usefulness of Foucault in non-European contexts, has remarked, he is better used for developing questions than answers. Two in particular come to mind. Firstly, should the echoes of Foucault in what African subjects of counselling experience be taken to imply that Africans are being made 'subject', in the sense of 'lacking sovereignty', in a new way? Do ART programmes imply their subjection to treatment regimes shaped by neoliberal agendas and ideologies of care determined elsewhere? Secondly, at the risk of sounding repetitive, where within persons do we find the Foucauldian kind of self? It is clear that we are looking at a phenomenon that can be 'called into being' by counselling encounters. How foundational is it?

The answer to the first question surely has to be 'yes'. Of course dependency on ART provision is about as stark as dependency can get, and enables the provider to impose conditions on the recipient. At the same time, providers want their drugs to be used; withholding them is self-harming punishment. There is thus an incentive and space to negotiate with as well as dictate to recipients. Besides, this level of dependency need not even be put in Foucauldian terms to be recognized as stark. The power to withhold life-saving treatment is 'biopower', power over life, in a very real sense, without therefore necessarily implying as sustained and intense an intervention into the individual person as Foucault proposed. ART programmes do imply subjection but the reference to Foucault does not in itself clarify how deeply this subjection reaches into a person's mind.

The second question can be answered partly with reference to Foucault's inattention to institutional weakness. While he is not terribly clear about it, his account of sexual selves in Europe includes long-term processes beginning in childhood and suggests that he is interested in a relatively strong notion of the self. He treats it as something deep-set, developed over the life-course, and once developed, not unlimitedly flexible. It takes a whole conjunction of influences, emanating from the institutions of control he discusses with, to bring this self into being.

The upshot of this is that it is good to distinguish between a strong and a weaker sense of self. In the former, the term denotes something a person acquires (evolves, perhaps even cultivates) over their life-course, that is poorly contained in verbal statements and is beyond the reach of change by intention. In the latter, it denotes what Dilger (2012) calls 'visions' of the self, projects or projections constructed with the help of current ideologies and in struggle with current challenges. The literature on ART and subject formation is concerned predominantly with the latter.

One thing that Weber and Foucault, the very different 'patron saints' of modernization theory and the notion of subject formation, have in common is that both warn against deriving the effects of texts or speech from their content. A discourse that is about liberation is not therefore liberating and the concrete ethical praxes that arise from a reorientation towards religious world views do not need to accord with the priorities stated in such a world view (the world rejection in Protestant Christianity engendered the decidedly this-worldly praxis of capitalism). In this sense, both the Weberian and the Foucauldian antecedents of the notion of subject formation caution against the acceptance of claims people make about themselves as 'truth', or assuming too much about the behavioural or social effects of conscious changes in attitudes. But how can we practise such scepticism without being condescending?

Speaking and Acting about AIDS and ART: A Question of Style?

If we accept the reach of the sorts of innovative personal commitments that observers like Burchardt observed in ART counselling sessions, their consequences for the speaker's life and sense of self cannot be taken for granted. The question then arises what these statements express – or indeed whether they are primarily 'expressive'. It is possible to take them not as expressions of an underlying identity, form of selfhood or process of self-fashioning, but as elements in a particular kind of trans- and interaction. In part, they are an exchange of commitments or confessions for material help, similar to 'performing survival' as Nguyen has suggested. But inasmuch as these performances are not one-offs but add up to persistent patterns, they go beyond exchange, towards the cultivation of forms of comportment that are both personal and interpersonal.

As discussed above, these patterns can be identified as *styles* in a manner derived from Ferguson's 1999 study of styles as a means of negotiating distinct yet deeply interdependent social contexts. Since speech is their cornerstone (but not their sum total), they may be called 'discursive styles'. The advantages of this notion have already been stated. Firstly, it allows for the acknowledgment of the incompleteness of commitments to reforming lives without designating it a sign of mere hypocrisy or pragmatism. Secondly, the term reflects well the interplay of creativity and necessity, and of individual and collective processes at work in the rhetoric of self-reform, which is shaped by urgent needs, the set rhetoric of donor institutions and institutional demands as well as by individual initiative. Particularly important in the present context, the concept of style acknowledges the role of non-verbal, bodily and performative aspects of the interaction between ART or aid recipients and donor organizations. It thus points beyond the verbal interactions that, albeit crucial to the understanding of changing visions of self, can be misleading on their own.

Ferguson employs his concept of style to understand how Zambian miners negotiate between the closely related but very different cultural spheres of the rural home village and mining town. He insists that miners do not simply 'switch' between pre-existing, fixed cultural codes like you change coats, but rather that they have to work towards 'pulling off' specific urban and rural styles. There is room for creativity in adopting either style, but there is also the possibility of failure, and a need for improvisation, for putting oneself across one way or the other and often with slightly unpredictable results. As Ferguson (1999: 96) puts it, 'the doer may be constituted in the deed', but the actions become meaningful within structures not of the actors' choosing.

Transferred to the situation of African ART recipients, we can then propose that patients who adopt new stances on the care of the self as part of their treatment regime are in the process of developing a 'compliant patient' style. They are learning, by trial and error, how to behave in a manner that not only facilitates their passage through the ART clinic but, in a less instrumental sense, makes them a person, and an intelligible and welcome person, in this context. Such a style would be more persistent and less situational than Nguyen's expression 'performing survival' suggests. At the same time, it may still be less pervasive and personal than descriptions based on the terms 'self' or 'subject' suggest. Moreover, such a style would be context-specific, appropriate for the ART clinic environment, and could extend more or less far into a patient's life outside it. It would also be the outcome of a process of negotiation, trial and error, whereby the patient develops an appropriate register of behaviour in a context shot through with both opportunity and constraint.

It is worth pointing out that the aim, in proposing this concept of evolving 'styles' at work among Africans affected by AIDS, ART and counselling, is not to contrast these styles with older, authentic ways of acting and reasoning. The argument could be made that the performance of social roles and allegiances through elements of style has been part of the African experience since before colonialism. But the elements of style and their significances change: Hadhrami silver daggers and cowboy hats, for instance, have come and gone. Some practices may become routinized and be thrown back into question later, like certain forms of veiling among Muslim women. A long argument, paralleling the one over the extent to which selves have changed in the twentieth century, could be had about how much more varied and self-reflexive style choices for Africans have become. At any rate, it is not a case of 'traditional' aetiologies of AIDS on the one hand and 'ART-focused' ones on the other.

A Case Study in Style: Dar es Salaam's Muslim Campaigners

For this observer, the potential usefulness of the notion of style first became tangible at a meeting in Dar es Salaam in late October 2008. At stake was a style relevant not for ART recipients directly but for Africans involved in ART provision; what one could call a 'reliable funding recipient' style. Representatives of 20-odd Tanzanian Muslim groups gathered for this meeting at the Starlight Hotel, a Muslim-owned business in the Muslim-dominated Kariakoo District, to discuss the development of a mechanism for receiving financial assistance from TACAIDS, the Tanzanian Commission on AIDS. This was an attempt by Muslim organizations to draw even with Christian organizations that had already submitted proposals for such mechanisms to TACAIDS. The commission itself had declared that it was moving towards providing its funding exclusively through these channels. Muslims would, therefore, risk losing access to TACAIDS funding if they did not set up such a recipient and distributing structure.

In this sense, the meeting was kindred to a process that Green, Mercer and Mesaki (2010) discussed critically as the 'production' of civil-society organizations, including faith-based ones, through donor programmes that focus on supporting such organizations. While the rhetoric of such programmes, they show, typically presupposed the existence of these groups, they are often only 'called forth' by them; brought into being specifically as mechanisms for the absorption and redistribution of the cash provided by donor programmes. In the present case, though, whatever mechanism would result from TACAIDS's demand and this meeting was not to be created from scratch but would be a spin-off of existing Muslim organizations. Nevertheless, its tone and modus operandi would be heavily influenced by the stated expectations of TACAIDS.

This does not imply that such an organization would be entirely a creature of TACAIDS. Rather, the Muslim organizations involved already existed and were discussing establishing a spin-off organization. Moreover, they had strong points of view of their own. I had been invited to attend the wrap-up of the conference by one of its organizers, with the prospect of interviewing some of those present. Instead, I became the interviewee: my seven interlocutors asked me to speak at length about my research to date, and particularly about my insights into the history of Muslim congregations within Tanzania. In effect, the organizers were making sure that I appreciated their view of their own history, as a group with deep roots not only on the Swahili Coast, but also elsewhere on the mainland, and one that had been deeply involved in opposition to colonialism. They wanted me to acknowledge the role of Muslims in achieving political independence and the legitimacy of their grievances about the under-representation of Muslims in higher education and in the upper levels of the administration in the post-colonial state (see also Loimeier 2007; Becker 2008).

At the same time, in posing their questions, my interlocutors emphasized the ethical character of Islam and its status as a 'complete way of life' (a turn of phrase much used both by academic observers of Islam and Islamic reformists; see Eickelman and Piscatori 1996). This emphasis is significant in more ways than one. In part, these references had a political import. In keeping with the rhetoric of many political Islamists, the activists suggested a connection between the obstacles that they claimed the contemporary Tanzanian polity posed to Muslims leading fully Islamic lives, and Muslims' perceived helplessness in the face of the AIDS emergency. Again and again, they pointed out that AIDS control was a political issue and that the requisite ethical and practical changes could only occur if they were given due scope within the Tanzanian polity.

Simultaneously, the ethical emphasis chimed with the parallel interest of the activists in religious reform. At this level, it bears resemblance to the Christian-inspired discourses of ethical living described, for example, by Burchardt, albeit with more emphasis on community than individual relations with the creator.

The way I was spoken to at this meeting was clearly shaped by my status as a Western, non-Muslim outsider with academic credentials in the subject of history. But once satisfied with my appreciation of their history, the activists treated me as an audience for historically based stances that were both ethical and political, and that they viewed as inseparable from the issue of AIDS control. They combined this rhetoric seamlessly with elements of the medical/technocratic language of AIDS education and ART provision. In a politic and rhetorically skilful way, my interlocutors handed me a message to take home to my assumed European interlocutors, adapted to my interests and skills. Such redeployment of the terms of our encounter is arguably a fairly routine event between European researchers and African subjects (Bayart 1993; Ellis 2011; Vaughan 1991).

Though clearly opportune to propose when speaking to an outsider, the nexus between the political, the medical and the ethical that these activists proposed was not only a rhetorical ploy. The case can be argued that the educational weakness and political marginality of the Muslim community in Tanzania adds to its difficulties in organizing to face the threats of AIDS, and in maintaining those standards of controlled sexual behaviour that might contribute to limiting the spread of the disease. Moreover, further interaction with some of the activists present at this meeting showed them to be quite consistent in their views. Nevertheless, the way they put their stance to me was deeply shaped by the activists' understanding of the institutional and political context of both AIDS control and the politics of religion in Tanzania.

In particular, they had developed a vocabulary that combined elements of reformist and political Islam with a donor-friendly, Anglophone language of public health education. It was the work of relatively young sheikhs with experience of living abroad[2] and a perfect command of English. Their personas, or in Fergusonian terms their style, were altogether more donor-friendly than that of the older generations of typically exclusively Swahili-speaking Muslim notables. Yet it was also clearly kindred to the style of this older generation. For instance, they wore the *kanzu* gowns and *kofia* caps favoured by the older generation and in their Swahili-language discussions used a similarly ceremonial turn of phrase.

Many of the views stated and the comportment on display in the Starlight Hotel meeting room were not specific to that occasion. The people assembled formed part of a milieu where *kanzu* and *kofia*, Arabic-language interjections

---

[2] One of them claimed to have a wife in Plymouth, the site of exile of the last Sultan of Zanzibar.

in everyday speech and complaints of discrimination against Muslims are part of a settled and ordinary, rather than activist, way of life. Arguably, this complex could itself be identified as a Fergusonian style, in the sense that it is a half-conscious, half-intuitive form of negotiation between different spheres of life and cultural influences. At the same time, the people at this meeting had an agenda and a rhetoric that went beyond this settled way of life. They fell into a spectrum of popular Muslim reform that has in other contexts been convincingly described as an ethical project calling on members of its audience to reform themselves (Hirschkind 2006). It is impossible to distinguish the 'activist' from the 'settled' practitioners of this style except by detailed knowledge of their life and affairs.

The meeting at the Starlight Hotel however also displayed a more specific permutation of this form of 'demonstratively Muslim' comportment, whose hallmark was the combination of what might be called 'moderate Muslim reformist' language with medical-technocratic 'donor speak'. This observation does not imply that the people present were either disingenuously manipulative or naïve and manipulated by donors. Rather, they were trying to make the best of the constraints imposed by TACAIDS's proposed funding regime, while also pursuing a much wider religious, political (and for some of them, very likely, ethical) project. In so doing, they were developing a 'trustworthy Muslim funding recipient' style intended to provide them with credibility both in interaction with donor agencies and with fellow Muslims.

Events in the years since this meeting suggest that this project, while demanding constant attention, works. The trajectory, people and institutions involved in the original meeting show both how individuals move between different personalized styles and how different styles meet in institutional settings. One of the results has been the setting-up of the Tanzania Muslim Welfare Network (TMWN), with the help and constant involvement of TACAIDS. While it has focused so far on the 'mainstreaming' of AIDS education into the regular educational activities of its constituent organizations (rather than setting up AIDS-specific projects), it is intended as a means of extending such activities and making them more specific.[3]

Among TMWN's central office-holders are at least two of the people I interacted with at the 2008 meeting (TMWN 2010: 22). One of them, Sheikh Muhammad Bashir, demonstrated the possibilities of 'style-switching' to me as we met in a succession of different contexts.[4] At an initial meeting in a smart suburban Dar es Salaam hotel, he emphasized his ability to function in Anglophone aid-focused contexts: speaking English by default, mentioning

[3] Interview with Hashim Kalinga, Dar es Salaam, 28 July 2012.

[4] As I have not been able to confirm with this sheikh that he is comfortable with being mentioned by name, I have used a pseudonym here.

his extended stay in the UK, and discussing his past role as an adviser to an aid organization developing a guide to women's rights and gender relations for Muslim women. When we met again at the Starlight Hotel, the default language was Swahili. The discussion, as mentioned above, was much more focused on Muslims' problems, and the rhetoric used was suffused with expressions of piety. The mixture has been effective inasmuch as it has enabled the sheikh to pursue an active career on the interface of religious activism and AIDS-related consulting.

Hashim Kalinga of TACAIDS assesses the progress of TMWN very cautiously, in large measure because of the different organizational traditions, interests and religious stances that have to be accommodated. He described a sheikh from the periphery of Dar es Salaam who had been sniping from the sidelines at TMWN as obsolete and self-seeking, intent on directing funds to his own mosque only. This man had clearly failed to project a 'trustworthy recipient' persona, but Kalinga and his colleagues felt that they were succeeding, if gradually, with others in TMWN. While dedicated, institutionally separate AIDS-related projects remain few in number, TMWN supports the mainstreaming of AIDS education in the schools and mosques run by its members.

To expand these activities, TACAIDS is now actively encouraging TMWN participants to develop their aptitude in the production of donor-friendly rhetoric by way of bidding for funds from donors. At a time of dwindling state funds, Kalinga is explicit that learning to convince non-state donors to provide funds was part of TMWN members' brief. The engagement between parastatal TACAIDS and Muslims has thus become a three-way conversation in which non-state donors set some of the parameters, which reinforces the importance of speaking their language.

The first source of such funds mentioned by Kalinga, the Rapid Funding Envelope (RFE) for HIV/AIDS in Tanzania, is not strictly speaking private but is distinctive in the way it presents itself as the equivalent of an issues-focused private philanthropy.[5] Concomitantly, it demands a particular kind of self-presentation from its grantees. RFE is a consortium of several European donor nations with Tanzanian government participation on its board, and administration provided *pro bono* by a management consultancy firm. Rather than hand funds to government or state institutions, it makes grants to so-called civil-society groups ranging from mission hospitals to women's self-help groups.

There are just a handful of Muslim groups among its grantees so far (RFE 2010). Yet the RFE is a practical reflection of current donor emphasis on interaction with civil-society partners, the importance of engaging stakeholders and partnership in development (Mercer 2003). The efforts of TACAID and the Muslim activists in TMWN show some of the ironies of this approach. Representatives of Muslim groups are learning to project a particular kind of

---

5 See http://www.rapidfundingenvelope.org (accessed 22 November 2012).

persona, with help from an arm of the Tanzanian state, so as to obtain funds that are aimed at pre-existing (non-state) civil-society groups. Yet as the notion of civil-society groups as partners in AIDS activism becomes entrenched, this style of self-presentation is likely to endure (PEPFAR 2010).

'The Sated Infect the Hungry': Popular Perceptions of ART and Political Power

If we identify this demeanour as a 'style' in the sense discussed above, it has to be acceptable, tolerable or intelligible to a variety of constituencies, not all of them Muslim, in order to be viable. Moreover, it is less a planned stratagem than an exercise in tentative and intuitive meaning-making. The wild variety of narratives and stances on AIDS that has to be negotiated is in evidence up and down the country (Iliffe 2006). Arguably, it provides further pointers towards understanding why my interlocutors at the Starlight Hotel were committed to a narrative on AIDS that had a strong political element and questioned the ethical commitments of representatives of the state: it also resonates with popular perceptions.

The slogan 'AIDS: those who have eaten their fill infect the hungry' was on display for some time along one of Dar es Salaam's main bus routes in a religiously mixed neighbourhood. It is a pithy summary of a popular understanding of AIDS that connects it to a broader account of the strong in Tanzania increasingly taking advantage, or disregarding the needs, of the weak. 'Strong' in this case typically stands for privately wealthy, politically well-connected or – increasingly – both. There is some indication that this view of the character of Tanzanian society is spreading in connection with the increasing brazenness of advantage-seeking among political and commercial elites (Kelsall 2002; Jim Giblin, personal communication).

This perception also resonates with attitudes in the provincial town of Lindi where Muslims on the whole have limited sympathies for the reformist convictions and rhetoric of my Dar es Salaam interlocutors. Reformists here tend to be perceived as young troublemakers (Becker 2008). When the existence of ART first became known here, a couple of years before it was affordable for the less affluent, it raised comment not due to any conceivable religious implication or association, but rather because access constituted another instantiation of affluence or privilege. Before AIDS began to carry off precarious young petty traders in large numbers, it was sometimes spoken of as a disease of the affluent who could buy sex (Becker 2009) and now, it was again the affluent who could buy a reprieve from death. 'Some fat people would grow very thin', this line went, 'and then suddenly they start growing fat again. Then you know they're on ART.'

In this line of reasoning, access to ART was effectively located in a space that is antithetical to the main concerns of religious practice. As I have argued elsewhere, Islamic allegiance in Lindi and similar towns is very much about participation and equality (Becker 2008). The personal wealth of the cliché of an ART recipient invoked here is, however, widely associated with the ruthless pursuit of personal advantage and ascendancy. Unfortunately, the arrival of ART provision through government channels has not made this cliché entirely obsolete. A doctor working in Lindi reports rigid bureaucratic insistence on the part of the staff running the treatment programme that treatment must not be started until a specific CD4 cell count is reached. In some cases, clearly needy patients, including a two-year-old girl, were denied treatment because such a count could not be established, even if this was merely due to technical difficulties. The doctor felt that the two-year-old might have had a better chance of obtaining the drugs if she had had connections or money.

With occurrences such as this, the ART programme does not dispel but in fact reinforces the wider perception of an ongoing convergence of political and economic power in the hands of a few, to the detriment of the majority of Tanzanians. If ART access appears to be a privilege, it becomes associated, in the minds of observers if not recipients, with the opposite of ethical restraint, namely with influence-peddling, greed and dissipation. Such clichés, of course, recall those previously associated with HIV infection, which are a well-known part of the problem faced by people living with HIV/ART. But now they are coming to be directed against the medical establishment that deals with AIDS.

The Persistence of Early Established Narratives about HIV/AIDS

This insertion of ART into an older moral narrative on HIV/AIDS suggests the possibility of recuperating the new medical practice of ART into established ways of thinking. There is some evidence of such recuperation: ART may be spoken of as a 'strong medicine' with its attendant dangers, much like other substances obtained from both healers and biomedical practitioners (Becker 2009; Dilger and Luig 2010). If, in turn, ART joins the category of strong medicine, it also becomes amenable to the sort of personal negotiation that characterizes the interaction between healer and patient. Of course, the institutional structures that provide ART are nowhere near as flexible as healers are. But this does not stop patients from looking upon the substances they provide as part of a broader quest for healing rather than as a drug to be taken in one way only and superseding all other treatment.

The spectrum of 'traditional' healing practice also comprises Muslim specialists among its most respected members (Langwick 2001, 2011). Islamic, particularly Quranic, healing is an important part of medical practice for

Muslims, but we have almost no information about how Quranic healers are contributing to efforts to confront AIDS. It is worth noting though that Muslim reformists have been cautious about speaking out against Quranic healing (Becker 2009). They have generally limited themselves to condemning its dark side, witchcraft, and some reformists endorse Quranic healing. Reformists' acquiescence in Quranic healing shows that an explicit orientation towards ethical self-fashioning – setting aside the question of how it is lived – can coexist with an understanding of healing as part of a mutual interaction between patient and practitioner, rather than the process of self-regulation where maintenance of an ART regime is most readily presented.

Taken together, the phenomena identified in this section suggest possibilities of an understanding of HIV/ART that is informed by Islam, and may even coexist with reformist, ethical religious orientations, yet does not constitute an individualized process of religiously inspired ethical self-fashioning of the kind that other observers have suggested. Instead it appears that concerns surrounding AIDS and ART can be integrated into hybrid ways of reasoning that now have a long history in Africa. There is a large body of literature on the way African mission Christians redeployed missionaries' teachings on the devil and on spirits, integrating witchcraft and spirit beliefs into their Christianity (Meyer 1999). There is evidence that HIV too may be likened to an evil spirit, to be countered not only with the cultivation of religious commitment but also with prayer (Dilger 2007).

Some of the earliest literature on Africans' intellectual responses to HIV/AIDS showed that indigenous notions of health and pollution were deeply involved in the conceptualization of AIDS, concomitantly allowing for the devising of responses to the epidemic that showed clear similarities with ways of countering more traditional epidemics (Schoffeleers 1999). More recent work, already encompassing the implications of ART, is still finding similar dynamics at work: anthropologists have had recourse to such staples of ethnography as pollution fears (focused on death at least as much as sexual transgression) to interpret the way people think about AIDS, in the presence of ART, in the twenty-first century (Dilger and Luig 2010).

All this suggests that discourses indicative of ethical self-fashioning can coexist with, and perhaps even mimic and redeploy not just fairly standardized international religious discourse (both Christian born-again and Muslim reformist) but also long-standing African views on virtue, self-cultivation and self-control. Similarly, it is likely that the relationship between ART recipient and counsellor, or between international donor and a local faith-based provider echoes not only interactions in educational seminars held in Western contexts but also that between healer and patient/customer in African healing practice.

Conclusions

Reviewing the observations so far, we face the following situation: the interpretation of the ramifications of AIDS education and, even more, ART provision in terms of self-fashioning or subject formation is immediately plausible. It captures both the self-reflective nature of the process of learning to live with an HIV-positive diagnosis and the strongly prescriptive elements in AIDS education and ART patient-compliance education or monitoring programmes. At the same time, though, due to the intractability of the object of discussion – the self – such interpretations are hard to elaborate on with specificity and certainty.

In other words, it is possible, even likely, that for many people, an HIV-positive diagnosis and integration into an ART programme constitute a profound reorientation that by some standards merits description as self-fashioning. But it is also possible that subjects of counselling simply 'go through the motions', saying what they think they should be saying. Privately, they may persist in drawing on accounts of HIV/AIDS as well as ART that are closer to the refashioned traditional aetiologies and narratives of social anomie already known from earlier literature on cultural responses to AIDS in Africa. This leaves us with the question of how to characterize such pragmatic responses. It is dissatisfying to characterize them as hypocrisy, not only because of the judgmental nature of this term but also because it insinuates a degree of conscious reflection and planning that cannot be taken for granted in people facing a life-threatening and life-altering situation.

Moreover, even where transformations do occur, they are liable to be ambivalent and partial, leading Dilger (2012: 85) to assert that 'these different types of gendered subjectivities and concepts of the person ... are not mutually exclusive'. Africans, it appears from this point of view, are growing *multiple* selves. This state of affairs gives added urgency to the question about whether or in what sense these subjectivities are specific to Africans, which they would have to be unless we accept that all of us juggle multiple subjectivities. This is a tenable position but not one to be taken for granted. Moreover, accounts of subject formation invite questions as to what previous kind of self Africans' 'new' selves are supposed to be changing from.

It is possible to construct answers that avoid modernization-theorist clichés of transition from pre-modern, purely relational, or somehow sectional and multiple 'African' selves. Still, there is a rat's tail of problems attached to the proposition of changing selves in the context of AIDS and ART provision. The main reason why the concept is readily used appears to be its ability to highlight the machinations of 'soft', non-state, interpersonal rather than official forms of power. This capacity, in turn, is due to the significance invested in the complex of subject formation, care of the self and biopower by the writings and readers of Michel Foucault.

However, as signposted above, state institutions as well as international donors and NGOs in Africa have a tendency towards impermanence, ineffectualness and even evanescence that sits poorly with Foucauldian descriptions of the 'capillary power' inherent in things such as discourses of self-care as an *extension* of more solid, institutional forms of power. In the African case, aid programmes and civil-society or faith-based organizations are often substitutes or competitors for state institutions and the whole ensemble does not form a solid block. Prince's work, for example, suggests that these discontinuities deserve more attention than the routine deployment of Foucauldian language draws to them.

Against this background, thinking of the processes under discussion as the cultivation of discursive styles is helpful because it focuses attention on the observable. It also allows for the possibility that in a group of people professing similar commitments to self-care, there may be sharply varying degrees of commitment to these commitments, not because some people are hypocrites and others are not, but because styles become internalized, personalized and habitual to varying degrees. The cultivation of 'compliant ART patient' or 'competent aid recipient' discursive styles, in other words, can be thought of as a medium in which the fashioning of new kinds of selves can happen, but does not have to. In this sense, it is not an alternative to subject formation but its kindred.

The notion of discursive styles also entails a different way of thinking about the tension between the liberation often professedly experienced by subjects of counselling, and the subjection that observers trace in the same process. Cultivating a style always means dealing creatively with necessity. It is an improvised process of trial and error, part reflective and part intuitive, and not necessarily verbalized. The slippage between emancipation and subjection is in-built, and which element predominates is contingent upon a person's situation more widely.

Tatu Mohamedi and her scrapbook, mentioned at the outset, form a good illustration of this. She moved on from dutiful daughter to dutiful wife, endorsing close regulation of her personal behaviour in the scrapbook and using it to demonstrate her readiness to make the transition. In a sense, she is a case study in subject formation, the capillary power of a religious discourse expanding into the intimate details of her life. But in her everyday life, quite different elements of her experience were in the foreground. Thanks to her marriage, she had company she liked, two rooms to herself (shared with her husband but beyond the control of her birth family), the relative calm that came with the absence of her effervescent stepmother, and even enough respectability, as a married woman, to take a job without setting tongues wagging.

Her experience thus highlights the close relationship between oppressive and emancipatory elements in the development of AIDS-related styles. It also points to an apparent contrast between Muslim and Christian styles: the former focus more on collective control of individual morality, the latter on emotionally charged personal relationships (with others as well as with God). In part, this reflects the greater attention to politics that their discomfort in the contemporary polities forces on Muslims. It is also a permutation of a long-standing contrast (in the modern East African setting, not globally) between legalism on the Muslim side and prophecy on the Christian one. But perhaps both languages focused on law and those focused on prophecy can be understood also as a means to devise *collective* responses, and hence pointers to the persistence of the 'networked' individual in Africa.

References

Bayart, J.F. 1993. *The State in Africa: The Politics of the Belly*. London: Polity Press.

Becker, F. 2007. The virus and the scriptures: Muslims and AIDS in Tanzania. *Journal of Religion in Africa*, 37, 16–40.

Becker, F. 2008. *Becoming Muslim in Mainland Tanzania*. Oxford and London: Oxford University Press.

Becker, F. 2009. Competing explanations and treatment choices: Muslims, AIDS and ARVs in Tanzania, in *AIDS and Religious Practice in Africa*, edited by F. Becker and P.W. Geissler. Leiden: Brill, 155–88.

Beckmann, N. 2009. AIDS and the power of God: Narratives of decline and coping strategies in Zanzibar, in *AIDS and Religious Practice in Africa*, edited by F. Becker and P.W. Geissler. Leiden: Brill, 119–54.

Bhabha, H. 1995. In a spirit of calm violence, in *After Colonialism: Imperial Histories and Post-Colonial Displacements*, edited by G. Prakash. Princeton, NJ: Princeton University Press, 326–44.

Bosma, H. and Gerlsma, C. 2003. From early attachment relations to the adolescent and adult organisation of self, in *Handbook of Developmental Psychology*, edited by J. Valsiner and K. Connolly. London: Sage, 450–90.

Burchardt, M. 2009. Subjects of counselling, in *AIDS and Religious Practice in Africa*, edited by F. Becker and P.W. Geissler. Leiden: Brill, 333–58.

Comaroff, J. and Comaroff, J. 1993. *Modernity and its Malcontents: Ritual and Power in Post-Colonial Africa*. Chicago, IL: University of Chicago Press.

Dilger, H. 2007. Healing the wounds of modernity: Community, salvation and care in a neo-Pentecostal church in Dar es Salaam, Tanzania. *Journal of Religion in Africa*, 37(1), 59–83.

Dilger, H. 2012. Targeting the empowered individual: Transnational policy-making, the global economy of aid and the limitation of 'biopower' in the neoliberal era, in *Medicine, Mobility, and Power in Global Africa:*

Transnational Health and Healing, edited by H. Dilger, A. Kane and S. Langwick. Bloomington, IN: Indiana University Press, 60–91.

Dilger, H. and Luig, U. 2010. *Morality, Hope and Grief: Anthropologies of AIDS in Africa*. Oxford: Berghahn.

Eickelman, D. and Piscatori, J. 1996. *Muslim Politics*. Princeton, NJ: Princeton University Press.

Ellis, S. 2011. *Season of Rains: Africa in the World*. London: Hurst.

Falk Moore, S. 1996. Post-socialist micro-politics: Kilimanjaro. *Africa*, 66, 587–606.

Ferguson, J. 1999. *Expectations of Modernity: Myths and Meanings of Urban Life on the Zambian Copperbelt*. Berkeley, CA: University of California Press.

Foucault, M. 2008. *The Birth of Biopolitics: Lectures at the College de France, 1978–79*. London: Palgrave Macmillan.

Geissler, P.W. and Prince, R.J. 2010. *The Land is Dying: Contingency, Creativity and Conflict in Western Kenya*. Oxford: Berghahn.

Glassman, J. 1995. *Feasts and Riot: Revelry, Rebellion and Popular Consciousness on the Swahili Coast, 1856–88*. Oxford: James Currey.

Glassman, J. 2011. *War of Words, War of Stones: Racial Thought and Violence in Colonial Zanzibar*. Bloomington, IN: Indiana University Press.

Green, M., Mercer, C. and Mesaki, S. 2010. *The Development Activities, Values and Performance of Non-governmental and Faith-Based Organisations in Magu and Newala Districts, Tanzania*. Birmingham: Religions and Development Research Consortium, Working Paper No. 49.

Gulliver, P. 1971. *Neighbours and Networks: The Idiom of Kinship in Social Action among the Ndendeuli in Tanzania*. Berkeley, CA: University of California Press.

Hirschkind, C. 2006. *The Ethical Soundscape: Cassette Sermons and Islamic Counterpublics*. New York: Columbia University Press.

Iliffe, J. 2006. *The African AIDS Epidemic: A History*. Cambridge: Cambridge University Press.

Irigaray, L. 1985. *Speculum of the Other Woman*. Ithaca, NY: Cornell University Press.

Kelsall, T. 2002. Shop windows and smoke-filled rooms: Governance and the re-politicization of Tanzania. *Journal of Modern African Studies*, 40, 597–616.

Kresse, K. 2007. *Philosophising in Mombasa*. Edinburgh: Edinburgh University Press.

Langwick, S. 2001. Devils and development. PhD thesis, Department of Anthropology, Chapel Hill, University of North Carolina.

Langwick, S. 2011. *Bodies, Politics and African Healing: The Matter of Maladies in Tanzania*. Bloomington, IN: Indiana University Press.

Lockman, Z. 2004. *Contending Visions of the Middle East: The History and Politics of Orientalism*. Cambridge: Cambridge University Press.

Loimeier, R. 2007. Perceptions of marginalization: Muslims in contemporary Tanzania, in *Islam and Muslim Politics in Africa*, edited by R. Otayek and B. Soares. London: Palgrave Macmillan, 137–56.

Mbiti, J. 1969. *African Religions and Philosophy*. Portsmouth, NH: Heinemann.

Mercer, C. 2003. Performing partnership: civil society and the illusions of good governance in Tanzania. *Political Geography*, 22, 741–63.

Meyer, B. 1999. *Translating the Devil: Religion and Modernity among the Ewe in Ghana*. Edinburgh: Edinburgh University Press.

Mitchell, J C. 1956. *The Yao Village: A Study in the Social Structure of a Malawian Tribe*. Manchester: Manchester University Press.

Nguyen, V.-K. 2009. Therapeutic evangelism: Confessional technologies, antiretrovirals and biospiritual transformation in the fight against AIDS in West Africa, in *AIDS and Religious Practice in Africa*, edited by F. Becker and P.W. Geissler. Leiden: Brill, 359–78

PEPFAR (Presidential Emergency Program for AIDS Research) 2010. *Tanzania Operational Plan Report, FY 2010*. [Online]. Available at: http://www.pepfar.gov/documents/organization/145736.pdf [accessed 18 February 2012].

Prince, R. 2012. The moral economy of survival in an East African city. *Medical Anthropology Quarterly*, 26(4), 534–56.

RFE (Rapid Funding Envelope for HIV/AIDS) Tanzania 2010. *Project summaries, round 0–4*. [Online]. Available at: http://www.rapidfundingenvelope.org/documents/grantee/RFE_Award_Summaries.pdf [accessed: 18 February 2013].

Schoffeleers, M. 1999. The AIDS pandemic, the prophet Billy Chisupe, and the democratization process in Malawi. *Journal of Religion in Africa*, 29, 406–21.

Stoler, A.L. 2010. *Carnal Knowledge and Imperial Power: Race and the Intimate in Colonial Rule*. Berkeley, CA: University of California Press.

TMWN (Tanzania Muslim Welfare Network) 2010. *Tanzania Muslim Welfare Network (TMWN – Mtandao Wa Ustawi Wa Uislamu Tanzania): Katiba*. Dar es Salaam: No publisher given.

Van Dijk, R. 2009. Gloves in times of AIDS: Pentecostalism, hair and social distancing in Botswana, in *AIDS and Religious Practice in Africa*, edited by F. Becker and W. Geissler. Leiden: Brill, 283–308.

Vaughan, M. 1991. *Curing their Ills: Colonial Power and African Illness*. Cambridge and Oxford: Polity Press and Blackwell.

Weber, M. 1988 [1920/21]. *Gesammelte* Aufsaetze zur Religionssoziologie. Tuebingen: UTB.

Chapter 2

The Logic of Therapeutic Habitus: Culture, Religion and Biomedical AIDS Treatments in South Africa

Marian Burchardt

Introduction

The history of HIV/AIDS in South Africa is complex, with the most contradictory and politically contentious part being the history of the scientific search for biomedical treatment (Nattrass 2008). Well into the second part of the last decade, the government remained critical of ARVs, with this rejection forming a central part of its 'AIDS denialism' (Posel 2005; Fassin 2007). By 2011, however, South Africa boasted the largest ARV programme in the world with an enrolment of more than 1.8 million people. As a result, ARVs are now mediating the survival, health and well-being of huge numbers of people, turning patients into drug users and 'programme clients', and rendering their lives contingent upon the sustainability of the financing mechanisms of global and national public health systems and medical humanitarianism.

Despite the sweeping biomedicalization of HIV/AIDS treatment in Africa, which the spread of ARVs highlights with the concomitant 'pharmaceuticalization of public health' (Biehl 2007), studies by medical anthropologists have demonstrated that, at least for those diagnosed as HIV-positive and enrolled in a treatment programme, AIDS is often far from normalized (Mattes 2011). On the contrary, collective negotiations of the meanings of ARVs in many African countries reveal features of a multilayered politics of cultural reproduction, in which pharmaceuticals are sometimes seen as contesting the authority of traditional healers, are interpreted through religious idioms or are otherwise placed within local universes of therapeutic significations. They also constitute a new step in the long history of engagements with biomedicine (Vaughan 1991), a step that reveals the specificities of the cultural politics surrounding HIV/AIDS that, in the eyes of many observers, marked the disease as being unique from the beginning, and are now returning in contestations over therapeutic practices regarding ARVs. Moreover, ARVs do not seem to be dramatically altering or diminishing the experience of existential contingency attached to infection and diagnosis, and that is typically expressed in the question 'Why me?'.

Questions like this point to the problem of suffering and remind us of Geertz's (1973: 104) claim regarding the links between religion, well-being and pain:

> As a religious problem, the problem of suffering is, paradoxically, not about avoiding to suffer but how to suffer, how to make of physical pain, personal loss, worldly defeat, or the helpless contemplation of others' agony something bearable, supportable – something, as we say, sufferable.

This proposition was derived from an engagement with Weber's concerns with theodicy and the observation that preoccupations with the contingency of suffering and injustices in a world, supposedly created by a higher or even perfect being, were at the very bottom of the world religions. Weber (1972: 318) began his sociology of religion with the suggestion that religious or magically motivated action is a rational practice guided by the rules of experience, directed at this-worldly affairs and aiming to enhance well-being and long life. Despite some differences in nuance, Geertz's rendition of the religious problem shares Weber's view that religion is less about solving than formulating problems and suggesting ways of dealing with them.

Some anthropologists have observed powerful articulations of religion with biomedical treatment for HIV/AIDS in the way patients deploy religious vocabularies and ideas in expressing and conceptualizing the transcendent experiences of recovery following enrolment. Robins (2004) shows how patients who are recovering draw on the discursive repertoires of charismatic Christianity in assimilating their recoveries to, or even identifying them with, spiritual states of salvation in terms of being 'born again'. In a different vein, Nguyen (2009) explores the striking similarities between religious forms and biomedical HIV/AIDS prevention and treatment campaigns with regard to the confessional technologies employed in both, so as to target 'the self as substrate' (ibid.: 360) and to produce experiences of conversion. Kalofonos (2010), albeit focusing on different questions, captures another important aspect of the links between religion and biomedical pharmaceuticals in the title of his article 'All I eat is ARVs', namely the sacralization of ARVs as life-giving and life-sustaining substances and their prioritization within broader hierarchies of need and human value in local and transnational therapeutic discourses.

Some broader theoretical concerns at stake here, however, are most productively addressed by emphasizing the way religion is associated with the contingency of living with HIV/AIDS, as Geertz suggested. Taking contingency as a vantage point, this chapter outlines the relevance of three key theoretical concepts for studying religion and biomedical HIV/AIDS treatments: the functional differentiation of knowledge, the idea of self-formation, and the notion of therapeutic habitus, which is akin to what Becker (this volume), drawing on Ferguson, terms 'discursive styles'. I begin with an ethnographic sketch of religious treatment activism in Cape Town, from which I develop these concepts. Next, I elaborate on how they help to shape a notion of 'therapeutic habitus' that can be conceptualized in Bourdieu's (1977) terms. The final part of the chapter analyses how therapeutic choices are shaped by therapeutic habitus. Drawing on two autobiographical accounts and ethnographic data linked to them, I explicate distinct forms whereby HIV-positive people construe the meanings of treatment while navigating religious fields.

Religion and Biomedical Activism in Cape Town

In 2005, a small group of HIV-positive people began to meet regularly on Saturday afternoons in a small community hall in Town II in the township of Khayelitsha. Most were women and they followed the initiative of Melisizwe, a 45-year-old self-inspired AIDS activist.[1] Until the end of apartheid, Melisizwe had spent most of his life in training camps run by the ANC's military wing in Angola and in the apartheid government's political prisons in the Western Cape Province. Gradually withdrawing from politics, he converted to Pentecostal Christianity in the late 1990s and became acquainted with a Baptist pastor from the U.S. This pastor not only trained him in theology and later ordained him, but also helped to establish close contacts between his American Baptist congregation and the Pentecostal community called El Shaddai that Melisizwe had meanwhile founded. These contacts eventually materialized in a monthly stipend of US$200 from the American Baptists, with the idea that this would enable him to pursue his HIV/AIDS projects.

Médecins Sans Frontières (MSF), in close cooperation with the Treatment Action Campaign (TAC), has been implementing an ARV treatment programme at four pilot sites in South Africa since 2003, one of which was located in Khayelitsha (Robins 2004). Several of the members of Melisizwe's group were enrolled in the MSF programme and thus belonged to the first (small) cohort of South Africans to become ARV users. The same people also participated as activists in TAC's mobilization and awareness campaigns, demanding universal access to free treatment but also hoping to found their own initiative in the context of Melisizwe's Pentecostal church. Drawing on their training with TAC, which was instrumental in disseminating knowledge

[1] Melisizwe is the leader of the group but is not HIV-positive himself. Leading by example, he goes for HIV tests every two months. All the names used in this chapter have been changed to protect the informants' identity.

about the buzzwords, organizational forms and practices of the transnational assemblage of biomedical humanitarianism dominating the global AIDS industry, they labelled their group a 'support group' and began carrying out a host of different activities. They organized anti-stigma fun walks through the neighbourhood and distributed condoms in *shebeens*, taverns, youth clubs and private houses in door-to-door campaigns and also distributed leaflets about the support group as a way of self-promotion, rallying financial support and trying to appeal to new members. In 2006 they also started organizing workshop trips to the Eastern Cape Province where they would tour villages and small towns to raise awareness and spread progressive messages about HIV prevention, educate villagers, whom the activists were inclined to deem retrograde, and, most importantly, to spread the news that, with the arrival of ARVs, South Africa and its people were at the dawn of a new era.[2] At some point, the group established formal ties with a local governmental clinic in Khayelitsha that would send people with an HIV-positive diagnosis to them through a referral system. Those group members who were activists were open about their status inside as well as outside group meetings, while other members developed a more differentiated pattern of disclosure.

One of the most striking features of Melisizwe's group was the overwhelming preoccupation with ARV treatment, especially since it occurred at a time when most church-based groups were still focusing on practical and spiritual support. What is more, most Pentecostal churches were still squarely opposed to HIV/AIDS work, which they deemed ambivalent, if not dangerous, because it seemed to support sinners. In fact, the earliest of Melisizwe's activities was to visit dozens of the small Pentecostal and African-initiated churches in Khayelitsha and other townships to pray with their pastors and enlighten them, as he saw it, on sexuality, HIV infection and Jesus Christ's 'real' message to an AIDS-ridden society. For the group, this message centred on love and support for the excluded. Here, as in the villages and small towns visited during the workshop trips in Eastern Cape Province, pastors were encouraged to found their own support groups so that these standardized practices would spread in a snowball system of sorts.

Just as ARVs started to become available for a small number of people in Khayelitsha through the MSF pilot programme, various Pentecostal pastors began to agitate against these medicines in their congregations. Palesa, a young female group member, reported that her pastor had asked her to stop taking ARVs, which he condemned as demonic substances. From this and similar occurrences, a clear pattern emerges, namely that Pentecostals reject ARVs to the extent that their use is perceived as undermining absolute faith in the

[2] In 2003, the South African government had, after a protracted legal struggle with the TAC, eventually decided on a comprehensive treatment programme on the basis of free universal access.

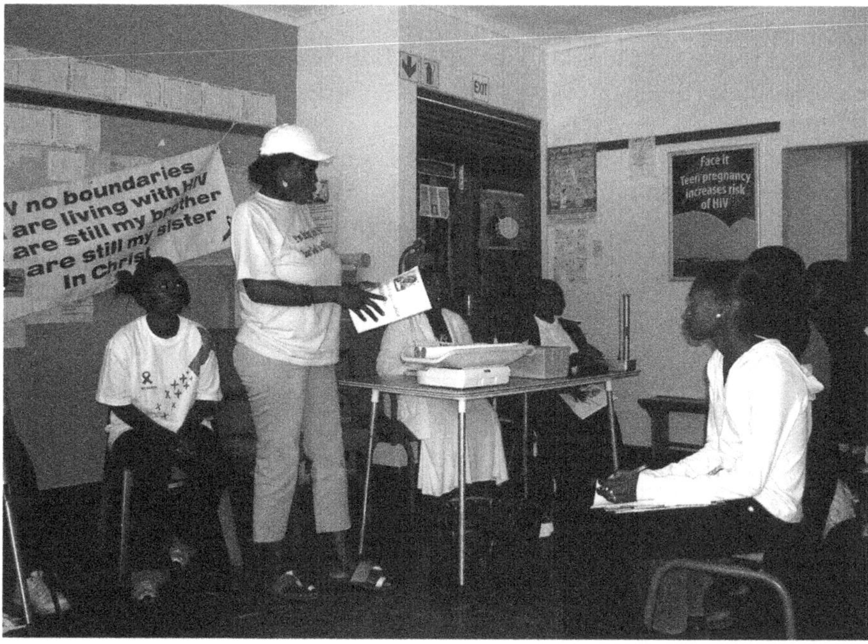
no boundaries
are living with HIV
are still my brother
are still my sister
EXIT
Face it
Teen pregnancy
increases risk
of HIV

Figure 2.1 South African HIV/AIDS treatment activists in a village clinic in the Eastern Cape Province (Source: Marian Burchardt)

healing power of the Holy Spirit and the ways in which this power can be accessed through prayer alone. Prayers, however, demand and presuppose an inner state of belief, and the conviction that 'the Holy Spirit can do *everything*', as Pentecostals never tire of mentioning, is viewed as incompatible with the mental state underlying the use of biomedical drugs. The same kind of religiously inspired humanitarian progressivism that drove Melisizwe to agitate amongst Pentecostal pastors against the simple equation of HIV/AIDS with sin now motivated him to visit these pastors again to convince them of the need to fight for universal access to treatment. Importantly, these conversations rarely involved any theological reasoning on the divine nature of pharmaceuticals. He would usually talk to the pastors about his activities, tell them how much people enjoyed sharing the Christian spirit in meetings and how desperately people needed ARVs to survive. In addition, there was a substrate belief that a positive spirit would be disseminated amongst these pastors most effectively through collective effervescence spawned by common prayers.

Yet the concerns among some Pentecostal pastors over ARVs not only reflected their theologies of the Holy Spirit but were also closely entangled with sexual moralities. Similar to many of the larger Evangelical churches, they worried that advances in medical treatment would undermine their efforts to frame solutions to the HIV/AIDS crisis exclusively in terms of sexual restraint (Burchardt 2011). They thought that the more easily accessible medical treatment for AIDS was, the less likely it would be that people would adhere to abstinence and the 'be faithful' messages on which their entire HIV/AIDS work was based. More broadly, such concerns epitomized fears of a general normalization and de-dramatization of the HIV/AIDS epidemic after which people would return to careless, irresponsible and un-Christian sexual practices. Interestingly, some secular public health officials shared these concerns, arguing that only a fear of death would motivate people to adhere to prevention messages. However, social scientists (Nattrass 2008) claimed that the availability of treatment would encourage people to test precisely because HIV infection was not tantamount to impending death anymore, and that higher testing rates would allow for better prevention. With the reductive effect of ARVs on the infection rates of potential patients at moments of unprotected sex, these positive aspects would far outweigh the negative ones.

Melisizwe was not, however, only concerned about the spiritual value pastors were ready to afford life-sustaining drugs against AIDS but also about the everyday pragmatics of treatment adherence, whose failure he could frequently observe amongst his friends, his congregation and support-group members. In 2008, pillboxes were increasingly promoted by TAC and other HIV/AIDS organizations as a new medical technology to improve adherence. Referred to as 'medication organizers' in public health discourse, these are flat plastic boxes with a transparent cap and differently coloured cases for pills that are arranged into weeks, days and hours. The idea was that taking medication on time would be done more reliably by using these boxes. Melisizwe took up this idea, used his connections in TAC to obtain a few initial boxes for free and began promoting them in the neighbourhood. After a few months, he and the group began to raise funds for more trips to the Eastern Cape villages with the sole aim of promoting this technology. As he had done on other occasions before, he asked me to support him by generating lists with addresses of charismatic churches in Europe and to pass on his fundraising letters to them, believing they would be ready to jump on the bandwagon and sponsor his pillbox activism. Melisizwe and the group members shared the assumption that, apart from charitable impulses, common Pentecostal sentiments in terms of a concept of global Pentecostal brother- and sisterhood would facilitate flows of resources. While most of this came to nothing, the pillboxes and the idea that they would help save lives in Africa mediated a complex set of clientelist relationships between Cape Town, Berlin and other places in Europe for a few months.

ARVs were thus a key theme in the group's 'therapeutic evangelism' (Nguyen 2009) and outreach activities, and also in the group's regular meetings. These meetings were replete with conversations about medical drugs, the importance and complexity of treatment adherence, and concerns about what was best for members in terms of 'healthy lifestyles'. Often members would engage in lengthy discussions on the benefits and risks of ARVs, immune boosters and their possible side-effects. These themes were elaborated on in great technical detail that would have been barely intelligible to outsiders. At one level, these discussions were meant to disseminate the latest highly relevant medical knowledge, pointing to support groups as cultural arenas for negotiating therapeutic choices and brokering therapeutic resources in the context of widespread therapeutic uncertainty.[3] At another level, however, there was a great deal of redundancy in these discussions and many seemed to rehearse what everybody already knew. As a result, it was clear that the members simply liked addressing these issues. What emerged was a medical sociality of sorts, wrought from the common biological condition, with pharmaceuticals as one of the group's preferred subjects: it was distinctly *their* subject. For this reason, I argue that this support group can be construed as a production site of medicalized subjectivities, in which biomedical meanings of living with HIV/AIDS were systematically organized into the frames of perception and progressively also into the daily routines of patients. It was in this kind of support group that, in a strictly sociological rendition, people became HIV-positive in that HIV positivity was collectively and interactively produced as a common aspect of their life histories, experiences and expectations.

I suggest that the controversies surrounding ARVs and religion addressed above, just as the proclivities within Melisizwe's faith-based support group to discuss ARVs and organize its discourse and practices around issues of biomedicine, should be interpreted in the light of theoretical concerns associated with the functional differentiations of knowledge, the formation of subjects and the differential cultural logics of therapeutic habitus and practice.

Differentiation, Self-Formation and Therapeutic Habitus: Elements for a Theorization

Functional Differentiation and Knowledge

The refusal by some Pentecostal pastors to accept ARVs as a legitimate response and treatment for HIV/AIDS implies the contention that biomedicine and science challenge religious authority on issues of illness. Such controversies over the nature of religion and science therefore reflect concerns over functional differentiation. In social theory, functional differentiation is closely associated with the advent of modernity and has been addressed by thinkers such as

---

3 On the notion of brokering therapeutic resources, see Luedke and West (2005: 6).

Durkheim, Weber and Simmel.[4] Basically, functional differentiation means the process whereby social domains, such as religion, politics, and law, are increasingly less organized through hierarchical relationships of authority and become more independent of one another. Whereas before modernity the centres of political power were to a large degree fused or even identical with sacred authority and constituted prime sources of law, these domains or social spheres have gradually become more autonomous. In the process, they have developed their own internal practical logics through which institutional boundaries have been established.

These concerns were famously addressed in Weber's 'Intermediate Reflections' on the stages and directions of religious rejections of the world. According to Bellah (1999: 279):

> *the* key text in Weber's entire corpus. For the subject is not, or not simply, religious rejections of the world, but the differentiation of what Weber calls value spheres (*Wertsphären*), and the increasingly irreconcilable conflict between them, a differentiation which leads to the 'polytheism' of modernity, a 'war of the gods', which is the result of the entire process of rationalization, Weber's central preoccupation ... [italics in original].

Central to this chapter is an analysis of tensions between religion and the world. Arising from both, Bellah further notes (ibid.: 281) religious rejections of the world and worldly rejections of religion. Amongst the tensions between religion and different 'life orders' that Weber discusses, the tensions between religion and the intellect, which is in its most rationalized form the production of scientific knowledge, is crucial to the central topic in this volume.[5] In many instances, religious concerns over ARVs, described for instance in the chapters by Oxlund and Mattes (this volume), focus on connections to asceticism and mysticism as two fundamental forms of religious rejection of the powers of biomedicine.

This is by no means a routine pattern for people with strong beliefs in Africa or elsewhere. Weber argues that religion and science are also routinely seen as producing different epistemologies and ontologies but that these differences may allow for the cohabitation of the different gods of, and in, modernity. While science seeks explanations of phenomena in the world, religion affords them meaning. In various conversations, Pentecostals from Melisizwe's support group told me of their conversations with God about HIV/AIDS

---

[4] In his recent theorization of 'Modernity as Experience and Interpretation', Wagner (2008) traces modern differentiations back to the series of revolutions (intellectual, political, industrial and so on) that mark the beginnings of modernity.

[5] Differentiation theory has primarily been developed in sociology. For a productive anthropological engagement with Weber's version of it, see Robbins (2009).

therapies in their prayers. Many construed praying as an important mode of negotiating therapeutic options. But in these prayers, biomedical options were not questioned per se; members were looking for answers to questions such as 'When should I begin ARV therapy?' and 'Should I try immune boosters first?' For this group of people, there was little in the way of tension between religion and biomedicine but rather a confluence of religious and secular practices and discourses. However, scientific medicine can fully dispense with religious ideas as a set of explanatory formula about the human body and human life that denies the agency of spirits. It is indeed one of the midwives of the 'disenchantment of the world', and has also been denounced as such by religious authorities.

This approach, however, has difficulties capturing the specificities linked not to the 'world religions' but to the largely fictitious boundaries between 'African culture', 'African tradition', 'African traditional religion' and witchcraft. There is in fact an important undercurrent of conflict between world religions and inherited African thought and ritual practice in contestations over HIV/AIDS treatments. In South Africa, for instance, a Christian physicians' association protested against the integration of traditional healing into the public health sector in the wake of the Traditional Healers' Act of 2004, arguing that traditional healers were the priests of 'African Traditional Religion' and that their recognition as health providers violated the secular nature of South Africa's Constitution. Among the numerous twists in this argument, one is attached to the differentiation of 'religion' and 'culture' as official categories that are associated with specific rights and authorizations of medical and other forms of knowledge. In fact, this seems to be an example of functional differentiation that is more telling of social dynamics of post-apartheid South Africa than of religion and science.

On the flip side, however, differentiation theory seems to rely on categorizations and epistemic separations that may be largely irrelevant or alien within everyday life contexts in many African settings. There is something important to be learnt from the fact that biomedicine may be working to disenchant the world but that it can also itself be re-enchanted, and this is where the concerns over ARVs in the prayers of members of Melisizwe's group are a prime example. As a sensitizing concept, however, functional differentiation has much to commend it when analysing the ways people navigate religious worlds in their search for therapies.

Reforming Subjects as Selves

There are remarkable confluences of religious discourses with biomedical, psychological and other pedagogical vocabularies in the institutional ARV assistance (Nguyen 2009; Burchardt 2009). In their discussions, members of Melisizwe's support group reconstructed their lives around an emphatic notion of being ARV users. In their debates about CD4 counts, viral loads and so on, these medical parameters turned into values and ARVs into sacralized substances. In addition, the exigencies imposed on ARV patients often morph into projects of personal reform that are structurally akin to those suggested by Pentecostal Christianity. This is evident, for instance, in the notion of breaking with one's former daily routines, which is central to Pentecostal ideology surrounding conversion (van Dijk 1997) as it is to biomedical discourse on ARV adherence. This raises questions about the concepts of the 'self' called forth in these arenas and the ways in which they operate to mediate such projects of personal reform and transformation.

This second set of issues strongly resonates with questions of governmentality and the Foucauldian problematic of the subject in relation to the power/knowledge nexus. Governmentality refers to the technologies 'through which human beings had been made subjects of diverse "techniques of the self"', technologies that concerned the ways in which one should undertake the practical organization of one's daily business of living, in relation to considerations as to the kind of person one should aspire to be and the kind of life one should lead' (Rose 1996: 297). For Foucault, transformations of the self are thus construed in terms of self-relationships within diverse historical power relations, that is, at the intersection of practices of government and ethical self-formation (Foucault 1988: 19; Dean 1994: 147). Ethical self-formation can be seen as reflecting technologies of moral regulation that aim at shaping the conduct of individuals and are the domain of pedagogical and medical agencies, churches as well social work institutions of all kinds.

In ARV treatment discourse, patients are enrolled in order to learn new ways of being. This involves all sorts of practices that promote treatment adherence but also dietary programmes, abstinence from alcohol and other ideas about promoting good health. These are invariably presented as healthy choices and associated with strong moral values. Through moralization, discourses surrounding ARVs seek to shape the needs and preferences of patients and enjoin upon them an ethics of individual responsibility. Becker (this volume) makes the important point though that, when addressing issues of self-formation, one must carefully analyse where power is based, and how it operates. We should thus distinguish between the ways in which forms of the self can be identified in the routine patterns of social practice of ARV users, and the ways in which the self is imagined in the institutional apparatuses of the AIDS world.

While this analytical perspective draws attention to the different notions of self that are projected in hierarchies of discourse, it is less geared towards capturing the horizontal differences of therapeutic concepts and practices circulating amongst groups of HIV-positive people. These differences can be conceptualized in terms of cultural propensities that reproduce different logics of practice.

Therapeutic Habitus: Religion, ARVs and the Logics of Practice

It is no exaggeration to say that members of Melisizwe's support group really believed in ARVs and in the mantras surrounding biomedical treatment that TAC has popularized over the years. Importantly, the dramatization of attitudes towards these drugs amongst their promoters and users in terms of belief was an effect of the government's ostentatious disbelief in them. For members, it was clear that they differed in important ways from both official, that is governmental, disbelievers and Christian disbelievers in ARVs. This raises questions as to whether there is some sort of cultural habitus in Bourdieu's sense (1977) amongst the members of the group that shapes their navigations of the religious and medical worlds surrounding them; a systematic orientation that implies a therapeutic habitus and distinguishes them from other groups in more than their therapeutic orientations. Following Bourdieu (ibid.: 78):

> the habitus, the durably installed generative principle of regulated improvisations, produces practices which tend to reproduce the regularities immanent in the objective conditions the production of their generative principle.

The notion of therapeutic habitus can be defined as the embodied generative principles that mediate the complex relationships between the objective circumstances of patients and their therapeutic ideas, beliefs orientations and practices.

Two elements of cultural explanation need to be distinguished in this regard. First, cultures constitute, in phenomenological understanding, universes of meaning; meanings that are organized into discourses that endow actors and events with specific qualities, linking knowledge to social ontology and to practices. Through this link, culture is thought to shape action. Second, culture is understood as underlying the formation of social relations. These can be based on religion and lifestyle but also on biological condition. The assumption is that culture expresses what the people connected through social relations have in common and that those connected act similarly. Here, the totalizing notion of discourse being characteristic of total social formations breaks down into a plurality of cultural orientations characteristic of groups, defining for their members what can be thought and done. Taken together, these cultural, epistemological and ontological orientations form the habitus.

The remaining part of this chapter takes this perspective to show that individual practices regarding HIV/AIDS treatment are embedded in wider routines of action and differential universes of meaning. To this end, I offer an analysis of the autobiographical accounts of two HIV-positive people, showing how they make sense of and rework the cultural scripts for dealing with HIV/AIDS offered to them from different sources and examining how these reworkings resonate with their religious trajectories. The two cases have been chosen according to the methodology of maximum contrast, depicting two typical ways of navigating religious worlds in the era of ARV treatment. The first case examines the interface of religion and ARVs in the world of Pentecostalism; the second one explains the eclipse of any religious meaning in the life of a young HIV-positive woman who is struggling to remain in the margins of churches and the HIV/AIDS world.[6] Both contrast with the religious activist group.

Healing through Conversion: ARVs and Pentecostalism

Maggie is a 36-year-old woman working for the faith-based organization Living Hope Community Centre (LHCC). She was born in the Eastern Cape Province and grew up experiencing relatively little parental control. After apartheid she was 'crazy about life'. But her conversion to Pentecostalism generates ambivalences: 'We were doing things that were not suitable for life,' she recalled. 'It was really bad ... It was just partying. We just had a really good time.'

The time of 'care-less' youth ended when she became pregnant at the age of 23. Although the pregnancy came as a surprise, she was prepared to raise the child alone with the help of her mother and immediately foreclosed the idea of marrying the child's father. She acknowledged that the relationship did not reflect deep personal commitment. The father's lack of care for the baby and his refusal to provide material support, however, left her disappointed. Fortunately, her mother's support in raising her daughter allowed her to complete her secondary education. Yet after a whole year of looking for a job in her native town, she saw no other option than to move to Cape Town, leaving her child with her mother.

On her arrival in Cape Town, she first moved in with an aunt. Soon afterwards and through contacts she made through her church, she started working in an orphanage run by the international NGO SOS Children's Home. She worked there for about eight years. In the meantime her father passed away. 'And then,' she continued, 'I met this guy and we fell in love. And I ended up pregnant again in 2002.' Their relationship was consolidated and, like many other South African women, Maggie was tested for HIV during her antenatal exams. Not surprisingly, her HIV-positive diagnosis came as a shock. The first thought she had was simply: 'This is the end of my life' and her feelings of frustration were exacerbated when the doctor told her about the risks of mother-to-child transmission. In addition, she had to change her job as employees in the orphanage were not supposed to have children. 'I didn't know what to do with

[6] The dynamics of HIV/AIDS and religion are in an important sense gender-specific. For a detailed discussion, see Burchardt (2010).

my life anymore,' she said and decided to have an abortion. For reasons she did not elaborate on, she later changed this decision and kept the child.

Maggie was then channelled into psychological recovery projects and participated in the meetings of an HIV/AIDS support group. Seeing people coping with HIV/AIDS in a positive way and identifying with them by finding out that 'we are the same' were important in helping her recover from depression. As a result of participating in these care programmes, her emotional situation gradually stabilized. In medical terms as well, her situation appeared increasingly positive: her CD4 count increased and she was generally satisfied with the treatment and medical services she had access to through her health insurance. Despite some second thoughts, she agreed to enrol in ARV treatment therapy and her second child was born healthy. And after the delivery she moved in with the child's father.

She gradually began distancing herself from her past, a process that eventually culminated in her conversion to Pentecostal Christianity. After 18 months of cohabitation, she started feeling uncomfortable and decided to move out while still maintaining her relationship as this decision was motivated by issues relating to the organization of everyday life. At another level, this illegitimate cohabitation already signalled much of what she later perceived as essentially un-Christian behaviour. Moving from the joint flat was therefore a first act in spatially and socially distancing herself from the world she used to inhabit.

Around 2004, soon after she moved out, a friend took her on an Evangelical crusade. This is where, as she put it, 'she found God'. What followed was a process of acting out her religious conversion, which provided her with an elaborate web of categories through which to understand and act: 'My life totally changed. I began loving and accepting myself. I grew spiritually. I didn't know anything about my life but now I know that Jesus admonished me and I changed my whole lifestyle.' Some of the most important lifestyle changes she made concerned her relationships with men, her views on sexuality and her gender identity. Immediately after her conversion, she decided to leave her partner. In this context, she explicitly stressed that the reason for breaking up with him was not that she did not love him anymore. 'I just left him after I converted,' she recalled, indicating that her reasons for quitting were essentially external to the relationship itself. What is more, she eventually opted for a lifestyle of total sexual abstinence. Asked whether she would be interested in marrying she stated:

> Now I don't even care about guys anymore and Jesus is helping me every day ... But because I am a born-again child I am saved, I am a child of God. So I don't even care, I don't even think about marriage. I am only focusing on my life in Jesus. That's it. As long as I am getting into my promised land, that is all that concerns me. Marriage will come if God wants it. I don't think about it.

What we see here is a narrative of radical disjuncture. It seems that the belief in being saved and thus not 'having to care' was an experience of liberation for Maggie. Yet what precisely is it that she does not care about when saying she 'does not care about guys anymore'? We might suggest that it is the whole drama of intimate female-male interaction, especially of achieving personal fulfilment, and of finding help in a partnership that is much more reliably provided by Jesus Christ. Conversion to Pentecostal Christianity removed all these concerns and substituted them with a single destiny, that is, a focus on her faith in Jesus. This argument confirms the findings of other studies into the gender dynamics of Pentecostal Christianity in Africa and Latin America that point out that conversion often comes to signify a process of purification, in which relations with men are symbolically replaced by a relationship with Jesus Christ. This dynamic thwarts the otherwise existing pressures on Pentecostal women to get married and assume subservient positions in the household (Rasing 2007). Not sharing the same religious conviction may also have undermined her relationship, which reinforces the idea that the separation was indeed necessary.

This raises the question of whether it was dissatisfaction with her partner or with men in general that pointed to the benefits of conversion for Maggie in this regard, or whether it was rather the religious conversion that imposed a different set of interpretative categories and moral norms regarding interaction with men. The question is difficult to answer. It would seem that the abandoning of intimate relationships and her religious conversion are mutually entangled in terms of cumulative evidence: both are parts of a more encompassing process of distancing oneself from the past. This process had already begun well before Maggie's religious conversion. She recounted that, through some medical inquiries she did following her diagnosis, she found out that abstaining from sexual intercourse would be beneficial to her health.[7] As a result, she stopped having sex right after the diagnosis. Thus we could argue that her religious conversion ratified an ongoing process of personal transformation rather than ritually initiating it, while certainly bestowing the practice of sexual abstinence with new personal meaning.

Eventually, the conversion had profound implications on the way she dealt with her HIV status. The following passage illustrates how her understanding of HIV and ARV treatment was affected by that process:

> Doctors are not God, they just give you the results of scientific exams but that's a lie. They tell you, you are gonna die. But you are still alive. They are not God. So why should I bother? They just use their machines. You never know, today my

---

[7] Having unprotected sexual intercourse when HIV positive carries the risk of so-called superinfection and of increasing the viral load of the blood. It seems plausible that, in the given context, Maggie was referring to this theory.

> CD4 count is low, maybe tomorrow it is up again. I was well treated but it is my understanding. You don't know what God is doing overnight. HIV doesn't exist in my blood. That is what I believe.

Maggie firmly believed that her life was ultimately in the hands of God and took the changing results of medical tests as evidence of this. Her conversion, it would appear, confirmed her profound mistrust of medical definitions of HIV/AIDS, a development that is especially reflected in the fact that she stopped taking anti-retroviral drugs in spite of receiving them free of charge through her health insurance. She removed her body from the medical machineries to put it in the hands of God. And in this act, we find a striking analogy with the way she removed herself from men to dedicate her life to Jesus Christ. Her faith in biomedicine is replaced by faith in God. Pointing again to the link between her religiosity and her disease she explained:

> I got spiritual healing and I could feel that I am healed. So for me, HIV is not in my mind, it is not in my brain because I understand that I am healed and I believe that I am healed through Jesus Christ.

The notion of spiritual healing in Pentecostal Christianity is often an intrinsic element of conversion and of being saved and, in some contexts, all these ritual practices acquire an almost synonymous meaning. Spiritual healing is a practice that typically denotes the ritual treatment of afflictions ranging from spirit possession, disturbed kin and other social relations to physical ailments such as infertility and impotence. It is thus often used when addressing concerns about endangered social reproduction and a wider understanding of social and cultural suffering. Against this backdrop, Maggie's remark strikingly captures how this notion can be employed in the context of HIV/AIDS, in other words, how the selective appropriation of elements from the available repertoire of religious vocabularies helped her deal with her disease. While she had earlier claimed that Jesus had literally removed the virus from her blood, in the sequence above she draws attention to how spiritual healing was helpful in removing HIV from her thoughts (see Oxlund, this volume). HIV infection thus emerges as a psychological disease, as an affliction that impairs life by constantly reminding the infected person of possible future suffering, the corresponding breakdown of life routines and impending death. It is also, therefore, these mental impairments that are remedied by the spiritual healing she received. In this sense, 'healing through conversion' should be understood both as a ritual passage linked to critical biographical experience and as a practice of care that is in some sociological proximity to notions of psychotherapy. At once we find here a form of self-care that allows her, as she put it, 'not to care' because many of the contingencies of life with HIV are bracketed in the phenomenological sense through religious conversion.

Painful Memories: Sexual Violence, HIV/AIDS and the Longing for Normality

At the time of the interview, Thembisa was 22. Just as Maggie, she was born in the Eastern Cape Province where she lived with all kinds of relatives. When she was 8, she and her mother moved to Cape Town where they lived with her mother's new husband and her younger brother in a small backyard shack in the township of Gugulethu. At the time, her mother's husband was working at an industrial plant while her mother worked as a nurse at the local clinic. With a sudden absence of parental care, Thembisa construed this as the time 'when the problem started'. A man from the neighbourhood was supposed to take care of her and a few other children but for more than two years this person repeatedly abused her sexually, initiating Thembisa into a life marked by abuse, violence and coercion.

This history of violence and abuse, however, pertains to the dark side of her life, and while delivering her autobiographical account, she constantly dragged these negative events from her subjective experience into the light of narrative representation. However, she took pains to present herself as someone who has had a normal social life. In this sense, she was quick to add: 'But in short, I grew up like any other kid.' It seems that to understand her account, we should construe such suggestions of normalcy as introducing a fundamental distinction between what is visible and what remains hidden; between what one discloses to others and what constitutes the elements interwoven into one's social identity on the one hand, and what remains within the confines of subjective experience on the other. These latter aspects were then, as she observed, what she was trying to deal with by 'wiping it out of my mind'. I would argue that relating a biography replete with dire experiences as if it were a normal one, and constantly attempting to locate herself with the terrain of normality, is constitutive of Thembisa's way of dealing with uncertainty and is endemic to her biographical experience. It was also this search for normality that later motivated her to forego ARV treatment. As a teenager, 'growing up like any other kid' meant that in her view in order 'to get by' one had to choose between a number of alternative pathways:

> And well, to live in an area where I live, you have to ... it's either you get yourself into a church, get yourself a very well-known boyfriend or get yourself a gangster. There are three options. You get yourself an ordinary guy and he's gonna end up dead or something. So I got myself this well-known gangster. But I didn't know at the moment actually.

Ensuing from this, there is a life story that revolves around profoundly disturbing relationships with men. At the age of 14 she started dating 'this well-known gangster'. This relationship she perceived as essentially *formative* for years to come: he introduced her to alcohol and drugs; he taught her how to use guns; and eventually she insisted that it was him who taught her 'everything I know'. After two years, her boyfriend was shot dead in one of the township taverns in an act of revenge for a murder he had committed shortly before. Instead of being repelled by this event or encouraged to change her social milieu, she was suddenly afforded some kind of fame out of 'having survived' in the eyes of the township youth. Her life became ever more excessive and I could sense some degree of pride when she related how, even after a series of consecutive nights of parties, she would invariably prevail in brandy drinking competitions with her male peers.

The fact that she was abused during this period must have given her the idea that a relationship with a man was a way of circumventing many of the potential dangers single young women living in the townships of Cape Town are exposed to. This belief was to be painfully consolidated soon afterwards. During one of the weekends of partying she followed a group of friends, this time without her boyfriend, to the neighbouring township of Nyanga where they got to know another person in a tavern who invited them to his house to continue the 'night out'. It was just after the men had left the house to purchase more drinks, leaving her behind alone, that 'some gang pushed the door open. And I was gang-raped'. She recounted how she was lying on the floor covered in blood with her face all swollen up when her friends eventually returned.

Out of fear of being reprimanded for putting herself into such dangerous situations in the first place, she decided not to disclose this to her family: 'I went home and I got scolded for being away from home for the whole weekend and that was it.' What emerged was a pattern of organizing her everyday life in which she constantly moved between the cultural milieu of township gangsterism and youth adventurism on the one hand, and her family on the other, without feeling safe in either. While being in the terrains of peer sociality certainly provided her with the kind of excitement she was looking for at the time, it also created a strong sense of uncertainty against which the family could have been a haven of security and trust. However, it appeared though that none of her youthful adventures would have been tolerable to her mother. On various occasions, Thembisa's mother actually admitted that she had been too harsh on her daughter, thereby possibly having contributed to the difficulties in familial relationships and, by implication, to her daughter's hardships. These feelings, however, were only revealed to her much later. This harsh treatment had left Thembisa with no other option than to perpetually strive to polish her image as a good daughter in the familial context. The gap between this image and the sense of self she had meanwhile acquired within her peer circles virtually split her personal identity and progressively prevented the family from helping her move out of the violent environment of township youth culture. And yet it must be noted that adventurism was at once an instantiation of an emphatic idea of uncertainty, the fact of freedom as she repeatedly stressed.

In the years to come, she went through a series of intimate relationships with men, all of which were marked by experiences of intra-relationship violence, sexual coercion and disappointment over her partners' unfaithfulness. Repeatedly, even when realizing the detrimental effects these relationships were having on her life, she had trouble actually ending them. For months, sometimes years, she continued to be harassed by former partners. While the experience of being abused by her partners had shown her that, for a young township woman, 'getting yourself a boyfriend' was far from being a satisfactory strategy in pursuing a secure life, she also understood that having a partner did not save her from abuse outside the relationship either. On one occasion, she was kidnapped on a street in the neighbourhood and taken by car to another city where she was gang-raped again. Amidst these recurring experiences of debasement, she tried leaving the pathways of alcohol, substance abuse and gangsterism, first by joining a Christian church community, and later by enrolling in a rehabilitation process in a therapeutic institution. On several occasions, she even told me that her grandfather had been a prophet, founded a church and that religion had played a huge role in her family history. But in some way she felt disconnected from that history. Through continued social connections with former friends, she always returned to the beaten tracks after trying the 'Christian way'.

After telling me the story of just another episode of abuse, she concluded in retrospect that:

> at this point, being raped was not an issue anymore. It wasn't such a deal that I would say, 'OK, this happened, I am crying'. Think of it like, 'I have been raped again'. I just said, 'OK, fine'. But of course, it was anything but fine.

Four years ago, she began to feel suicidal and reported having tried to kill herself several times, but always half-heartedly. Eventually, in late 2005, she decided to seek help from a professional social worker to whom she disclosed her entire story. At the time of the interview, she was still living in a shelter for abused women that was run by the public health system to which the social worker had referred her.

Her autobiographical account had reached the present without her having mentioned her HIV infection once. It was only now that she explicitly addressed this history:

> Oh, and then I got sick ... I was dating this guy from work. And we hadn't slept together. From Pick'n'Pay. Before I worked for the organization, I worked for Pick'n'Pay.[8] And I decided to date this guy at work. And we haven't slept together.

---

[8] A big South African supermarket chain.

> And I am thinking, my life is finally on track. Got back to school, have a boyfriend, good times with my mum. Life couldn't be happier. And I got sick.

She was in hospital for three weeks while the doctors did various medical examinations. One of them showed that Thembisa was HIV-positive. Vividly she recalled how, after having received the news from the HIV counsellor, her hearing was impaired: she could see the counsellor's lips moving without hearing a word of what was said. The subsequent descriptions of her experiences over the following weeks show a typical reaction to the diagnosis of chronic disease:

> I am dead. I am dead. My life ended and I have no children, no husband, no nothing. And I am dead. And I am thinking this guy, when I got sick, he actually stuck with me. And I am thinking this is the one who actually did like me and I am going to lose him, I am losing him, I am losing him. Cause I know the moment I am telling, look I am HIV positive, he's gone. And I decided OK, I have to tell him as soon as I get better. So my mind was, I am thinking I can't go back to school, I can't work, I can't do anything because I will be dead in a few months, or few years probably.

There is, first of all, a tremendous experience of loss, namely of everything in the future, because the diagnosis has rendered virtually everything beyond the actual moment of survival radically uncertain and her capacity to plan had been undermined. Only now she began, step by step, revealing her entire story to her mother. In an attempt to resume the role of the primary caretaker, her mother advised her to give up working and return to the family home. However, after recovering, Thembisa soon realized that much of the care she was given somehow pushed her towards adopting aspects of an HIV-positive identity that she was not ready to accept. Instead of accepting her HIV status as an important or even defining aspect of her sense of self, she invested much of her energy in creating a sense of continuity in her life, even if this implied rejecting the care and affection she was offered by others:

> I don't like people that sympathize with me. I am a normal human being. And sometimes I get on people's nerves. I like people who are honest, you know, don't judge me by my disease but for myself. So I don't tell a lot of people.

Ambivalence was one way her HIV infection worked to reconfigure her relationship with men. First of all, she related that her current relationship did not survive the difficulties imposed by her disease. Her boyfriend took great pains to be careful and supportive but, precisely by doing so, he appeared to tie her to her disease in a way she was not prepared to accept. Matters became even more complicated: on the one hand, her HIV infection seemed to provide her with a nearly perfect solution to her troubles with men. Whenever she faces unwelcome approaches, she mentions being HIV-positive 'and they run away'. On the other hand, however, when meeting a man she is interested in, there is no way of circumventing disclosure. With frustration in her voice, she mentioned: 'I am stopped by ten guys a day. It gets tiring saying, I am HIV-positive. And they are always like, I'll call you, I'll call you. And they never do.'

At yet another level, her difficulties in accepting the role of an 'HIV patient' may be unpacked through paying attention to her attitude towards anti-retroviral treatment. Unlike Maggie, for whom conversion to Pentecostalism was pivotal for retrieving some level of biographical stability, Thembisa emphasized her determination to stay healthy without neither biomedicine nor religious commitment. In her view, ARVs, because of the need of life-long daily adherence to the treatment regime after initial enrolment, signified the opposite of living the kind of normal life that she longed for. Thembisa's story shows that the formation of a therapeutic habitus in the context of religion and biomedical treatment does not revolve around binary choices. For her life, religion was largely irrelevant, and even more so for her therapeutic choices.

Conclusions

These two autobiographical stories show that, instead of a fixed medico-social assemblage, HIV positivity is a highly flexible marker of self-identification and acquires its cultural specificity through its position in the web of meanings characteristic of distinct cultural worlds. In this way, we can construe Pentecostalism, progressive HIV/AIDS activism (as exemplified in Melisizwe's group) and township youth culture as three cultural worlds offering distinct symbolic and material resources to HIV-positive people to allow them to construct a therapeutic habitus. Each of the resulting forms of therapeutic habitus involves ideas about biomedicine and is shaped through specific relationships to religious practice and ideology.

The most striking dimension differentiating the cases concerns the perceived significance of the disease and treatment in individual life. In Maggie's Pentecostal circles, social ties and practices are facilitated through the common belief in the presence of the Holy Spirit as a social substance, which led to her belief that ARV's were a chimera. In the cultural world of AIDS activism, which I discussed with regard to Melisizwe's support group at the beginning, on the contrary, ARVs are essentially understood as social substances in that these drugs and the activism surrounding them mediate social relations to others who are perceived as members of the same therapeutic community, and hence as people of the same kind. These activists spent most of her time with HIV/AIDS-related activities. Much of their social life revolved around issues of AIDS and it is this kind of subjective appropriation of HIV/AIDS as a vocation that sustains much of the activism and political mobilizations. Importantly, it is linked to a highly positive perception of ARVs; for these activists, these drugs are sacred substances; for in their eyes they give life. Particularly among patients-turned-activists, adherence to the mantras of ARV treatment created a profound perception of commonality, not only in the sense of taking the same treatment but as a principle marker of common sense. Belonging to the therapeutic community of ARV users was seen as imparting the credentials of cultural competence against which those who had doubts about biomedicine were branded as 'denialists', if not as uneducated and backward people.

Maggie and Thembisa both refused to take ARVs but these refusals followed different practical logics. Thembisa's main wish after diagnosis was to live 'as if nothing had happened'. Much to her frustration, this goal was constantly being undermined by the need to disclose her HIV status to partners. In much the same way, she saw ARVs as undermining her fantasies of continuity. Looking for spiritual support in church always signalled new discontinuities in her life that she could not accept. After all, her trajectory led her to a point in which religion had lost all practical relevance in her life. She was living within an 'immanent frame' (Taylor 2007) in which her notion of human flourishing had been closed to the idea that any god could be of help.

For Maggie, the practical logic of organizing the construction of a therapeutic habitus was not one of continuity but of a radical break. 'Healing through conversion' in its most radical form forecloses positive approaches to biomedicine. Here, the changing results of medical exams were taken as evidence of their unreliability and hence rendered invalid. What matters is that the links between conversion and the refusal to take ARVs are not arbitrary. 'Healing through conversion' makes sense in the world of Pentecostalism for HIV-positive converts because of their emphasis on the healing power of prayer. This emphasis does not force people to rely on prayers alone but patients who do so are typically Pentecostals. ARVs and religion can thus be seen to be playing into the ways different forms of therapeutic habitus are sustained through logics connecting assumptions of disease, healing and agency.

References

Bellah, R.N. 1999. Max Weber and world-denying love: A look at the historical sociology of religion. *Journal of the American Academy of Religion*, 67(2), 277–304.

Biehl, J. 2007. Pharmaceuticalization: Aids treatment and global health politics. *Anthropological Quarterly*, 80(4), 1083–1126.

Bourdieu, P. 1977. *Outline of a Theory of Practice*. Cambridge: Cambridge University Press.

Burchardt, M. 2009. Subjects of counselling: HIV/AIDS, religion and the management of everyday life in South Africa, in *Aids and Religious Practice in Africa*, edited by P.W. Geissler and F. Becker. Leiden: Brill, 333–58.

Burchardt, M. 2010. Ironies of subordination: Ambivalences of gender in religious AIDS interventions in South Africa. *Oxford Development Studies*, 38(1), 63–82.

Burchardt, M. 2011. Missionaries and social workers: Visions of sexuality in religious discourse, in *Religion and Social Problems*, edited by T. Hjelm. London and New York: Routledge, 142–56.

Dean, M. 1994. 'A social structure of many souls': Moral regulation, government, and self-formation. *Canadian Journal of Sociology*, 19(2), 145–68.

Fassin, D. 2007. *When Bodies Remember: Experiences and Politics of AIDS in South Africa*. Berkeley and Los Angeles, CA, and London: University of California Press.

Foucault, M. 1988. The political technology of individuals, in *Technologies of the Self: A Seminar with Michel Foucault*, edited by M.H. Luther, H. Gutman and P.H. Hutton. Amherst, MA: University of Massachusetts Press, 145–62.

Geertz, C. 1973. *The Interpretation of Cultures*. New York: Basic Books.

Kalofonos, I.A. 2010. 'All I eat is ARVs': The paradox of AIDS treatment interventions in central Mozambique. *Medical Anthropology Quarterly*, 24(3), 363–80.

Luedke, T. and West, H. 2005. Healing divides: Therapeutic border work in South East Africa, in *Borders and Healers: Brokering Therapeutic Resources in Southeast Africa*, edited by T. Luedke and H. West. Indianapolis, IN: Indiana University Press, 1–20.

Mattes, D. 2011. 'Just like buying sweets at the store?' Antiretroviral treatment and the ambiguity of normalcy in urban Tanzania. Paper to the American Anthropological Association Conference: Traces, Tidemarks and Legacies, Montreal, Canada, 18 November.

Nattrass, N. 2008. AIDS and the scientific governance of medicine in post-apartheid South Africa. *African Affairs*, 107(427), 157–76.

Nguyen, V-K. 2009. Therapeutic Evangelism: confessional technologies, antiretrovirals and biospiritual transformation in the fight against AIDS in West Africa, in *AIDS and Religious Practice in Africa*, edited by F. Becker and P.W. Geissler. Boston, MA, and Leiden: Brill, 359–78.

Posel, D. 2005. Sex, death and the fate of the nation: Reflections on the politicization of sexuality in post-apartheid South Africa. *Africa*, 75(2), 125–53.

Rasing, T. 2007. The role of Christianity in the context of HIV/AIDS: Dealing with HIV/AIDS in Pentecostal churches and mainstream churches in Zambia. *Word and Context*, 6, 33–49.
Robbins, J. 2009. Morality, value and radical cultural change, in *The Anthropology of Moralities*, edited by M. Heintz. Oxford: Berghahn, 62–80.
Robins, S. 2004. 'Long live Zackie, long live': AIDS activism, science, and citizenship after apartheid. *Journal of Southern African Studies*, 30, 651–72.
Robins, S. 2006. From 'rights' to 'ritual': AIDS activism in South Africa. *American Anthropologist*, 108(2), 312–23.
Rose, N. 1996. Authority and the genealogy of subjectivity, in *Detraditionalization: Critical Reflections on Authority and Identity*, edited by P. Heelas, S. Lash and P. Morris. Cambridge and Oxford: Blackwell, 294–327.
Taylor, C. 2007. *A Secular Age*. Cambridge, MA: Harvard University Press.
Van Dijk, R. 1997. From camp to encompassment: Discourses of transsubjectivity in the Ghanaian Pentecostal diaspora. *Journal of Religion in Africa*, 27(2), 135–69.
Vaughan, M. 1991. *Curing Their Ills: Colonial Power and African Illness*. Cambridge: Polity Press.
Wagner, P. 2008. *Modernity as Experience and Interpretation: A New Sociology of Modernity*. Cambridge: Polity Press.
Weber, M. 1948. Religious rejections of the world and their directions, in *From Max Weber: Essays in Sociology*, edited and translated by H.H. Gerth and C.W. Mills. New York: Oxford University Press, 323–59.
Weber, M. 1972. *Wirtschaft und Gesellschaft. Grundriß einer verstehenden Soziologie*. Tübingen: Mohr.

Chapter 3

'A Blessing in Disguise': The Art of Surviving HIV/AIDS as a Member of the Zionist Christian Church in South Africa

Bjarke Oxlund

Introduction

The Zionist Christian Church (ZCC) in South Africa has a following of approximately 5 million, which is the same as the number of people living with HIV/AIDS there. As a healing-oriented African Independent Church that embraces ancestor worship and the belief in witchcraft, the ZCC does not subscribe to a viral aetiology of HIV/AIDS (Niehaus 2009: 316). And in accordance with a more general rejection of and ambivalence towards Western biomedicine, it does not recommend anti-retroviral therapy (cf. Anderson 1999: 208). The symptoms often associated with HIV/AIDS meanwhile lend themselves to a ZCC interpretation of misfortune brought about by breaches of moral rules and social taboos. This chapter analyses the influence that the ZCC exercises in relation to local understandings of HIV/AIDS in the social context of the Turfloop Campus at the University of Limpopo. Moving from a general analysis of social meanings of HIV/AIDS in South Africa, it deals with two separate cases of ZCC converts. The first is a male student who converted to the ZCC as part of a process of questioning misfortune, while the second considers a man who was simultaneously a ZCC follower, a prominent PLWHA[1] community leader and an HIV/AIDS counsellor at the University of Limpopo. In the second case, it questions how he tried to balance a life caught between worship, kinship and therapeutic citizenship. The case highlights how the individual ZCC member living with HIV has had to manoeuvre a highly contradictory environment where divine healing, care and support from the ZCC congregation came to stand in opposition to the pursuance of anti-retroviral therapy (ART). The article is based on a one-year period of ethnographic fieldwork at the Turfloop Campus of the University of Limpopo (2006–2007), which is only seven km from the ZCC religious city of Moria.

1 PLWHA (People Living With HIV/AIDS).

The fieldwork took place at a time when the South African government's HIV/AIDS policies were being heavily criticized at the international level because of the so-called dissident stance adopted by former President Thabo Mbeki and his Minister of Health, Manto Tshabalala-Msimang. Their ban on the use of anti-retroviral medicines in the prevention of mother-to-child transmission, in conjunction with their promotion of beetroot, African potatoes, garlic and vitamins as a treatment regime, caused an unprecedented international focus on the management of health issues in a sovereign state (Nattrass 2007: 8–14). At the Toronto AIDS Conference in 2006, the UN Special Envoy for AIDS, Stephen Lewis, thus broke with conventions of international diplomacy when he dubbed the South African government's promotion of vegetables as a treatment regime 'more worthy of a lunatic fringe than of a concerned and compassionate state' (Posel 2008: 13; Thornton 2008: 174). In short, the fieldwork took place in a political milieu where the orthodox scientific understanding of HIV/AIDS was challenged from the highest echelons of South African society, which had severe implications for the implementation of programmes to distribute anti-retroviral medicines.

Zionist Christians at Turfloop Campus

During my stay at the University of Limpopo, I became familiar with the practices and beliefs of the followers of the ZCC. Among the first-year students, a total of 25.6 per cent[2] belonged to the ZCC,[3] which is known to proscribe such phenomena as alcohol, pork, smoking and sex outside marriage. Kuperus (2011: 23) describes the ZCC as being founded on both African traditional and Pentecostal-type traits, while Sundkler (1961: 55), in his classic work on Bantu prophets, noted that across the board of African Independent Churches:

> Theologically the Zionists are now a syncretistic Bantu movement with healing, speaking with tongues, purifications rites, and taboos as the main expressions of their faith. There are numerous denominational, local, and individual variations in Zionist groups and every Zionist prophet is anxious to point out some speciality through which his Church stands out from the rest.

Today the ZCC is the largest and fastest-growing of the African Independent Churches in South Africa, and so the huge following of the ZCC at Turfloop

---

[2] n = 1,823 first-year students (questionnaire completed during Orientation Week in 2004, 2005, 2006 and 2007).

[3] Followed by Roman Catholic: 22.3 per cent; Protestant: 8.8 per cent; Apostolic: 8.1 per cent; African Tradition: 7.1 per cent; Other: 22 per cent; Atheist: 3.3 per cent.

Campus is not only explained by the close proximity of the ZCC religious city of Moria but also by the fact that, overall, this particular denomination among the African Independent Churches proved to be the most successful in the long run. The ZCC was founded in 1910 by a farm worker, Engenas Lekganyane,[4] who laid the ground for this Zion city about 40 km from the provincial capital of Polokwane (then Pietersburg) in Limpopo Province (formerly Northern Transvaal) (Anderson 1999: 287). Educated by Scottish Evangelist missionaries, Lekganyane drew on this learning in developing the ZCC liturgy, although he did so in an eclectic fashion that allowed the ZCC to embrace beliefs in ancestral spirits and their powers to intercede on behalf of humans. Arguably, it was because of his 'powers to heal the sick' that Lekganyane succeeded in building up a successful church (Lukhaimane quoted in Anderson 1999: 290). The ZCC preaches 'deliverance from sickness and the oppression of evil spirits' by receiving the Holy Spirit (ibid.: 285), generally without the use of biomedicine (ibid.: 308).

When it comes to assessing the success of the ZCC in comparison with other African Independent Churches, Jean Comaroff (1985: 238) wrote the following about Moria:

> By constructing a particularly powerful central place, which administers a fund of spiritual, material, and symbolic power, the Z.C.C. has managed to counteract, for the most part, the inherent tendency toward fission and secession in such movements.

I went to Moria several times to accompany one of my closest interlocutors who converted to the ZCC in December 2006, and on other occasions I followed him there to purchase blessed items, to be cleansed and to attend sermons or overnight prayers. Through this acquaintance and by virtue of having acquired the research assistance of a ZCC follower, Bernhard Mphalele, I also started attending ZCC services on campus (Turfloop hosts a very active ZCC group) and the *mkhukhu* dance on dusty ground in the nearby township of Toronto. The *mkhukhu* is a dancing style exercised by male ZCC members wearing khaki uniforms and large boots that make them 'all feet', with the actions of the dance mainly involving pounding the bare ground so as to 'stamp evil underground' (Comaroff 1985: 244). In its capacity as a healing church, the ZCC is of crucial importance in relation to HIV/AIDS, which was poignantly brought home to me at Turfloop Campus by the fact that the University Health Promoter, a ZCC convert, was living positively with the virus. My research, and this chapter, however, does in

[4] At first, his brother was part of the movement but later broke away and formed a separate Zionist Christian Movement with its headquarters near the religious city of Moria. In the wider South African public, they are understood to form one movement.

no way qualify as an exhaustive account of the beliefs and practices of the ZCC, although they do pose a number of pertinent questions about the ZCC and the practices and beliefs of its followers in relation to HIV/AIDS.

HIV/AIDS in South Africa

Students at the University of Limpopo have more often than not come of age in an environment marked by poverty and hardship, which is exacerbated by the harsh realities of the South African HIV/AIDS pandemic. According to a national survey, Limpopo Province had an antenatal sero-prevalence rate in 2005 of 21.5 per cent (low estimate: 18.5 per cent – high estimate: 24.6 per cent) (DoH 2006: 11). In spite of high prevalence rates, communication about HIV/AIDS at the interpersonal level is clouded in secrecy and denial. Writing about nearby Bushbuckridge, Niehaus (2007: 845) suggested that people living with AIDS are locally seen to be caught 'in the anomalous domain betwixt-and-between life and death' and therefore constructed as 'dead before dying'. Because they are still young, Limpopo students have also come to see an HIV diagnosis as being 'dead before living', reflecting an understanding that their social becoming is terminated before it has ever taken off.

In the light of the political turmoil that has followed in the wake of the South African AIDS pandemic, a considerable amount of AIDS-related research has focused on these political battles (Nattrass 2007; Forsyth et al. 2008; Fourie 2006), while too little attention has been paid to the more immediate threats that people are experiencing on a personal and bodily level (cf. Kleinman 2006). With reference to classic anthropological concepts such as purity and danger, it could be argued that what people are trying to avoid is social death (cf. Vigh 2006: 103) rather than simply HIV infection. In the Northern Sotho semantic field, a person is seen to be made up of the four different components of blood (including semen), flesh, spirit and shadow (*madi, mmele, moya* and *seriti*), where it is the spirit and the shadow that are the real life-giving entities. The shadow (*seriti*) is a soul-like concept understood as the personality and moral strength of a person, while the spirit (*moya*) has been interpreted as a 'life force' that has 'suffused throughout the whole body' and is 'associated with the lungs, liver, genitals, head and hair' that are all 'organs believed to be especially susceptible to disease' (Hammond-Tooke 1993: 149; Niehaus 2009: 325). The *seriti* makes a person open and permeable to others, and one therefore has to enhance or protect the strength of one's *seriti* because others can weaken it with harmful intent (Mönnig 1967: 51). In particular, it is when the exchange of bodily fluids places a person in contact with a polluting *seriti* and bad blood, when the exchange takes place in a condition of ritual impurity or when somebody is trying to harm a person's *seriti* that health problems or misfortune are likely to follow.

To many student followers of the ZCC it made sense to question his/her situation pragmatically by drawing on the explanatory powers of witchcraft, pollution and biology at the same time. This is reminiscent of Evans-Pritchard's (1936: 23) observations about the way in which the Zande use witchcraft as an explanatory idiom to make sense of two chains of causation intersecting at a certain time and place. One of the examples he presented was that of a granary that collapsed because the supports were undermined by termites. Evans-Pritchard's interlocutors acknowledged this cause but questioned why it happened while people were sitting beneath the granary. In the same vein, the students at Turfloop queried why HIV was transmitted on some occasions while not on others, that is that two men may sleep with the same HIV-positive woman but only one of them becomes infected. Although most of the students believed the modes of HIV transmission presented in the biomedical accounts promoted in the national prevention campaigns, many simultaneously alluded to the influence of witchcraft. Students who were studying for degrees in biology and nursing, however, found it hard to reconcile their scientific knowledge about HIV/AIDS with local aetiologies of illness, whereas students of Northern Sotho and political science, clearly taking inspiration from President Thabo Mbeki, seemed to take pride in presenting 'African solutions to African problems', thereby implying that the South African HIV/AIDS pandemic could best be understood separately from the global epidemic.

Overall, it is not difficult to appreciate how the gradual and uneven process of deteriorating health associated with the weakening of the immune system due to the viral load in the blood can be cast as the interplay of a seriously weakened *seriti* and the subsequent weakening of the *moya*. In this account, knowing conclusively that one is living with HIV will fundamentally erode one's *seriti* and lead to a quick death, which many students quoted as a reason for postponing an HIV test until the symptoms became visible. Since an HIV test also has the potential to rewrite a person's moral past and significantly influence his/her social future (Oxlund 2009: 144; Burchardt 2009: 342), there are naturally reasons over and above the level of aetiology for students to prefer not knowing their HIV status. For instance, some students feared that their parents would then get to know that, contrary to discourse, they were actually pursuing an active sex life (cf. Burchardt 2011: 671), while others worried that their extended families would claim that the huge investment in their education had been made in vain. Consequently, a lot of HIV/AIDS communication in Limpopo was quite aloof and left many things open. The next section details how ZCC messages on HIV/AIDS have been carefully crafted to be so enveloped and imprecise that they succeed in not challenging differing aetiologies of HIV and AIDS, while still acknowledging the suffering that many members of the ZCC congregation are experiencing.

The ZCC's AIDS Message

Over the years, observers have commented on the political acquiescence and public silence of the ZCC in political matters (Anderson 1999: 294; Ashforth 2005: 192; Schoffeleers 1991: 4–16). At a time when HIV/AIDS was the most politically charged topic in South African politics, due to the dissident views of then President Thabo Mbeki and his Minister of Health Mantho Tshabalala-Msimang, the ZCC stance on HIV/AIDS was not simply a matter of aetiology but also of political manoeuvring. At the widely attended annual September Conference held in Moria City in September 2007 and with Thabo Mbeki in the audience, the ZCC bishop B.E. Lekganyane made reference to AIDS when he stated:

> As your spiritual leader, I encourage our youth to abstain from 'adult activities'. There is no cure for HIV-AIDS. Please stop misleading our children that there is a cure. ('Knowledge is Power', *Sowetan*, 6 September 2007)

When reading this passage in the full transcript of his speech in the newspaper, I was astonished as it was the first time I had heard a ZCC official talk about HIV/AIDS in a manner that implied that the pandemic existed at all. In relation to making explicit mention of HIV/AIDS, I would have expected the bishop to make the case for divine healing and immunity by faith (cf. Dilger, Burchardt and van Dijk 2010: 374–5) but he simply stated that 'there is no cure'. At second glance, however, the bishop characteristically did not make any mention of the prospects of going on ART, which was at the time available from many health facilities in South Africa, including the local Mankweng Hospital that was only 10 km from the city of Moria. Arguably, the bishop's open-ended wording can be partly explained by the ZCC tradition of being 'aloof' (Kuperus 2011: 22) and shying away from making bold statements (Ashforth 2005: 192) on politically sensitive matters, that is that the way of characterizing the challenge posed by HIV/AIDS was not going to fly in the face of either the state president or the ZCC followers at large. On the other hand, avoidance of any explicit mention of ART is also explained by the ZCC's reliance on other explanatory idioms. In this regard, Niehaus (2009: 324) noted that:

> The very same symptoms that biomedical practitioners interpret as evidence of AIDS, [Zionist] Christian healers interpret as evidence that that [*sic*] witches are trying to transform the sick person into a zombie.

Viewed from this perspective, it is no surprise that the bishop's statement did not go into a specification of the aetiology of HIV/AIDS but was instead kept short, distanced and uncharged. Instead of exploring the delicate question of what HIV/AIDS is and how it comes about, the bishop used the sentences quoted as a smokescreen to turn an awkward question into an opportunity to preach to the youth that they should abstain from sexual activities before marriage. The leader of South Africa's largest healing church thus used the attention offered to him on this occasion to deliver the well-known moral rule of sexual abstinence rather than making any promises of a cure, care or healing for those infected. There was thus no mention of either ARTs or divine intervention by the Holy Spirit. Instead, the bishop emphasized the need for young people not to engage in adult activities, thereby implying two things: first that HIV is related to sexual activity; and second that married adults are not at risk. In some ways this line of thinking has translated into a ZCC trademark as, according to the young and dedicated ZCC members that I interviewed, one of the benefits of being a Zionist Christian was that the strict discipline of the Church made sexual abstinence possible.

The great majority of peer educators at the University of Limpopo were members of the ZCC, which was intriguing in view of the ZCC's strict prohibition on premarital sex. When I asked one of my key interlocutors in his capacity as peer educator and ZCC member why this was so, he said that it was because the ZCC bishop had encouraged young members of the ZCC to take part in community work so as to avoid teenage pregnancies in their areas:

> It is a word from our God that we must go and help the community. We mustn't stay and help ourselves, so you find that we are dominant [ZCC members within the group of peer educators].

Peer education is generally promoted because it is believed that, through peer-to-peer interaction, health messages can be delivered in an interactive environment in which the involvement of young people should help bring about 'a critical renegotiation of young people's gender and sexual identities' (Campbell 2003: 133). However, Campbell (ibid.: 134–6) found that peer educational activities often did not succeed in generating this kind of renegotiation. The peer educators at Turfloop who were also followers of the ZCC were under strict instructions to abstain from sexual activities themselves, and if they violated the 'rules and regulations' of the church, they 'had to confess'. Thus, 21-year-old Sithole explained the strict principles of the ZCC to me:

> It is difficult to be a Christian, more especially a ZCC member, if you are not going to cooperate. If you are willing to cooperate, it is not difficult. And it is even more difficult if you don't understand some of these things. And if you are not on

> good terms at all times, some of these people will end up misleading you – saying – no – like I told you before that a baby kiss ... it's not a problem. The pastor will tell you that a kiss is a problem at all times. But if you listen to the people, they will tell you that a baby kiss is not a problem. You can hug your girlfriend. The pastor will tell you that you must stay away from those people.

Sithole was already used to hugging his girlfriend Thabang and giving her a kiss on the cheek. One day his roommate was away and he found himself alone with her in the room and they began kissing and hugging. Sithole started to have an erection and felt in a special mood, so he explained to his girlfriend:

> Thabang! Can you feel what I am feeling? And she will say, yes. Then I say – no – if we continue – we are going to end up having sex. Then we stay away from each other. Then we were on the way out, she will go and see the church and that is how we stop it, because sitting with her – just playing with her – we end up getting excited ... I go to the pastor and confess. One, two, three, one, two, three, and the pastor will guide me as a parent. The pastor will tell me to keep some distance [from Thabang]. He's saying, if you can continue like this, one day you will end up doing that – you're going to regret it for the rest of your life.

Sithole told me how the ZCC takes pride in promoting the notion that 'with the ZCC, abstinence is possible'. The authority exercised by the ZCC in this regard reminds me of what Foucault (1997: 246) calls 'the monastic technology of the self', which rests on the obedience and willingness of the subject to sacrifice one's self. If one does not manage to obey fully, the only way out is to renounce oneself through disclosure and confession (ibid.: 249). Building on Sundkler's (1961) work, Jean Comaroff (1985: 229) likewise described how, through confession (*bolela*), members were expected to recall 'a string of personal misdeeds, centering around sexual "looseness" and the "eating of filth", acts which in the Zionist scheme typify defiling transaction with an alien world'. Obviously, this is what happened in Sithole's story above but it also shows that, in order to abstain from sex, one has to work hard on the self. From studies of Pentecostal youth in Khayelitsha, Cape Town, Burchardt (2011: 671) has noted that the everyday intimate practices of Pentecostal youths do not seem to tally with discourses of sexual abstinence. Likewise, the ABC model of HIV/AIDS prevention presents abstinence as simply an absence of actions, but this is to invoke far too passive an imagery when one takes into account the active efforts made by Sithole and Thabang in trying to avoid having sex before marriage. Meanwhile, in his capacity as one of the university's peer educators, Sithole facilitated workshops in which he instructed other people about safe sex and HIV/AIDS prevention. In this way, the ZCC used the tricky situation brought about by a large-scale sexually transmitted infection to propagate their usual safeguards against dirt and pollution, namely sexual abstinence outside marriage. By acknowledging in his widely broadcast speech that even the ZCC could not cure those infected with the virus, the bishop was probably trying to be politically versatile and not raise expectations of a cure and treatment by divine healing that his church would eventually not be able to fulfil. Yet, the bishop's statement revealed curiously little information about HIV/AIDS, which left ZCC members that I spoke to bewildered and trying to make sense of these matters themselves.

George's Conversion to the ZCC

The process of trying to figure out what is behind the failures of health or misfortune came to the fore when students discussed the likely involvement of *muthi*[5] and the agency of witches in their daily lives, although I never heard students claim that HIV/AIDS was directly attributable to witchcraft as such. In a few instances, some quoted other sources as saying that HIV was about bewitchment, as was the case when a male student stated during a group discussion that:

> You'll find some of the pastors saying that sometimes AIDS is not really like a physical disease – is not a disease of the physical, it's more of a spiritual thing. They can say witches they attack you, you see – one mentioned you get bitten by a frog and they say you have AIDS and you've never slept with anyone or been in an accident. So it's a belief that ... witchcraft does also form part of the – the – of transmitting HIV.

Another male participant said that, from a cultural point of view, it had also been taken as a curse and was still regarded as something bad or bewitched. Likewise, a 22-year-old student, Makgotla, whom I played soccer with said in an individual interview:

> The thing is – more especially with we black people – we believe too much in witchcraft – you see – so if somebody is sick – the first thing that one suspects is that that person is bewitched. I guess you know that one. We would say that person – what people know is that Mr So and So didn't like him or her. That person that I said didn't like him – did what? – is the first suspect.

Some students drew on their natural-science training in rejecting such notions entirely, while others grappled with questions of misfortune at a more generalized

[5] A traditional herbal medicine in Southern Africa derived from the Zulu word for tree (Ngubane 1977: 22).

level. George, a 22-year-old social-sciences student who converted to and was baptized in the ZCC in December 2006 after I got to know him, narrated how his rationale for joining the ZCC (as the first member of his family to do so) was that relatives in his extended family had been behind a number of ailments suffered by himself and his sister. In 2004, when he was writing his matriculation exam, George fell seriously ill for the first time and was taken by his parents to see a female *sangoma* (diviner healer), who tried to heal him using a range of different herbal remedies.[6] George explains how:

> She was doing her things, but I could see that she wouldn't be able to help me because she wasn't sure that – my state – I'm in danger – I know danger because the people who are doing this, they are around my family, so they've been doing it long time before. So their objective was to make sure that I don't matriculate.

In a pragmatic attempt at seeking curative services from more than one provider, George was also taken to a medical practitioner who diagnosed his coughing as ordinary influenza and prescribed some tablets that did not help. He therefore felt that the condition was much more serious and complex than the practitioner was saying:

> It was like a flu of some sort – yeah – but I was coughing constantly. I used to know that the flu they have to take you two weeks, not more than that, but it was taking me more than that – of which was uncommon. That's why sometimes I couldn't cope – say no – it's over ... my health is vulnerable, because those witchcrafts they are dangerous.

In considering the aims of the perpetrators behind his identified bewitchment, George suspected that the families of his father's sisters were actively trying to prevent his family from prospering and being successful in their endeavours:

> Actually, they wanted to turn the family into a laughing stock because it's what is happening to many families where I come from. Most people, they are not achieving. It's not they are not clever or what – there are many clever people around – but this thing – witchcraft – is stopping them – it's the big stumbling block around our area because you can see a person whose having potential – but when he writes his matric, many things happen around that particular person. He can start drinking and doing many things – negative things – and that particular person ends up failing to reach his potential.

---

[6] Niehaus (1997: 261) similarly reports on how matriculation examinations play a role in producing envy between neighbours that may lead to witchcraft accusations in the Lowveld.

George explained how his failing health made his mother fear that he was about to suffer the same fate as his late sister. Unfortunately, having delivered a baby that died shortly after birth of an unspecified illness, she herself died following a brief illness in 2000. In view of the South African HIV/AIDS prevalence rate, it is not unlikely that, biomedically speaking, George's sister died from AIDS-related symptoms, whereas, in George's view, the death was attributed to the envy of relatives and the witchcraft that they had exercised. In relation to his own illness, I asked George whether he had ever feared that it was related to TB or HIV/AIDS but after the medical practitioner failed to cure his cough, he felt that it was a different phenomenon altogether:

> I had the feeling that this was too much – it wasn't flu – because I was having stomach cramps sometimes, so I assumed that I'd been cursed for some reason. It's just that these things – there are dangers in society.

George's outlook on the nature of his illnesses was tangled up with the fact that, subsequent to his conversion to the ZCC in December 2006, he had more or less abandoned biomedical understandings of illness. In view of the ZCC conceptualization of disease as a matter of witchcraft, spirit possession or pollution (Sundkler 1961: 226–7, Comaroff 1985: 201), my question about TB and HIV/AIDS was somewhat ambiguous or even futile. Since his conversion, George claimed to have experienced an improvement in his health, and he also spent part of his university winter break at the ZCC religious city of Moria to undergo cleansing and purification through deep prayers and the ingestion of lots of tea and water. The ZCC defines good health as the free flow of body fluids, which is greatly assisted by an excessive consumption of cold tea and water, 'quenching thirst and cooling the heated blood that is incapable of smooth flow' (Comaroff 1985: 234). On later occasions, I accompanied George to Moria so he could purchase tea, coffee and cooking oil that had been blessed by ZCC ministers and were therefore understood to possess curative qualities (see also Anderson 1999: 290). Before entering Moria, visitors have to undergo cleansing and purification rituals in which a ZCC minister sprinkles them with water, burns little pieces of paper around their body, beats them gently with a piece of wood and serves them vast amounts of tea. Furthermore, the gatekeepers have to ensure that people do not bring items such as weapons, cameras and biomedical drugs into the religious city because these are prohibited. In some cases, I heard ZCC members talk of pastors allowing essential medicines to be brought into Moria but I have never been able to verify this, and it was not something that ZCC officials were willing to talk about. At the sermons held during the week at the ZCC structure on Turfloop Campus, water was also sprinkled, since the underlying notion is that human beings are 'dirty' in the sense of being hot and polluted, and are therefore in need of 'cooling' through cleansing with water (cf. Hammond-Tooke 1993: 181–2, cf. Douglas 1966: 171). In keeping with Sotho concepts of pollution, there is a taboo against going to church if you are in a state of pollution or hotness, which is the case if you have recently had sex, if you are menstruating or if you have just attended a funeral or have recently been bereaved. It is significant that excessive sexual desire is understood to result in the infringement of moral norms associated in Northern Sotho with heat (*fiša*). In this regard, Hammond-Tooke (1993: 181) wrote that:

> Literally translated, *fiša* meant a state of hotness. This might be brought on by a number of factors, chief of which was contact with death or with a woman who was in an 'abnormal' sexual condition ... The term *go fiša* meant 'to be hot'. It could be used both in a literal sense, as when someone was suffering from a fever, or in a figurative one ... The symbolic meaning of *fiša*, however, was much more extensive. (original emphasis)

Being hot produces a condition of impurity (*ditšhila*) that will eventually make a person fade away (Mönnig 1967: 67, Hammond-Tooke 1981: 121), which resembles the process of bodily decline when faced with a weakened immune system.

During weekly ZCC sermons, individual members become prophets through an immediate process of spirit possession, where the possessed persons point out the recipient of a message by clapping their hands right in front of the person. Since the prophet often speaks in tongues, a third-party interpreter is also appointed to act as an intermediary. At the Turfloop structure of the ZCC, one is then taken to a small room at the back of the building where, surrounded by other prophets, recipients and intermediaries, the three of you form a small circle on the ground and lean forward on your knees with your hands held out in front of you, while the prophet delivers his/her message in an exhilarated tone through the possessed person. The interpreter performs simultaneous translations and has the subsequent task of noting on a small piece of paper the prescriptions of ZCC remedies to be purchased and the rituals to be performed to alleviate or prevent the condition identified by the prophet.[7] The ZCC service comes across as a rather open-ended process, with considerable space for individual involvement and intersubjective interpretation in the construction of knowledge about a condition. The diagnoses do not seem to produce certainty vis-à-vis the causes of ailments as such, but instead the messages received from

---

7 I attended a series of ZCC services with a Dutch student, Anne van de Sande, who was studying HIV/AIDS communication for her MA thesis. Probably due to the fact that we were the only white people attending the ZCC sermons at Turfloop, we received overwhelming attention and were called by numerous prophets and given detailed prescriptions to alleviate a number of ailments identified in us.

prophets generate a different kind of certainty in terms of providing an outline of the necessary steps and actions that one has to take. As noted by Comaroff (1985: 232), 'Zionist testimonies are the immediate expression of a reality holistically perceived, of a system of meaning that does not distinguish knowledge from experience'. In itself, the continual process of questioning and trying out new healthcare providers and healers, as was evident in George's narrative, highlights the fact that the meanings and understandings of failures of health are not fixed or static. This suggests that people do not simply evoke diagnoses from a given frame of knowledge or social meaning but that they can enter into a process of active sense-making, drawing on multiple sources and frames of meaning, and trying out different healthcare providers until they reach a satisfactory level of comfort or of certainty and alleviation. In some circumstances, 'the openness of uncertainty may be preferred to certainty and control', to quote the introduction to an edited volume containing ethnographic studies of illness, risk and the struggle for control (Jenkins, Jessen and Steffen 2005: 9). In the same volume, Whyte (2005: 251) suggests that, in a world of uncertainty, the concept of subjunctivity may be analytically useful to denote 'the mood of doubt, hope, will, and potential' in which people go about dealing with the problems that matter to them most.

In the years when the South African Ministry of Health refused to make anti-retrovirals available in public health facilities (Nattrass 2007: 91–127, Thornton 2008: 171–93, Fourie 2006: 162–6), the argument was often advanced that people felt it was useless to know their status, given that treatment options and anti-retrovirals were not available at public facilities (cf. Le Marcis and Ebrahim-Valley 2005: 217). According to the body of my ethnographic material, there is more at stake here than the contested roll-out of anti-retroviral therapy (see also Steinberg 2009). Many Limpopo students insisted that a person does not die from the virus itself, but that once you know that you are living with it, you will 'die from worrying' and that the certainty of having the virus will make the process of dying much more expedient. Makgotla, who was also quoted above, thus explained that:

> The thing is – like our youth especially – thinks that if somebody is HIV positive, it's simply that the guy is dying ... and that person is not going to live much longer. All their assumptions are that if you are HIV-positive, a year for you is too long. The minute you hear you are HIV-positive – then that thing lie in your heart – that thing is in your heart – you're gonna die, of course.

A similar point was made by Tlhokomelo, a 20-year-old female student, when she said that:

> No, we are not afraid to go to the Health Centre – we are afraid of the results – because we end up dying of stress that [is] carr[ied] by HIV. We are not afraid of HIV, but the fear, you see.[8]

Students often reported having gone for a test without going back for the results, a pattern confirmed by the Student Health Centre at Turfloop Campus, where only one in five came back for their results after having been tested in 2004 (*Limpopo Leader* 2004: 31). Among the first-year students at the University of Limpopo, it was therefore only 17.5 per cent of the young women and 17.2 per cent of the young men that had ever been tested for HIV.[9] It seems, therefore, that the subjunctive mode of not knowing one's HIV status enabled a person to continue to strengthen or protect his/her *seriti*, while the certainty of a positive HIV test barred one from doing so. Viewed from this angle, the importance of the roll-out of anti-retroviral treatment came second to a person's local social standing, since an HIV test was understood to have the potential to rewrite a person's past and future. This aspect will be illuminated below since this is what happened to the only person who was living openly and positively with the virus on Turfloop Campus, namely the university's health promoter.

'A Blessing in Disguise'

The smiling face of Dios Moagi was well known to everybody on Turfloop Campus. Plastered all over campus, posters inviting students to come for voluntary counselling and testing carried his photo and the message: 'I know my status – do you know yours?', followed by the sentence: 'I have been living with HIV since 1993 – come and hear how!'. Curiously, I do not think that anybody knows exactly how Dios managed to live positively for so long given that he claimed not to be following anti-retroviral treatment. In a feature article in the university magazine published shortly after Dios had been appointed as health promoter and HIV/AIDS counsellor in 2004, he was quoted as follows:

> I have been living with the virus for 11 years. My CD4 count is down to 99 ... But I am still feeling strong. No, I am not yet ready to take anti-retrovirals. They say that once you start taking them, it is for life. (*Limpopo Leader* 2004: 31)

For several years Dios was tasked with the HIV/AIDS briefing that took place during Orientation Week when students first came to Turfloop in February every year. Students often mentioned Dios as the only person they knew to be

---

8 The concept of stress was also highlighted by interviewees in Niehaus's study.

9 n = 1,823 first-year students in 2004, 2005, 2006 and 2007.

living with HIV when they were prompted about their familiarity with people living positively. Generally, when asking about HIV/AIDS in the province, it was as if there was a magnetic force drawing every programmer, researcher or foreign student interested in HIV/AIDS straight to Dios, whose story had been widely published, not only in the *Limpopo Leader* but also in a French magazine[10] and in several anthropological texts.[11] Although I think that every life story has a repetitive touch, Dios's story had been told so often that it could be seen as an active project of self-making. When I first met him in 2006, he had just married his wife, who was also living positively, and Dios told me with pride that this was his 'best campaign ever, since people do not think that people living with HIV/AIDS can marry'. It was telling that Dios spoke of the intimate parts of his life in the language of HIV/AIDS campaigning, and I think it is fair to say that he was someone who, in the wake of having contracted HIV, had taken it upon himself to become a new kind of person, in line with the prescriptions of rights-based citizenship promoted by organizations such as the Treatment Action Campaign (TAC) and Doctors Without Borders (MSF). In his work on West Africa, Nguyen (2010: 99) has convincingly argued that those who can tell their story of HIV/AIDS well in resource-poor settings will be singled out for treatment through a process of triage, which makes telling one's story successfully a matter of survival. Since Dios claimed not to be taking medicine, it would perhaps be reasonable to say that his story-telling skills earned him social and material support rather than medical support. At the same time, however, the vocabulary of AIDS activism offered a new language of confessional technologies that enabled him to conjure a new self (ibid.: 38–40), thereby producing what Burchardt (2009: 335) has dubbed 'HIV positivity'. In this regard, Robins (2006: 312) has claimed that:

> Although these activist organizations are generally understood as rights-based social movements, the illness narratives and treatment testimonies ... suggest that experiences of illness, treatment, and participation in TAC and MSF can produce radical transformations in subjectivity and identity that go well beyond conventional liberal democratic conceptions of 'rights' and 'citizenship'.

In the same article, Robins (ibid.: 316) describes how an HIV-positive woman in her thirties who was a TAC activist in Cape Town claimed that 'AIDS has been a "blessing in disguise"' in view of the opportunities that her positive status

---

[10] http://www.liberation.fr/cahier-special/0101422900-denuement-durable, Accessed 28 April 2009.

[11] All names in the text are pseudonyms except for Dios who not only figures prominently in other anthropological texts as well – a fact that has been confirmed by Dios himself – but who also specifically requested that he be named in full, which I have respected.

had given her access to. Strikingly, Dios used exactly the same words when he explained how he never expected to reach the level of professional status and position that he had acquired at the age of 35:

> B: What did you think your life would look like when you were ten?
>
> D: Ehm – when I was ten, because you know I was coming from my disadvantaged family, I never thought that one of the good days I could be working in the university advising educated people – learned people like professors and doctors about the programme I am doing. I wasn't thinking of that. You know, most of the time when we are young, we are sticking to the culture and beliefs of our current communities, you understand, so we don't think big. You see, but now I have realized that maybe it's a blessing in disguise I'm having this virus ... just because I got an opportunity to come and work in the university where I am advising university students.

According to his often-narrated life story, Dios moved to Johannesburg in 1991 at the age of 20 to become a 'fly-by-night[12] businessman'. He delivered packages all over South Africa and made a good salary, which he often used to buy sex from sex workers. In 1993 he was tested for HIV and found out that he was positive but he had difficulty accepting this and continued to go around the country, where he deliberately had unprotected sex so as to infect others because, as he put it: 'I was having this anger that I didn't want to die alone'. At the same time, he was rejected by his family back home in Limpopo, and therefore simply continued his lifestyle until 1998 when his steady girlfriend became pregnant and gave birth to a baby girl. Unfortunately, Dios's daughter died in 2000 and he wanted to bury the baby girl at the family home in Tzaneen in accordance with Northern Sotho customs. Yet, once again, he was rejected by his family:

> [They said:] 'Look – you know we told you that we don't like this AIDS of yours here.' And you know it was very difficult. As a man I had to take responsibility. I had to make sure that – you know – I dig that grave myself. Without the help of them, you know, they were folding hands saying: 'We don't want to touch this AIDS of yours.' So then I happened to dig everything and you know wash the baby and put on another cloth and lay her in that small grave.

One can only guess what led family members to cut off relations with Dios but judging from his own account of his life, there may have been other reasons than HIV alone for them to pass moral judgements on him. Subsequently, Dios and

---

[12] In one of the focus-group discussions at Turfloop, 'fly by night' was said to be one of the phrases used to describe one-night sexual encounters.

his girlfriend broke up, and Dios decided to go back to Tzaneen to be part of the local branch of the National Association of People Living With HIV/AIDS. He became a provincial chairman in 2003 and met Mogadi (who he would later marry) through one of the counselling groups for people living positively with HIV. For a while, Dios's family allowed him to stay on their plot and he had contact with his mother at this point, but eventually he was kicked out again and had nowhere to stay. Luckily, in recognition of his volunteer work as an HIV/AIDS activist, he was granted an RDP[13] house by the local council, so he and Mogadi eventually had a place to stay.

About the same time, Mogadi persuaded Dios to convert to the Zionist Christian Church, which meant that he was able to stop drinking and 'live a disciplined lifestyle', as he put it. Like George (in the previous section), Dios's view of illness and disease was tangled up with the ZCC view that bad health or misfortune are brought about by witchcraft, spirit possession or pollution and that biomedicine has nothing or very little to offer. This goes a long way towards explaining why he was not taking any anti-retroviral medication, but is odd given that he was employed in a public health facility as a full-time health promoter in charge of the voluntary counselling and testing programme at a university with 14,000 students where one of his responsibilities was to refer students for anti-retroviral therapy. In spite of his expressed wish not to take anti-retroviral medicine, Dios always had up-to-date knowledge of his viral load and his CD4 count, which was usually below 100. Although a CD4 count below 200 would qualify him for a disability grant of about Rand 800 from the South African government (cf. Robins 2006: 320) should his short-term contract with the university not be extended, it is not plausible that this alone would have kept him from taking life-prolonging medicine that was otherwise available to him. In the field, I grappled with the question of whether Dios was shying away from medication because of the possibility of receiving social welfare grants or as a matter of aetiology following his conversion to Zionist Christianity, or for both reasons. At one point, while driving to his place in Tzaneen, I asked him whether or not the ZCC would allow members to go into anti-retroviral therapy and if the ZCC ministers could 'bless' the pills the way they bless tea, cooking oil, coffee and water. Dios answered in an aloof manner, not unlike that of the ZCC bishop when he stated that while on the one hand medicines are not strictly forbidden by the ZCC, they cannot be blessed or embraced. Similarly, although it was his job to distribute thousands of condoms on campus every week, he maintained that, according to the ZCC, this should not be necessary given that young people are supposed to abstain from sex until marriage. In an interview in the *Limpopo Leader*, he explained that: 'I am giving the message of abstinence and positive

---

13 Low-cost housing constructed for marginalized population groups under the Rural Development Program initiated by the ANC government.

living' (2004: 31), without making any mention of safe-sex practices or the prospect of living positively with ART. So, irrespective of his radical identity as an AIDS activist, Dios managed, just like the ZCC bishop, to leave the matter of the aetiology of HIV/AIDS open and instead stress the importance of adherence to moral rules. I do not know what he said to students who tested positive when he met them in his counselling room, and it remains unclear to what extent he would be able to univocally refer them to the nearby facility offering anti-retroviral therapy given that he clearly did not believe in it himself. My claim is that in relation to ART and his own body, he was more influenced by the ZCC stance on HIV (informed by local aetiologies of witchcraft and pollution) than he was by the orthodox rendering of the HIV/AIDS pandemic offered by the scientific community and the Student Health Centre in which he was employed. Still, he used his CD4 count to keep track of his bodily status and to make nutritional adjustments to improve his condition at any given time.

Dios's story bears testimony to the intricate ways in which the HIV/AIDS pandemic is unfolding and influencing people's lives in South Africa. At face value, it may be read as the story of a young man who contracted HIV/AIDS and experienced severe stigmatization and rejection by his family, which resulted in him becoming part of an open and supportive HIV/AIDS community that enabled him to build a successful new life for himself, with a job, a wife and a house. This narrative fits nicely with the vision of HIV/AIDS campaigners that, in the face of stigma, people living positively should be empowered to reclaim their lives in an environment that offers treatment, care and support. Yet, it is also a story about a landscape characterized by a multiplicity of contradictory meanings and beliefs, where people carve out new lives and livelihoods for themselves along lines made possible by specialized funding. Such new spaces in relation to health crises have recently been dubbed biological citizenship or therapeutic citizenship involving 'selective access to social welfare based on scientific and legal criteria that both acknowledge ... injury and provide ... compensation for it' (Robins 2006: 320). Dios's story shows that in looking to harvest the benefits offered by these new forms of citizenship, one does not necessarily have to subscribe wholesale to the ideas on which they rest. So although Dios rebuilt his life through the opportunities that opened up for him in relation to HIV/AIDS campaigns, and even though he found a job as a health promoter in a public health facility, this did not mean that he fully subscribed to a viral aetiology of HIV/AIDS or that he necessarily believed in the curative power of anti-retroviral medicines. It would therefore appear that, in their understanding of HIV/AIDS, Dios and his wife Mogadi were influenced more by their engagement with the ZCC than by their involvement with the HIV/AIDS community. This resonates with the fact that, at the practical level, Dios and Mogadi relied on members of the ZCC congregation for assistance. Thus, when Mogadi was too weak to fetch water from the well or to take care of the garden when Dios was away from home, it was their fellow believers who could be called upon to assist, something that no amount of pills would ever be able to do for them. And not only did the ZCC congregation offer both material and social care and support, as part of a healing church it also helped Dios and Mogadi to 'maintain their spiritual strength' as they phrased it, in keeping with the interplay of *moya* and *seriti* in the Northern Sotho semantic outline of the body described above.

Conclusion

By bringing back perspectives drawn from the classic anthropology of misfortune, this chapter has sought to demonstrate how avoidance of testing for HIV/AIDS may serve to maintain or manage a desirable level of uncertainty that enables people to go about their lives for as long as possible. It has also demonstrated how students belonging to the ZCC invoke an understanding of the body, where a person is open and permeable to others through pollution brought about by moral transgression, spirit possession or witchcraft. Furthermore, students claimed that having knowledge of one's positive status would weaken one's life force and expedite the process of dying.

Curiously, when students went for a test at the Student Health Centre they were counselled by the health promoter, Dios Moagi, who had himself lived through the experience of being rejected by his family after testing positive. But the person that students thus encountered at the Voluntary Counselling and Testing Centre was far from subscribing to a viral aetiology. Rather, he was someone who was attempting to reconcile the two seemingly contradictory frameworks of HIV/AIDS campaigning and Zionist Christianity to reclaim personhood rather than to increase his CD4 count. The inherent contradictions and surprising developments in Dios's story are testimonies to just how complex the HIV/AIDS landscape in South Africa is. During my fieldwork, I only encountered one person living openly and positively with HIV/AIDS, and that was Dios. Yet, in spite of the fact that he was in charge of the voluntary counselling and testing programme at the university, he did not himself believe in the therapeutic prospects of anti-retroviral medicines, a point I infer from the fact that, having lived with HIV for 14 years and having a low CD4 count, he was still shying away from taking medication. In talking about his HIV status as a 'blessing in disguise', he pointed to the transformative experience that HIV had brought about. If being rejected by his family when he came home to lay his child to rest can be seen as the ultimate annihilation of his former personhood, then his simultaneous entry into the HIV/AIDS community and the ZCC congregation must be seen as the foundation for the new personhood he could achieve following his transformation. After joining both the National Association of People Living

Positively with HIV/AIDS and the Zionist Christian Church, Dios managed to remake his life according to the opportunities provided by his HIV-positive status when specialized funding for AIDS became available. It was, however, the way Dios managed to draw on the aetiologically contradictory but socially complementary frameworks of AIDS campaigns and Zionist Christianity that enabled him to restore his life world. Sadly, this restoration eventually proved to be of a temporary nature only. I spoke to Dios on the phone in March 2009 but two months later I received the distressing news that he had committed suicide in the wake of a housing scandal after he had allegedly sublet a university property made available to him as a staff member.

Through the ambiguity inherent in Dios's story, as well as in the other cases presented in this chapter, it should be clear that there is more to the South African HIV/AIDS issue than meets the eye. To my ZCC interlocutors, the art of surviving HIV/AIDS has more to do with avoiding social death and keeping the spirit high than it has with increasing CD4 counts aided by anti-retroviral therapy. For Dios, living with the virus was not a blessing in disguise in the long run. Meanwhile, it is worth pondering whether a bold statement by the ZCC bishop in support of anti-retroviral therapy could make a difference to the lives of those of his followers who are trying to excel in the art of surviving HIV/AIDS.

References

Anderson, A.H. 1999. The Lekganyanes and prophecy in the Zion Christian Church. *Journal of Religion in Africa*, 29(3), 285–312.

Ashforth, A. 2005. *Witchcraft, Violence, and Democracy in South Africa*. Chicago, IL: University of Chicago Press.

Burchardt, M. 2009. Subjects of counselling: HIV/AIDS, religion and the management of everyday life in South Africa, in *Aids and Religious Practice in Africa*, edited by F. Becker and P.W. Geissler. Leiden: Brill, 333–58.

Burchardt, M. 2011. Challenging Pentecostal moralism: Erotic geographies, religion and sexual practices among township youth in Cape Town. *Culture, Health and Sexuality*, 13(6), 669–84.

Campbell, C. 2003. *Letting them Die: Why HIV/AIDS Intervention Programmes Fail*. Oxford: International African Institute.

Comaroff, J. 1985. *Body of Power, Spirit of Resistance: The Culture and History of a South African People*. Chicago, IL: University of Chicago Press.

Dilger, H., Burchardt, M. and van Dijk, R. 2010. Introduction – The redemptive moment: HIV treatments and the production of new religious spaces. *African Journal of AIDS Research*, 9(4), 373–83.

DoH, 2006. *National HIV and Syphilis Ante-natal Sero-prevalence Survey in South Africa 2005*. Pretoria: Epidemiology and Surveillance, Department of Health, 1–20.

Douglas, M. 1966. *Purity and Danger: An Analysis of Concepts of Pollution and Taboo*. London: Routledge and Kegan Paul.

Evans-Pritchard, E. 1937. *Witchcraft, Oracles and Magic among the Azande*. Oxford: Oxford University Press.

Forsyth, B., Vandormael, A., Kershaw, T. and Grobbelaar, J. 2008. The political context of AIDS-related stigma and knowledge in a South African township. *Journal of Social Aspects of HIV/AIDS*, 5(2), 74–82.

Foucault, M. 1997. Technologies of the self, in *The Essential Works of Foucault, 1954–84*, edited by P. Rabinow. New York: The New Press, 223–52.

Fourie, P. 2006. *The Political Management of HIV and AIDS in South Africa*. Basingstoke: Palgrave Macmillan.

Hammond-Tooke, W.D. 1981. *Boundaries and Belief. The Structure of a Sotho Worldview*. Johannesburg: Witwatersrand University Press.

Hammond-Tooke, W.D. 1993. *The Roots of Black South Africa*. Johannesburg: Jonathan Ball Publishers.

Jenkins, R., Jessen, H. and Steffen, V. 2005. Matters of life and death, in *Managing Uncertainty: Ethnographic Studies of Illness, Risk and the Struggle for Control*, edited by R. Jenkins, H. Jessen and V. Steffen. Copenhagen: Museum Tusculanum Press, 9–30.

Kleinman, A. 2006. *What Really Matters: Living a Moral Life amidst Uncertainty and Danger*. Oxford and New York: Oxford University Press.

Kuperus, T. 2011. The political role and democratic contribution of churches in post-Apartheid South Africa. *Journal of Church and State*, 52(2), 1–29.

Le Marcis, F. and Ebrahim-Vally, R. 2005. People living with HIV and AIDS in everyday conditions of township life in South Africa: Between structural constraint and individual tactics. *Journal of Social Aspects of HIV/AIDS*, 2(1), 217–35.

Limpopo Leader 2004. Health in SA's higher education: Fighting AIDS at Turfloop. *Marketing and Communication Department*. Limpopo: University of the North, 2, 31–1.

Mönnig, H.O. 1967. *The Pedi*. Pretoria: J.L. van Schaik.

Nattrass, N. 2007. *Mortal Combat: AIDS Denialism and the Struggle for Antiretrovirals in South Africa*. Scottsville: University of KwaZulu-Natal Press.

Ngubane, H. 1977. *Body and Mind in Zulu Medicine: An Ethnography of Health and Disease in Nyuswa-Zulu Thought and Practice*. London and New York: Academic Press.

Nguyen, V.-K. 2010. *The Republic of Therapy: Triage and Sovereignty in West Africa's Time of AIDS*. Durham, NC: Duke University Press.

Niehaus, I. 1997. 'A witch has no horn': The subjective reality of witchcraft in the South African Lowveld. *African Studies*, 56(2), 251–78.

Niehaus, I. 2007. Death before dying: Understanding AIDS stigma in the South African Lowveld. *Journal of Southern African Studies*, 33(4), 845–60.

Niehaus, I. 2009. Leprosy of a deadlier kind: Christian conceptions of AIDS in the South African Lowveld, in *Aids and Religious Practice in Africa*, edited by F. Becker and P.W. Geissler. Leiden: Brill, 309–32.

Oxlund, B. 2009. Love in Limpopo. Becoming a man in a South African university campus. PhD thesis, Faculty of Social Science (Series no. 54, 1–265), University of Copenhagen.

Posel, D. 2008. AIDS, in *New South African Keywords*, edited by N. Shepherd and S. Robins. Johannesburg: Jacana Media, 13–24.

Robins, S.L. 2006. From 'rights' to 'ritual': AIDS activism in South Africa. *American Anthropologist*, 108(2), 312–23.

Schoffeleers, M. 1991. Ritual healing and political acquiescence: The case of the Zionist Churches in Southern Africa. *Africa*, 60(1), 1–25.

Steinberg, J. 2009. *Three Letter Plague: A Young Man's Journey through a Great Epidemic*. London: Vintage Books.

Sundkler, B. 1961. *Bantu Prophets in South Africa*. London and New York: Oxford University Press.

Thornton, R.J. 2008. *Unimagined Community Sex, Networks, and AIDS in Uganda and South Africa*. Berkeley, CA: University of California Press.

Vigh, H. 2006. *Navigating Terrains of War: Youth and Soldiering in Guinea-Bissau*. New York: Berghahn Books.

Whyte, S. 2005. Uncertain undertakings: Practising health care in the subjunctive mood, in *Managing Uncertainty: Ethnographic Studies of Illness, Risk and the Struggle for Control*, edited by R. Jenkins, H. Jessen and V. Steffen. Copenhagen: Museum Tusculanum Press, 245–64.

Chapter 4

'God has again remembered us!' Christian Identity and Men's Attitudes to Antiretroviral Therapy in Zambia[1]

Anthony Simpson

Introduction

With increasing access to antiretroviral therapy (ART), the HIV epidemic in sub-Saharan Africa has entered a new, and, many would agree, more hopeful phase. For many Zambians the 1980s and 1990s were times of fear and despair. The formula 'AIDS = death' proved to be tragically undeniable. HIV and AIDS understandably came to be perceived by young Africans as 'a disease without hope' (Smith 2003: 343). Yet for many Zambians pessimism has given way to the hope that there is a future available, as a life on ART is now possible (see Colson 2010: 145, who describes the mood of 'buoyant hope' she detected in Zambia among the Gwembe Tonga because of increasing access to ART in 2004.) In my own experience of continuing fieldwork, comments such as 'There's life now', 'You can live longer' and 'Why suffer? Just swallow [the medicine]' are commonly repeated in day-to-day life in Zambia. Such hope even extends to the idea that a cure may soon be found. Indeed, it seems that the restoration of body weight and energy convinces some observers that people are no longer sick, regardless of the treatment regime they must meticulously follow in order to maintain their health. However, as the editors of this volume, and commentators elsewhere (see Dilger 2010; Mogensen 2010) have pointed out, along with new opportunities come complex moral and ethical dilemmas. In the early stages of the pandemic, the dilemmas often centred on how to live in the face of what was understood to be a death sentence and how best to care for the dying. Paramount among contemporary concerns for the HIV-positive men discussed in this chapter is the dilemma of whether to disclose their status. I describe below what some of them perceive to be the risks of such disclosure. With the introduction of ART, the

[1] An earlier version of this chapter appeared in the *African Journal of AIDS Research* (AJAR) 9/4 (2010), in a special section on religion and antiretroviral therapy. Permission to reprint – in part or in whole – from that publication was kindly granted by AJAR.

care of the self and of others remains paramount. Entailed in this are questions of cultural and religious identity in African contexts in which churches continue to play major roles both in influencing values and attitudes, in the provision of treatment and care, and in the allocation of resources. Patterson (see Patterson this volume) has highlighted the expressly *political* nature of this involvement. This observation has particular resonance in Zambia where the first and second presidents, Kaunda and Chiluba, each espoused explicitly religious positions. Kaunda developed a notion of Christian humanism as his guiding political philosophy. He identified 'evil' as the 'animal in man' that needed to be eradicated. Following the announcement of the death of one of his sons, Masuzyo, from AIDS-related illness in 1986, he went on to promote the use of condoms as a means of HIV-prevention, arguing that their use was necessary because of the sinful nature of human beings. Chiluba attempted to go further by declaring Zambia a 'Christian nation'.

Recently, the apparent recoveries of many of the men and women with access to ART in Zambia have been little short of astonishing. The transformations of those thought to be on the brink of dying are often described by fellow Zambians as a process of bringing back to life those who were assumed to be, in local terminology, 'finished'. This has been aptly termed 'the Lazarus Effect'.[2] Chapter 11 of the Gospel of John tells how Jesus, moved to compassion by the grief of Martha and Mary (the sisters of Lazarus), raised his friend Lazarus from the dead. In Christian exegesis the episode is interpreted as a foreshadowing of Jesus' resurrection after his crucifixion. The aim of this chapter is to describe some aspects of the impact of such biomedical 'miracles' on the religious understandings and practices of a group of mission-educated men who self-identify as Catholic and the challenge that such phenomena pose for the Catholic Church.

For some years now, I have followed the lives of this group of Zambian men I first knew at a Catholic mission boarding school for boys (here called St Antony's) where I taught English and Literature in the 1970s, 1980s and early 1990s. I have analysed the mission education they received and their post-school lives in the shadow of HIV and AIDS (see Simpson 2003 and 2009). I first interviewed a cohort of students around the time they were completing their secondary education, and I recorded their life histories in 1983 and 1984. My interest was to explore the impact of Catholic mission education on their values

[2] See *The Lazarus Effect*, a film directed by Lance Bings, produced by Spike Jonze, and funded by the Red Campaign for the Elimination of AIDS in Africa. It was aired on the British television station, Channel 4, and on HBO, on 24 April 2010 (www. channel4.com/lazarus). The film documents the remarkable recoveries of a number of Zambians in the capital, Lusaka. A promotional note explains that the film 'follows the story of people who were at death's door and were restored to life in as few as 40 days thanks to access to [ARV] treatment' (see: http:// www.channel4.com/programmes/the–lazarus–effect/episode–guide/ series–1).

and beliefs. The young men were then mainly in their late teens or early twenties. My interviews with them covered a wide range of topics. The students recalled their childhood; they spoke about their religious beliefs and their hopes and fears for the future. They candidly described their childhood and adolescent sexual activity. In our early conversations the topic of HIV and AIDS did not figure: the epidemic was not yet on their horizon.

I had initially interviewed a cohort of 24 students in 1983 and 1984. I re-interviewed 12 of the surviving original cohort almost 20 years later, in 2002. I again collected their life histories and discussed their sexual activity. My interest was to explore how the former mission students conducted their adult lives in the context of the HIV epidemic. By 2002, eight of the original group had died, as had five of their wives – most of them, their friends and relatives assumed, from HIV-related conditions. One man declined to be interviewed and I was unable to locate three others. I contacted a further 18 former students who were school contemporaries of the original cohort. They were interviewed, as were 12 former students' wives, one widow, and other male and female household members.[3] During 12 months of ethnographic fieldwork I lived in the homes of some of the former students and participated in their everyday lives. My account is informed by this experience, as I draw upon my observations and on the many casual conversations that contributed to our shared sociality. I also draw upon additional contact with many of the men during stays with their families during brief research trips to Zambia each year, from 2004 to 2010.[4]

In 2002 the age range of the former students in this study was between 35 and their early 40s. They belonged to a number of ethnic groups, primarily Bemba and Tonga. Though very few of the men, unlike their wives, regularly attended church, all claimed a Christian identity, as they had done at secondary school, with the majority of them being Catholic, though their religious affiliation also included Seventh Day Adventist, United Church of Zambia, Jehovah's Witnesses, Assemblies of God and various Pentecostal churches. There was a wide range of income within the group of former students. Their occupations included the following: doctor, lawyer, manager, lecturer, teacher, engineer, petrol-pump attendant, security guard and 'businessman' (that is generally informal trading). Several respondents were unemployed. All 30 were resident in urban areas or provincial centres. All except two were married, and many of the marriages were inter-ethnic. They all had children of varying ages.

[3] The 2002 research effort, entitled 'Men and Masculinities in the Fight against HIV/AIDS in Zambia' (R00023493), was funded by a fellowship from the Economic and Social Research Council, United Kingdom. I am grateful to two local assistants, Dixter Kaluba and Chitalu Mumba, who interviewed school contemporaries of the original cohort and the wives of former students, and for their insightful discussion of the data. Interviews were taped with the interviewees' permission.

[4] Most of these research trips were part-financed by the University of Manchester.

In conversations with me, those men who feared they were HIV-positive told me that they hoped that they would live until such time as their children were old enough to fend for themselves. However, while they warned their teenage children of the dangers of HIV/AIDS and argued, with few exceptions, that the only message to give to their children was that of abstinence, few of them decided to forego unprotected extramarital sex because of the epidemic. Though they had not had an HIV test, for some of them, this decision was based on their assumption that they were already HIV-positive and, as they put it, it would now 'make no difference' whether they practised 'safe sex' or not. Some wives were in professional employment; some were marketers or traders; others were housewives with no employment beyond the household.

Several of the former students I contacted had been in poor health. One of them died from AIDS illness while I was writing up my recent research, and his widow had started ART shortly after his death. While the men often portrayed themselves as 'survivors' of Zambia's severe economic decline and the decimation of their generation by AIDS – the HIV epidemic threw its shadow over many of our encounters. All the men in this study had lost family members, friends or work colleagues to AIDS. Many of them suspected that they were HIV-positive. At times, grief and depression threatened to overwhelm them. Several had been entrusted with the support of a sibling's orphaned children. I discerned that all the men had the information and means at their disposal to protect themselves and their sexual partners from the risk of HIV infection. My ethnography (see Simpson 2009) is about why, in striving to appear 'a real man,' many of the men at times, in essence chose not to do so. I argue that, though there are a number of exceptions even within this small group of men, for many, masculinity may be best seen as a fragile entity, encompassed by a deep sense of insecurity that puts many men and their sexual partners at risk of exposure to HIV. They are at risk because they attempt to 'live up' to the image of 'real men' who are expected to have multiple concurrent extramarital sexual partners and who engage in unprotected sex.

In sexual matters, the example of their missionary teachers, Spanish Brothers vowed to a life of celibacy and dedicated to the Virgin Mary, appeared to have little or no impact on the majority of the cohort's conduct of their sexual lives, neither while they were at school nor in later life. Religious education at St Antony's taught students of the sinfulness of sex outside marriage. However, with few exceptions, as young men, they took an eager part in the play of sex. To be sexually active was simply to be human. They judged celibacy and virginity as 'unnatural' and equated them with impotence and infertility. With the exception of those former students who were born again, men's views of religion and of God appeared to remain very stable over the years. In sexual matters, as teenagers and as married men, their view appeared to be that the church had no place to speak to them about sexual matters. While they admired their missionary teachers' dedication to the school, what they valued most about their mission education was not the religious teaching they received but rather the excellence of the education provided for them as an elite-in-the-making. Most would leave St Antony's and go on, via university and further education, to well paid jobs and professions, offering them a certain status in Zambian society. It is this status that would be put at risk with the coming of AIDS and the risk of HIV infection.

Religious Ideas

I focus here mainly on former mission students who self-identified as Catholic. A number of commentators on Christian conversion in Africa have drawn attention to the question of identity. Peel (1978: 447) argued, 'It is often best to see conversion as the search for a new identity, embodied in the membership of an attractive reference group.' This remark has particular salience in Zambia where, I have argued elsewhere (Simpson 2003), self-denigration of things African and the association of Christianity with 'whiteness', education, modernity, and respectability are particularly strong (for Zambia see Taylor and Lehmann 1961; Scudder and Colson 1980; Fields 1985; for elsewhere in Africa, see Lienhardt 1982; Ruel 1982). Students at St Antony's willingly embraced the education provided by Catholic missionaries as a 'civilizing process', even while, at the same time, resisting other lessons that the institution had to offer, especially in relation to masculinity among educated men.

Having a chosen Catholic identity was no guide either to regularity of church attendance or to adherence to Catholic teaching on dogma or morals. For example, while there was great reluctance to use condoms, no Catholic former student suggested that this was because of Catholic teaching on contraception. They explained their reluctance in terms of the widely held Zambian male views that condoms 'robbed' men of pleasure, slowed intercourse, meant that sexual partners did not 'really meet' and hence were 'unnatural'.

Drawing attention to the historical and political circumstances that condition the 'meaning' of antiretroviral drugs (ARVs) in Zambia, Schumaker and Bond (2008: 2133) observe that 'talk about ARVs reflects the stages through which Zambians are now constructing a "cultural model" of ARVs'. Given the influence of Christianity in Zambia, religious understandings will also necessarily contribute to this model. Academic attention has increasingly turned to the role of religion, religious faith and practice in the HIV epidemic in Africa (for recent examples see Becker and Geissler 2007, 2009; Prince, Denis and Van Dijk 2009) Because of my privileged long-term involvement with this cohort of Catholic mission-educated men and their families, I have been able to witness and reflect upon the men's religious understandings over the course of their lives and over the recent history of the epidemic, which now includes increasing access to ART.

The men, like their wives, in their grief and loss, strove to understand the HIV epidemic in the context of their existential concerns and their religious understanding of human experience. As they had done at school, former students debated ideas of God. All the men I interviewed asserted some belief in God or a supreme being. Though third-generation Christians, for most of them Jesus was a shadowy figure. As Hodgson (2005: 224) has reported for Maasai Catholic women, these former mission students had a theocentric rather than Christocentric orientation. Indeed, what Christianity meant to the former students defies any easy summary. Self-identified as Catholics, for example, they rejected, or at least were sceptical about, many major aspects of Catholic doctrine. While the majority imagined some form of afterlife, few of them accepted the existence of heaven, hell or purgatory. They were puzzled by such doctrines as the resurrection of Jesus, and even more perplexed by the doctrine of the Virgin Birth. Those who attended Mass would take Communion while not assenting to the doctrine of transubstantiation. Their religious ideas might best be described with reference to Robbins's (2007: 14) distinction between 'belief in' and 'belief that'. Through their lived experience, they seldom doubted the existence of a male God. However, few saw any need to assent to the details of Catholic doctrine as a prerequisite for church membership.

The majority of the former students described God as a personal deity. Concepts of God are open to change, as people puzzle over the meaning of human life in light of their own experiences (see Colson 2004, and Hinfelaar 1994, for explorations of the history of Tonga and Bemba notions of God [*Leza*/*Lesa*]). Most of these men argued that God helped those human beings who sought his assistance. At school, and in later adulthood, many of the men offered me examples of when they thought that God had intervened in their lives. Several, especially the materially and financially successful born-again Christians, attributed their good fortune to divine assistance: they had given themselves to God; and God had given himself to them. Yet several students, while at school, said that God could also behave 'strangely' at times. One example often given was the existence of Satan, the devil. Why had God created the devil when He knew that human beings would thereby be tempted to commit wrongdoing and sin? The Catholics, like other denominations, also debated whether God could be both a loving God *and* a stern judge or even a vengeful deity. Was AIDS indeed a punishment from God, a sign of his displeasure?

Our discussions about HIV and AIDS in the early years of the new millennium frequently led to the topic of promiscuity, and reference, by former students of all Christian denominations, to God's destruction of the cities of Sodom and Gomorrah (in Genesis 19: 24). Their God was the God of the Old Testament. No one, for example, cited Jesus' compassionate encounter with the woman found guilty of adultery (in John 7:53–8:11).[5] Others, like many of their wives, wondered: Can faith in God cure AIDS? Two Catholic former students gave instances of where born-again pastors had persuaded women in their congregations to discontinue ART and place their 'faith' solely in God. In both cases, the women died. Yet the former Catholic students, who were now born again, sought assistance from all possible sources. For example, two siblings of one of these men had died from AIDS. While hoping and praying for God's intervention, he did all he could to provide them with the latest biomedical interventions in the hope that they might survive until the time when a cure could be found. In his own sexual conduct, like others who were born again, this man found that his conversion experience, together with his Pentecostal church's requirements regarding prayer and membership in church cells, assisted him in resisting sexual temptation and thereby exposure to HIV. However, he had recently embarked on an extramarital relationship and stopped attending church. (In general, however, church attendance was not a reliable indicator of which men were least likely to engage in extramarital affairs.)

Voluntary Counselling and Testing: Better to Know?

Through the early years of the new millennium there was extreme reluctance among most of the former students and some of their wives to attend voluntary counselling and testing (VCT) centres to discover their HIV status. For the majority of the former students, this reluctance at first continued even when ART became increasingly available in Zambia, especially in urban areas and provincial centres.[6] Wives did not insist on their husbands having an HIV test, despite fears about their extramarital, unprotected sexual activities. The sister of the man described in the paragraph above lamented:

---

[5] Jesuit commentators in Zambia, such as Dillon-Malone (2004) and Kelly (2008), have attempted to dispel the interpretation of HIV infection or AIDS illness as God's punishment.

[6] Access has been transformed in the last decade, as can be seen by the figures in the Zambia Country Report submitted to the United Nations General Assembly Special Session on AIDS in March 2010. By the end of December 2009, 283,863 adults and children with advanced HIV infection were reported to be on ART, out of 416,533 estimated to require such treatment (Government of the Republic of Zambia, 2010, p. 81, available at: <http://data.unaids.org/pub/Report/2010/zambia_2010_country_progress_ report_en.pdf>). By December 2010, the number on ART was estimated to be 344,407 (UNAIDS available at:unaids.org/en/media/unaids/contentassets/documents/unaidspublications/2011/JC2225_UNAIDS_datatables_en_pdf). The scaling up of providing access to treatment shows a remarkable increase from the 2005 figures when only 20,103 out of an estimated 368,406 adults and children with advanced HIV infection were reported to be receiving ART.

> Even though we have left our villages, we have not left certain cultural ideas – like men misbehaving. The husband is the boss. Women know but they stay. They don't say anything, even when they know that AIDS is coming ... It's very difficult to root out these ideas from our society. We bring these ideas with us. Even the young people, they have the same double standards.

Many of the men in this study trusted that 'tradition' and 'respect' would prevent their wives from demanding that their husbands must be tested for HIV. They anticipated that they would continue to draw upon the 'patriarchal dividend' (Connell 1995), demonstrating the ways in which sexual practices and the experience of HIV itself is profoundly gendered (see the editors' introduction to this volume; Sadgrove 2007; Burchardt 2010). Such gendered experience is particularly salient in matters of disclosure and the fear of stigma. (See Murray et al. 2009, for the role of stigma also as a barrier to acceptance and adherence of antiretroviral therapy among urban Zambian women.)

In 2002 none of the men in this study had access to ART. While wealthy businessmen and government officials often received the treatment in private clinics or travelled abroad for it, the costs were far beyond the means of the former students of St Antony's. Despite VCT slogans such as 'It's better to know', very few of the men and women interviewed at that time agreed.[7] They preferred the 'uncertainty' of not having their suspicions about their HIV status confirmed.[8] The majority of men and women in this study said they supported the idea of HIV testing in principle, but had no immediate plans to discover their serostatus. The fear of being stigmatized was uppermost in many minds because HIV and AIDS were associated with promiscuity, and promiscuous people lost the respect of others. Here there was a marked difference between the different Christian denominations. Those former students who were born again might confess the sin of sexual promiscuity as part of a conversion narrative – the public admission of such sins being a *sine qua non* for redemption. However, for most former students, many of whom no longer attended church but who self-identified as Catholic, HIV infection had the power to spoil their Christian identity.[9] One Catholic former student commented: '*When a man is found with HIV, well, this is interpreted as saying* – I am a sinner.' In addition, there was a widely held conviction among Zambians, also maintained by the former students, that an HIV-positive diagnosis would simply hasten death through ensuing depression and a sense of hopelessness. At the beginning of the new millennium, the former students found it difficult to imagine how, in

[7] I asked all former students in the study if they had had an HIV test, though I stressed that I was not seeking to know the result.

[8] See Whyte (1997) on the pragmatics of uncertainty in Uganda.

[9] On stigma and spoiled identity, see Goffman (1963).

the language of the HIV/AIDS awareness campaigns, they might find a way to 'live positively'. In the absence of ART, they asked me: 'What's the point?' Some men reflected upon past encounters when they had had unprotected sex and assumed the worst. They told me: 'The time for me to know will come' – that is, when they became sick with what they assumed would be an HIV-related illness. Besides, in the contemporary uncertainties of life in Zambia, many of the former students explained, they might well 'die another death'. For many of the men the limits of a particular construction of masculinity were revealed. They told me that they were not 'brave enough' to hear what they assumed would be a death sentence. Several of the former students were employed to deliver 'ABC' campaigns or to assist in HIV counselling and testing, though, with one exception, they had refused to be tested themselves. By 2003 only three of the 12 surviving former students had tested for HIV. Two of them and their wives had had HIV tests immediately before their weddings. Another, a bachelor, had been tested for HIV several times after a series of illnesses.

In 2002, one of the men who self-identified as a Catholic though he was no longer a churchgoer told me he had decided he would never have an HIV test. He had recently suffered from tuberculosis and it had taken him a long time to recover. He recalled his past sexual activity and assumed the worst, though he rarely explicitly expressed his fears. Because of his significant weight loss, he knew that other people assumed he was dying from AIDS:

> As you see, I am thin and it's a problem. It's a problem being thin in Zambia today because people suspect you have AIDS when you are thin. I wouldn't have a test ... There is no point in having a test. It won't help, no. Look, I know this. When I am happy, I am healthy. But when I start to worry, that's when I get sick. I won't have a test. Those years I was exposed, especially up to about 1996. You know whether you were exposed to HIV or not. I won't have a test, and among all my friends, not one of us will have a test. There is no point. There is no medicine. There is no help.

This man, Kangwa[10], wondered what would happen if his wife, who had been very sick, became aware of his HIV status, were he to test HIV-positive. Very few husbands and wives discussed whether or not they should test for HIV. Some of the former students anticipated a wife would react unsympathetically to a husband's HIV-positive diagnosis. They did not anticipate that their wives would leave them, but they feared that, while wives would keep 'the secrets of the house' and offer their husbands public respect by maintaining silence about the diagnosis, they would become 'difficult' and more demanding in the marriage.

---

10 All names in this chapter are pseudonyms.

Access to ART

Despite individuals' pessimism, ART became increasingly available in urban areas and specified health centres. By the end of 2003 approximately 3,000 people received ART in the public sector (National HIV/AIDS/STI/TB Council [NAC] 2006). In 2004 the government began to roll out ART in provincial hospitals. The cost of treatment was about US$10 a month. As funding became available through various agencies, notably from the United States President's Emergency Plan for AIDS Relief (PEPFAR) and from the Global Fund to Fight AIDS, Tuberculosis and Malaria, in June 2005 monthly treatment payments were abolished in Zambia. With my repeated encouragement,[11] Kangwa gave up his determination not to discover his HIV status. In mid 2005 he and his wife were both found to be HIV-positive. They began ART immediately, and five years later were continuing to respond well. With his access to ART and his return to health, he revised his ideas about God, declaring 'God loves me after all'. He could now plan ahead and look forward to watching the 2010 World Cup. Yet he did all he could to hide the fact that he was receiving ART. He was conscious of continuing HIV stigma and, like other men, argued that this stigma now targeted men to a much greater degree than women:

> Women go openly to collect their medication. They are even proud to go because everyone sees them as the victims. We men are now identified as the perpetrators and so we get much less sympathy.

His reported experience of stigma has parallels with other research elsewhere in the region (see Wyrod 2011; Colvin, Robins and Leavens 2010). Writing of men living with HIV in Swaziland and South Africa respectively, Shamos, Hartwig and Zindela (2009) and Simbayi et al. (2007) report that the men in their studies were more likely to internalize blame for becoming infected and expressed greater shame about living with HIV than women. I detected no such reactions among the cohort of former students. For self-identified Catholics this seemed to be in line with their earlier reluctance (see below), when at school, to avail themselves of the sacrament of Confession. My impression then, as now, was that they doubted that the Catholic Church had any right to dictate to them on matters of sexual experience. As adolescents, with few exceptions, they were eager for sexual experience. Playing sex (in cibemba *ukukwangala*) was exciting and mostly enjoyable. They considered that to be sexually active was simply to be human. Notably, in my later discussions about their extramarital unprotected sexual activity, many preferred to speak about being 'mischievous' and 'naughty',

---

[11] My involvement in encouraging the former students to discover their HIV status raises ethical and methodological issues which I have not space to discuss here.

in their account giving a lighter tone to these encounters and relationships. Perhaps some of reactions such as those recorded by Wyrod (2011) may, at least to some extent, be the product of the type of subjectivities produced in the discourses men become entrained in counselling and support groups. It would be instructive to compare the reported responses of men with experience in such groups with those who have no such experience. Kangwa's assertion that men at ART clinics were more stigmatized than women was contradicted by the experience of others who explained to me that, should they unavoidably become aware that an acquaintance was receiving ART, they felt unable to acknowledge this state of affairs. One man's wife recalled a recent visit to the outpatient department of her local hospital: 'I saw someone, a woman neighbour of mine, in the queue waiting for ARVs, but she didn't want me to see her – so we didn't greet one another. We just pretended that we had not seen one another … '.

By the end of 2009 several other former students had been tested and had begun treatment. I have seen the transformation that ART can achieve by observing a number of the former students and how they did indeed appear to 'come back to life' after seeming on the verge of dying just a few months before. Take, for example, Edgar, a practising Catholic, now a school administrator. In 2006, he at first rejected my suggestion that he should have an HIV test. From 2004 his health had begun to deteriorate. By 2006 he had suffered significant weight loss and a string of illnesses and infections. Lacking the energy to attend to his duties in a consistent fashion, he still doubted there was anything to be gained by discovering his HIV status. His first wife had died from AIDS in 2003 and he was left with five sons to take care of. He later married a widow with two children. By early 2007 his weight loss had become alarming. Most days, too weak to work, he discussed with me what he considered to be his imminent demise. When I tried further to encourage him to have an HIV test and to seek medication, his response was one of resignation: 'Look … I've reached forty! I never thought I would live so long after my first wife died. It's enough. It's okay to die now …'. Were he to have an HIV test, he did not trust the medical personnel at the nearby hospital to keep this matter confidential. Like some other former students, he considered the doctors and nurses at government hospitals to be 'childish' and prone to gossip. The last thing he wanted was for his pupils to discover that he was enduring 'this disease of these days'. He remained adamantly opposed to having an HIV test. Yet, I suggested to him that when he stood before his pupils at morning assembly his appearance would lead them to the conclusion that their headmaster was dying from AIDS.

Edgar finally relented. He and his second wife were tested at a nearby Catholic mission hospital and were both found to be HIV-positive. As a result of further tests, including the regular monitoring of his CD4 cell count, he was put on ART around the middle of 2008. He spoke repeatedly of the non-judgemental support and compassionate encouragement that he and his wife received from the Zambian Catholic nuns who were nurses at the hospital. With treatment, the changes in Edgar's appearance and general health were nothing short of dramatic. Most noticeable were his weight gain and improved energy levels. In 2009, he returned to work on a regular basis. In conversation with me, considering the numbers of Zambians now accessing ART, he commented:

> Now we are the majority! God has again remembered us! [by bringing free ART to Zambia] One day He will send a cure ... In future the *muti* [medicine] will be taken only once in a week – one pill in all.[12]

Hope had replaced resignation. Yet Edgar reflected on how HIV infection had driven him to prepare for an uncertain future:

> Since I discovered myself [to be HIV-positive], well, look at me! Look at my farm – thirty animals! If I wasn't sick, I wouldn't have done this – to leave something for my children – buying, raising, slaughtering animals, plus seventy hectares of land. The animals are there. Milk! More than twenty litres a day! My wife sells and I'm able to pay a worker at the farm. If I didn't have this thing [HIV], I wouldn't have done it.

Stigma, Shame and Silence

In 2009, the former students and their wives were divided on the extent of prevailing stigma around HIV/AIDS. While some thought the level of stigma had reduced, in part because of growing access to ART, others judged HIV stigma to be as strong as ever. There was a generally held view, shared by the former students and their wives, that the more educated people were, the more shame they experienced and consequently the greater desire they had to 'hide' their condition. Of course, many of the educated elite were the products of Christian mission schools and held fast to a Christian identity. As Edgar's wife remarked, 'They lose dignity and so they prefer to hide'. Christian churches in Zambia, including the Catholic Church, have played and continue to play a significant role in the provision of treatment and care for those with or affected by HIV or AIDS. The Catholic Church has officially continued to condemn contraception and in particular the use of condoms, which, as Pope Benedict has recently reaffirmed, are judged to promote the spread of HIV instead of acting

[12] Edgar's daily treatment regime entailed taking four pills in all, comprising zidovudine, lamivudine and nevirapine, two in the morning and two in the evening.

as a means to prevent infections.[13] I argue that the association between HIV infection, promiscuity, and condom use maintains stigma and has contributed to some men and women's decision to forego HIV testing, causing them to delay coming forward to access ART, with potentially fatal consequences.

While more and more Zambians are gaining access to ART, there remains some residual reluctance to seek treatment, especially among men. As noted above, for many of those who are on ART there is a strong desire to keep knowledge about this as private and secret as possible. Among the former students of St Antony's, no one wanted to be suspected of 'carelessness' and 'sinfulness'. Prior to awareness of HIV and AIDS, men with multiple sexual partners had been called 'champions' by their peers. But with the coming of the epidemic, men who did not know how to avoid HIV infection lost their respect and were accorded a discredited status. They were censured by fellow men, in the main, not because they were assumed to have had numerous premarital and extramarital partners, but because they had lacked wisdom. It was thought that they had not been clever enough to choose with sufficient care – that is, to choose women who were HIV-negative, those who were 'clean'. These men had not demonstrated the cunning of *Kalulu*, the hare, hero of so many Zambian folktales, adept at disentangling himself from seemingly impossible predicaments.

Despite the scale of the epidemic in Zambia, where seemingly every family has been, in the terminology of the campaigns, either infected or affected, few people speak openly about their HIV-positive status. While some parents may have made their children aware that they had been living with HIV, the popular view is that these are exceptions to the general practice. Several informants noted that although, from what they could tell, certain people had died of AIDS, at Catholic funerals no one identified the cause of death as AIDS-related illness. They suggested that such silence merely furthered stigma. One former student, critical of what he judged to be a conspiracy of silence, commented: 'Actually, you really have to face it. You really do.' Most exceptions were individuals employed by, or working as volunteers for, NGOs engaged in HIV-prevention campaigns or the promotion of counselling, testing, and treatment access. This silence is especially noticeable where those who are considered worthy of greater respect, such as religious ministers, are concerned. The Catholic Church is a case in point. Yet AIDS has taken a heavy, though undisclosed, toll among priests and members of religious orders and congregations. Earlier in the epidemic, the former students had generally commented disapprovingly upon the sexual

---

13 See the papal encyclical *Evangelium Vitae* (The Gospel of Life) on the 'contraceptive mentality.' There are, of course, dissenting voices among some Catholic clergy in Zambia regarding church teaching on condom use to prevent HIV transmission. In the region more generally, the South African bishop Kevin Dowling has been outspoken in acknowledging the role that condom use might play in HIV prevention.

activities of some of their priests (cf. Simpson 2009: 177; Setel 1999: 178). Yet they observed the prevailing etiquette of 'respect' – not speaking openly about the deaths of priests from what appeared to be AIDS.

In her work on HIV/AIDS in Botswana, Heald (2005) has usefully suggested that 'shame', rather than the universalizing term stigma, might well be more appropriate in African contexts. From my research I can see the value of employing the notion of shame. The term shame carries both connotations of pollution and implies a loss of 'respect', a central value in Zambian sociality and one that seems applicable to the silence that has obtained in the context of the Catholic Church in Zambia about accessing ART. Here silence and discretion shield local clergy from potentially shameful exposure as people with HIV. Undoubtedly compassion has been a major guiding principle in interacting with all those with AIDS illness in Zambia. This has often dictated how AIDS patients have been treated, especially in the early period of the epidemic when care and compassion appeared to be the sum total of what might be offered to those who were dying. In everyday social relations, those deemed worthy of greater respect should never be confronted with a situation that would cause them embarrassment and thereby threaten their social status.[14]

Some of the former students had noted a shift in Catholic preaching on the topic of HIV and AIDS. While congregations continued to be admonished to 'behave and be well', they were also encouraged as individuals to discover their HIV status and to seek ART. Joshua, a practising Catholic, noted a change in tone in Catholic priests' sermons on the topic of HIV and AIDS at Sunday Mass in his parish. In his opinion, preaching had recently become less judgemental; there was greater emphasis on care and compassion and the need to seek treatment and much less talk about the sinfulness of promiscuity. Joshua suggested that this change of emphasis was not without a measure of self-interest on the part of the preachers: 'Our priests now fear to preach about immorality because they know they will be accused of misbehaving [having sex].' He cited a recent incident in which a Zambian Catholic priest was required to pay 'damages' to the parents of a schoolgirl with whom he had had sexual intercourse. The parents and other parish council members who were aware of the incident all agreed to keep the matter secret, it seemed, to protect the reputation of the priest, rather than to protect the reputation of the schoolgirl.

Some of the former students also attributed the existence of such 'respectful', discreet conduct, especially where Catholic priests and nuns were concerned, to what they termed 'the African gift of silence' (see Simpson 2009: 39, 132). This was especially the case with those Catholic priests and nuns who, parishioners assumed, were infected with HIV and were on ART. While priests encouraged

[14] Students at St Antony's maintained that should a 'big' (elder) person break wind in company, the most junior in age should apologize as if he were the culprit.

their congregations to have HIV tests and to take advantage of the available treatment, they did not reveal that they themselves had embarked upon a course of such treatment. They were not seen in the queues at hospitals and clinics where ARVs were dispensed. The general suspicion was that such medical treatment was 'taken secretly to their homes'. Members of congregations observed subtle and not so subtle changes in the physical health and appearance of their pastors. For example, Edgar spoke of two priests of his acquaintance: 'You can see that they were almost going [dying], and yet suddenly they start to put on weight and to look healthy again.' This silence on the part of the Catholic Church appeared to resonate closely with local understandings of the proper conduct of social life, where confrontation should be normally avoided. Additionally, there was the general opinion that admitting wrongdoing was also particularly difficult for Zambians. Joshua's wife expressed a generally held opinion: 'We Zambians have a problem owning up. We fear the shame. This Africa! We fail to speak when we are involved in HIV ... '.

My own experience of dealing with discipline matters while teaching at St Antony's lent support to this view. When caught in the act of breaking school rules, such as smoking marijuana or being beyond the school boundary on visits to girlfriends in local villages, students would almost without exception refuse to admit their transgression. What puzzled me was that while they would deny their culpability, they would readily accept whatever punishment was imposed. It seemed to be the potential loss of face entailed in the admission of guilt that drove students to do everything in their power to avoid embarrassment. This was mirrored in religious practices. Despite regular priestly exhortations to avail themselves of absolution from their sins, Catholic students were extremely reluctant to confess their misdemeanours in the sacrament of Confession. They explained to me that not only was confession to a priest unnecessary (as God knew their sins already and would forgive them if they expressed remorse), but that it was 'embarrassing' to admit their wrongdoing to a priest who was, after all, 'just a person', like themselves. Additionally, it was unclear what the term 'sin' meant for them. As noted above, self-identified Catholic students, on the whole, told me that they refused to believe in the existence of hell, or purgatory. Several maintained that 'hell' had been invented by missionaries simply to frighten them. It was thus difficult to understand what the term 'sin' implied for them; they did not appear to think that such sin would have any lasting consequences. For most Catholic students, God was a loving, and above all, an understanding God.

Common strategies for avoiding speaking directly about HIV or AIDS included using such phrases as 'this disease of these days' and 'we are affected by this which has come'. The archive of anthropological research in Zambia offers relevant precedents with regard to the avoidance of confrontation and the use of euphemisms. Describing Bemba sociality in the 1930s, Richards (1982: 47) noted, 'Bemba admire ... the avoidance of quarrels, unpleasantness and "scenes" which might disturb the delicate balance of village relations ... They delight in circumlocutions ...' . Where religious matters were concerned, in the view of former students, congregations still earnestly desired to 'look up to' their priests and this would prove extremely difficult, if not impossible, should the presence of HIV be acknowledged. And yet as recent sexual abuse scandals in the Catholic Church in many parts of the world have demonstrated, in addition to the enduring harm, such silence threatens the authority of the church and its representatives in the longer term.

At the government school where Edgar was the principal, as at schools throughout Zambia, the topic of HIV and AIDS was brought into every aspect of the curriculum. Pupils were encouraged to learn about the HIV epidemic and to discuss prevention and care. This involved frank discussions about sex. Edgar had received training at a three-week workshop and highlighted what he considered were notable cultural differences between 'Africa' and the 'West' concerning when to be silent and when to speak. He recalled:

> We were taught – Let the children talk! It's better they share. These ideas come from your side [Europe] – I mean even discussing [sex] with a girl child. Ah! In my tradition it was not there! But you people [Europeans] – you came and said – You've got to open up!

Pupils were repeatedly told, 'Look after yourselves!' Yet Edgar observed that teachers, like himself, who were on ART were 'still hiding ... When we go to class we never self-disclose. We speak in general terms in talks prepared for assembly or class discussion.' He once again attributed this to stigma because of 'the association between AIDS and promiscuity'. He was convinced that pupils, witnessing their teachers' poor health, and concerned about their frequent absences from class because of sickness, were quite aware that the root cause was HIV-related illness. He commented:

> The pupils, especially Grade Sevens and above, they are sharp. They know! They can see from the hair and the loss of weight ... but what are they really thinking? Ah, it's impossible for us to know. They are Africans! They will discuss it among themselves. You see, they learn so much, they know so much about HIV/AIDS – so they can identify it among their teachers ... But me I eat! I eat! But some teachers start losing weight ... [15]

[15] Such silence does not always prevail among pupils themselves. In recent research in Zambian schools, I have recorded several instances of orphans being bullied and being told by other pupils, 'Go and ask Mr AIDS' to find out the reason why they have lost their parents. This may be an example of what is termed 'courtesy stigma' (Goffman 1963: 30), imposed not by teachers but by fellow pupils.

His first challenge was with his own children, as he explained in conversations with me. It was not uncommon for parents to hide their HIV-positive status from their children, though whether and what their children really knew remained an open question. Besides the potential loss of status that parents might feel, silence might well be considered the compassionate alternative – compassion being a 'local' as well as a Christian value – thereby relieving children of the burden of anxiety about the future, but also avoiding the attribution of blame. Edgar commented in one of our interviews:

> I have never shared with my children. I don't know how they are going to take it. Look at the way my son is [apparently suffering from severe depression]. I sometimes wonder if maybe he has heard – and that is why he is the way he is. Maybe he has heard from friends. Maybe they have whispered to him ... I've shared with the hospital, with my wife and with the deputy at work. She's also one [on ART] ...

Tony: 'Why not share with your children?' Edgar responded:

> Because I know how it came to me. It's my [first] wife. She went with another man. She married another man. Now when she came back, I didn't know ... Now, my five boys loved their mother so much. Now, if I tell them I've got this [AIDS] – Why? Should I cheat and say it's me who brought it? Why? Should I tell them that it's their mother who brought this? Ah, no, they won't believe me. So, let sleeping dogs lie. Maybe, when they grow older, maybe I'll take them one by one and tell them. It's very complicated – either accusing or you are accused ... It's a burden for me. It used to be a bigger burden for me when they were still small. I would look at them and think – Ah, am I going to live to see them grow? My wife, well, she left [died]. But now I can say – Ah, they can stand on their own now. I haven't asked my deputy if she has shared with her children. Her first husband, the one who died, he was very wealthy. She discovered his infidelity. Then he was a polygamist. The two wives lived here together. Then the other wife died. Then he died.

At schools throughout Zambia growing numbers of both self-identified Catholic teachers and pupils were receiving ART. This was usually only known to head teachers and selected teachers. Some young children on ART took their medication though they were given no explanation of why they needed to take it. Some older pupils, again because of what they had been taught about the link between 'promiscuity' and HIV/AIDS, refused treatment, saying that they had not 'misbehaved' and so how could they have this disease?

While among the former students of St Antony's and their families, access to ART had transformed the lives of many, there were still mixed opinions about the long-term effects on the success of HIV-prevention programmes. Some suggested that access to ART would encourage more 'carelessness' (the same argument often offered against the promotion of condoms), especially among the youth. One informant commented: 'The boys are still experimenting. Now there is the supply of ARVs. They think – Even if I have this thing, I'll still be able to live with it these days. So there is little fear.' Based on the adult men he knew, Edgar rejected this view, citing awareness of the possibilities of cross-infection:

> I am not aware of increased carelessness. You may have one strain of HIV but you can still be re-infected with another. Among most men I know, playing [extra-marital sex] has almost stopped completely.

Conclusions

Access to ART is transforming the landscape of the HIV epidemic in sub-Saharan Africa. In Zambia, people with HIV-related illnesses have recovered from near death. While remaining doubtful about Jesus' resurrection, many of the informants had experienced or witnessed such remarkable returns to normal living. Yet, despite the prevalence of HIV in Zambia, Christian identity for some appears to be fatally bound up with notions of 'respectability' and 'civilisation'. Additionally, there is the double jeopardy that men fear because of the threat to their loss of status as 'real men'. For some men, anything seems better than being labelled HIV-positive, even the prospect of death itself. As Twebaze (2009) has observed, HIV disclosure remains 'a navigation in a moral field'. Bond (2010), in her analysis of silence and limited HIV disclosure beyond a closed network in Zambia, argues that no single explanatory model seems to fit. She maintains that justifications for disclosure need to be considered very carefully. Apart from the right to privacy, she asks who would wish their identity to be restricted to PLWH (person living with HIV)?

The Catholic Church, like all churches, evidently needs to work much harder to avoid moralizing statements that bring shame on those who are HIV-positive. The Catholic Church in Zambia has recently made efforts to promote a type of masculinity, inspired by the figure of St Joachim (the father of Mary, the mother of Jesus). This figure is modelled on Catholic moral and spiritual values and intended to challenge prevailing hegemonic forms of masculinity that may assist the transmission of HIV (see Van Klinken 2011; Chitando and Chirongoma 2008). The fruits of such efforts will necessarily be difficult to measure. In the meantime, there is more that the Catholic Church might consider. A person's right to privacy must be acknowledged. However, public silence about priests and people in the religious community living with HIV may merely (if inadvertently) exacerbate the problems of HIV-infected people who delay seeking ART or who struggle to achieve good ARV adherence because of internalizing stigmatizing attitudes (see Nam et al. 2008). The sexual abuse scandals that have come to light in the Catholic Church in various parts of the world expose the dangers of a culture of silence (although we have yet to hear from the African continent about the extent of the sexual abuse of children, adolescents, and women by priests and members of religious orders and congregations there). The silence that continues around people with HIV among the Catholic clergy and the faithful militates against efforts to control the epidemic and to provide adequate care for those who continue to endure their condition in secret. Even when access to ART is achieved, individuals' perceived need to hide their treatment does little to normalize this 'disease of these days' and creates further barriers to a healthy society.

Men throughout the world are notoriously difficult to persuade to seek medical attention (Courtenay 2000; Sabo and Gordon 1995). However, faith-based secondary and tertiary education in Zambia, often associated with 'civilised Christianity', together with the demonization of men in the course of the HIV epidemic, provide further obstacles to accessing ART. For the former students of St Antony's, the education provided to them by Catholic missionaries vowed to a life of celibacy proved to be poor preparation for lives lived in the context of the HIV epidemic. Anecdotal evidence suggests that those who were not part of the 'fortunate few', as far as education is concerned, and hence not part of the Zambian elite, have in some instances found it easier both to acknowledge their HIV-positive status and to openly seek ART. For instance, some of the former mission students and their wives spoke about male and female relatives from rural areas coming to stay with them while they collected their medication and said that they were open about the reason for their visit. Of course, these individuals may travel in order to maintain some anonymity, but perhaps they also feel they have not as much to lose by publically disclosing their HIV-positive status. For some former students of Catholic mission schools like those from St Antony's, the cost of acknowledging an HIV-positive status still appears too high.

Acknowledgments

I would like to thank Marian Burchardt, Hansjörg Dilger and Rijk van Dijk who organized the 'Prolonging Life, Challenging Religion?' symposium held in Lusaka, Zambia, April 2009, and also the anonymous peer-reviewers of this paper.

References

Becker, F. and Geissler, P.W. (eds) 2007. *Faith and AIDS in East Africa [Special Issue]. Journal of Religion in Africa*, 37(1), 1–149.

Becker, F. and Geissler, P.W. (eds) 2009. *AIDS and Religious Practice in Africa*. Leiden and Boston: Brill.

Bond, V. 2010. 'It's not an easy decision on HIV, especially in Zambia': Opting for silence, limited disclosure and implicit understanding to retain a wider identity. *AIDS Care*, 22(1), 6–13.

Burchardt, M. 2010. Ironies of subordination: Ambivalences of Gender in religious AIDS-interventions in South Africa. *Oxford Development Studies*, 38(1), 63–82.

Chitando, E. and Chirongoma, S. 2008. Challenging Masculinities: Religious Studies, Men and HIV in Africa. *Journal of Constructive Theology*, 14(1), 55–69.

Colson, E. 2004. *Leza* into God – God into *Leza*, in *Religion and Education in Zambia*, edited by B. Carmody. Ndola: Mission Press, 1–7.

Colson, E. 2010. The Social History of an Epidemic: HIV/AIDS in Gwembe Valley, Zambia, 1982–2004, in *Morality, Hope and Grief: Anthropologies of AIDS in Africa*, edited by H. Dilger and U. Luig. New York and Oxford: Berghahn Books, 127–47.

Colvin, C., Robins, S. and Leavens, J. 2010. Grounding 'Responsibilisation Talk': Masculinities, Citizenship and HIV in Cape Town, South Africa. *Journal of Development Studies*, 46(7), 1179–95.

Connell, R. 1995. *Masculinities*. Cambridge: Polity Press.

Courtenay, W.H. 2000. Constructions of masculinity and their influence on men's well-being: A theory of gender and health. *Social Science and Medicine*, 50, 1385–401.

Dilger, H. 2010. Morality, Hope and Grief: Towards an Ethnographic Perspective in HIV/AIDS, in *Morality, Hope and Grief: Anthropologies of AIDS in Africa*, edited by H. Dilger and U. Luig. New York and Oxford: Berghahn Books, 1–18.

Dillon-Malone, C. 2004. Is HIV/AIDS a punishment from God? *Jesuit Centre for Theological Reflection Bulletin*, 59(1), 9–11.

Fields, K.E. 1985. *Revival and Rebellion in Colonial Central Africa*. Princeton, NJ: Princeton University Press.

Goffman, E. 1963. *Stigma: Notes on the Management of Spoiled Identity*. New York: Prentice-Hall.

Government of the Republic of Zambia 2010. *Zambia Country Report: Monitoring the Declaration of Commitment on HIV and AIDS and the Universal Access Biennial Report*. April 2010. Lusaka: Government of the Republic of Zambia.

Heald, S. 2005. 'Abstain or die': The development of HIV/AIDS policy in Botswana. *Journal of Biosocial Science*, 38(1), 29–41.

Hinfelaar, H.F. 1994. *Bemba-Speaking Women in Zambia in a Century of Religious Change*. Leiden: Brill.

Hodgson, D. 2005. *The Church of Women: Gendered Encounters between Maasai and Missionaries*. Bloomington, IN: Indiana University Press.

Kelly, M.J. 2008. *Education: For an Africa without AIDS*. Nairobi: Paulines Publications.

Lienhardt, R.G. 1982. The Dinka and Catholicism, in *Religious Organisation and Religious Expression*, edited by J. Davis. London: Academic Press, 81–96.

Mogensen, H.O. 2010. New Hopes and New Dilemmas: Disclosure and Recognition in the Time of Antiretroviral Treatment, in *Morality, Hope and Grief: Anthropologies of AIDS in Africa*, edited by H. Dilger and U. Luig. New York and Oxford: Berghahn Books, 61–79.

Murray, L.K., Semrau, K., McCurley, E., Thea, D.M., Scott, N., Mwiya, M., Kankasa, C., Bass, J. and Bolton, P. 2009. Barriers to acceptance and adherence of Antiretroviral therapy in urban Zambian women: A qualitative study. *AIDS Care*, 21(1), 78–96.

Nam, S.L., Fielding, K., Avalos, A., Dickinson, D., Gaolathe, T. and Geissler P.W. 2008. The relationship of acceptance or denial of HIV status to antiretroviral adherence among adult HIV patients in urban Botswana. *Social Science and Medicine*, 67, 301–10.

National HIV/AIDS/STI/TB Council (NAC) [Zambia]. 2006. *Follow-up to the Declaration of Commitment on HIV/AIDS (UNGASS) 2005 Zambia Country Report*. January 2005. Lusaka: NAC.

Peel, J.D.Y. 1978. The Christianization of African Society, in *Christianity in Independent Africa*, edited by E.W. Fasholé-Luke, R. Gray, A. Hastings and G. Tasie. Bloomington, IN: Indiana University Press, 443–54.

Prince, R., Denis, P. and Van Dijk, R. 2009. Introduction to Special Issue: Engaging Christianities: Negotiating HIV/AIDS, health, and social relations in east and southern Africa. *Africa Today*, 56(1), v–xviii.

Richards, A. 1982 [1956]. *Chisungu: A Girl's Initiation Ceremony among the Bemba of Zambia*. London: Tavistock Publications.

Robbins, J. 2007. Continuity thinking and problems of Christian culture: Belief, time and the anthropology of Christianity. *Current Anthropology*, 48(1), 5–17.

Ruel, M. 1982. Christians as Believers, in *Religious Organisation and Religious Experience*, edited by J. Davis. London: Academic Press, 9–31.

Sabo, D. and Gordon, D.F. 1995. *Masculinity, Health and Illness*. London: Sage.

Sadgrove, J. 2007. Keeping up appearances: sex and religion among university students in Uganda. *Journal of Religion in Africa*, 37(1), 116–44.

Schumaker, L. and Bond, V.A. 2008. Antiretroviral therapy in Zambia: Colours, 'spoiling,' 'talk' and the meaning of antiretrovirals. *Social Science and Medicine*, 67, 2126–34.
Scudder, T. and Colson, E. 1980. *Secondary Education and the Formation of an Elite: The Impact of Education on Gwembe District, Zambia*. New York: Academic Press.
Setel, P.W. 1999. *A Plague of Paradoxes: AIDS, Culture and Demography in Northern Tanzania*. Chicago, IL: University of Chicago Press.
Shamos, S., Hartwig, K. and Zindela, N. 2009. Men's and women's experiences with HIV and stigma in Swaziland. *Qualitative Health Research*, 19, 1678–89.
Simbayi, L.C., Kalichman, S., Strebel, A., Cloete, A., Henda, N. and Mqeketo, A. 2007. Internalised stigma, discrimination and depression among men and women living with HIV/AIDS in Cape Town, South Africa. *Social Science and Medicine*, 64, 1823–31.
Simpson, A. 2003. *'Half-London' in Zambia: Contested Identities in a Catholic Mission School*. Edinburgh: Edinburgh University Press/The International African Institute.
Simpson, A. 2009. *Boys to Men in the Shadow of AIDS: Masculinities and HIV Risk in Zambia*. New York: Palgrave Macmillan.
Smith, D.J. 2003. Imagining HIV/AIDS: Morality and perceptions of personal risk in Nigeria. *Medical Anthropology*, 22, 343–72.
Taylor, J.V. and Lehmann, D.A. 1961. *Christians of the Copperbelt*. London: SCM Press.
Twebaze, J. 2009. *Disclosure and Silence: Challenges to marital relationship in Uganda*. Paper given at the 'Prolonging Life, Challenging Religion?' symposium held in Lusaka, Zambia, 15–17 April 2009.
Van Klinken, A.S. 2011. St Joachim as a model of Catholic manhood in times of AIDS: A case study on masculinity in an African Christian context. *Cross Currents*, 61(4), 467–79.
Whyte, S.R. 1997. *Questioning Misfortune: The Pragmatics of Uncertainty in Eastern Uganda*. Cambridge: Cambridge University Press.
Wyrod, R. 2011. Masculinity and the persistence of AIDS stigma. *Culture, Health and Sexuality*, 13(4), 443–56.

PART II
Contesting Therapeutic Domains and Practices

Chapter 5

Prophetic Medicine, Antiretrovirals, and the Therapeutic Economy of HIV in Northern Nigeria[1]

Jack Ume Tocco

> The power of medicine stems not merely from the wonders of science. It stems, too, from the power of moral suasion.
>
> Paul Farmer, Infections and Inequalities

Introduction

Books and papers overtake Dr Inusa's desk and stack behind him from floor to ceiling.[2] Gilded inscriptions from the Qur'an, a photo of his staff with the emir of Kano, and several poster-size photos of the doctor in the long white robes of a Muslim pilgrim performing the *hajj* hang from the walls. Like other successful Islamic healers in Kano working in the tradition of prophetic medicine, Dr Inusa's parlour office is complete with carpet and plush couches. As is customary when entering someone's home, patients and other visitors remove their shoes at the door.

Dr Inusa directs a well-established Islamic health centre in northern Nigeria's most populous city of Kano, with branch offices in other northern cities and more recently an office opened in Lagos. He is not a biomedical doctor but is recognized locally as an expert in Islamic prophetic medicine, and began

[1] An earlier version of this chapter appeared in the *African Journal of AIDS Research* (AJAR) 9/4 (2010), in a special section on religion and antiretroviral therapy. Permission to reprint – in part or in whole – from that publication was kindly granted by AJAR. This chapter is based on research made possible by grants from the Institute of International Education Fulbright Program, and the Department of Afroamerican and African Studies, the International Institute, and the Global Health Research and Training Initiative at the University of Michigan. Thanks to Murray Last, Susan O'Brien, the editors of this volume, and two anonymous reviewers for comments on drafts.

[2] Names and certain identifiable characteristics have been changed to protect the anonymity of research participants.

consulting patients suffering from physical and spiritual afflictions decades ago. With the pledged support of several state government officials and religious leaders, he plans to expand his Kano office from an outpatient operation into a larger inpatient prophetic medicine hospital.

People seeking help at Dr Inusa's centre meet a receptionist in front of the building, where they explain their problem and wait on wooden benches to see Inusa or another staff member. Painted in large letters on the wall behind the receptionist's desk, a message in the local Hausa language informs that the centre helps people suffering from a range of maladies: 'sorcery, madness, polio, epilepsy, spirit possession, high blood pressure, asthma, hemorrhoids, AIDS, liver disease, respiratory problems, erectile dysfunction, low sex drive, infertility, lack of breast milk, menstrual cramps, indigestion, et cetera'.

Dr Inusa is reserved the first time we meet but becomes increasingly oratorical over the course of our first interview.[3] Explaining that the focus of my research is HIV/AIDS, I ask what treatments he gives to people living with the disease:

> We give them medicine that we make ourselves. We know the correct combinations. There are special herbs that we give them to eat, and we advise on a proper diet of vegetables to build their strength and increase the amount of blood in their bodies. If they have diarrhea, we give them herbs that will slow the problem and then stop it. Then we have another powerful medicine that helps us eliminate the virus, to make it leave the body.

Does this mean, I ask, that this powerful medicine is able to cure people of HIV completely? He responds emphatically:

> It can be cured completely! By the will of Allah, absolutely. In Islam, our belief is that there's no disease that doesn't have its medicine – absolutely. Allah sends the disease, and Allah does the curing. It's not people [who cure]. For Muslims, headaches, foot aches, stomach-aches, typhoid, asthma, diabetes, Allah sent them all – and so too HIV/AIDS. Allah sent them, and He is the one that cures them. We don't agree that someone with a headache will be cured, someone with a

[3] Most interviews cited in this chapter were conducted in Hausa and then translated by the author. All respondents quoted are men; there are three reasons for this. First, all *malamai* (Muslim scholars) and the overwhelming majority of medical doctors working in Kano are men, reflecting the gendered nature of medical and religious authority in Northern Nigeria. Second, it would be culturally inappropriate for a male researcher to ask women questions pertaining to personal health and sexuality given norms surrounding gender segregation. (For a recent account focusing on the experiences of HIV-positive women in Northern Nigeria, see Rhine 2009.) Third, while an explicit gender analysis is not the centrepiece of this chapter, the larger research project upon which the chapter draws focuses on the experiences of HIV-positive Muslim men.

> foot problem will be cured, someone with a stomach problem will be cured, but someone with HIV can't be cured. We can't agree – because all cures are from Allah.

In deeply religious societies, religious discourses on illness and healing play important roles in shaping practitioners' therapeutic approaches and patients' wellness-seeking. Based on fieldwork conducted in the late 2000s, this chapter compares approaches to HIV treatment in northern Nigeria from the perspectives of Islamic prophetic medicine and biomedicine. The research entailed participant-observation in settings including the HIV clinic of a large public hospital, Islamic health centres, the homes of Islamic scholars who provide care for people with HIV and other afflictions, and a support group for people living with HIV. I also conducted in-depth interviews with HIV-positive men[4] from diverse socioeconomic backgrounds and with different practitioners who treat them, including both biomedical practitioners and *malamai* (Muslim scholars) working in the traditions of prophetic medicine.

Following a brief overview of the social epidemiology of HIV/AIDS in the region, I trace the historical developments of biomedicine and prophetic medicine to address the following questions: How has the resurgence of Islamic conservatism affected healing practices in northern Nigeria? What etiological assumptions and therapeutic praxes do *malamai* working in prophetic traditions bring to HIV/AIDS? How has the massive influx of antiretroviral therapy (ART) altered the region's therapeutic economy? And how do Muslims living with HIV/AIDS and the practitioners who treat them evaluate different therapies with reference to scriptural pronouncements on illness and healing?

My analysis pivots on a tenet of Islamic faith: 'With every disease, Allah has also sent its cure'. Whereas, from the biomedical perspective, HIV is an affliction from which one cannot be completely cured, many *malamai* claim that their treatments cure HIV because the omnipotent and infallible word of Allah makes it so. By insisting upon the efficacy and safety of prophetic treatments and premising these assertions on widely agreed upon principles of Islamic faith, *malamai* attempt to shore up their own authority and render competing biomedical strategies less authoritative. Biomedical practitioners and people living with HIV also grapple to morally valuate ART and other therapies in light of religious doctrine and perceived efficacy. I argue that despite recent efforts by Nigerian Islamic organizations and the government to assert a unified, ART-centred Islamic perspective on HIV/AIDS, substantive disagreements persist in northern Nigeria over the causes, treatments, and curability of the disease.

---

[4] The HIV-positive men interviewed were recruited primarily from biomedical HIV clinics and HIV support groups (many of which are affiliated with hospitals and receive funding from Western donors). As such their responses were likely biased in favour of biomedical approaches to HIV and AIDS.

The Social Epidemiology of HIV in Northern Nigeria

With a population nearing 170 million and rapidly growing, Nigeria is by far Africa's most populous nation. The country's estimated adult HIV prevalence of 4.1 per cent is considerably lower than that of southern and eastern African countries, where the pandemic has been the worst. Yet given the sheer size of the country's population, Nigeria has over 3.4 million people living with HIV – the second highest HIV/AIDS burden in the world following South Africa (Federal Republic of Nigeria 2012).

Just over half of Nigerians are Muslims. HIV prevalence in predominantly Muslim societies is generally low, a fact which has been attributed to a range of possible factors including the universal circumcision of Muslim men, prohibitions against alcohol consumption, and restricted opportunities for socialization with the opposite sex (Gray 2004; Hasnain 2005). The Muslim communities of sub-Saharan Africa constitute the most HIV-affected majority Muslim societies worldwide.

Islam is practised throughout Nigeria, but the 12 states that comprise the northern region have by far the greatest Muslim majorities. While HIV prevalence in several northern states is below national prevalence, the northern region as a whole has an estimated adult HIV prevalence that is only slightly lower than the national average. As in other African countries, such as Chad and Tanzania, where populations of Muslims and Christians are roughly equivalent in number, there does not appear to be a substantial difference in HIV prevalence among the populations of Muslims and Christians in Nigeria.[5] In sum, northern Nigeria has among the highest HIV prevalence for predominantly Muslim societies.

Kano is the most populous of Nigeria's 36 states with over 9 million people, and has an estimated adult HIV prevalence of 3.4 per cent. Within the state, prevalence is generally lower in rural areas and higher in metropolitan Kano (Federal Republic of Nigeria 2012). The bustling and ancient metropolis of Kano (where I conducted most of my fieldwork) is Nigeria's second most populous city after Lagos. The de facto capital of northern Nigeria and Hausa society, Kano, is a major commercial hub and West Africa's largest Muslim majority city.

---

[5] It is not clear why this is the case, despite lower HIV prevalence among Muslims globally. Further research into why Muslims and Christians in countries like Nigeria face roughly equivalent levels of HIV prevalence might consider factors such as equivalent rates of male circumcision among Christians, intra-national mobility and inter-religious 'culture contact,' and the effects of national HIV/AIDS campaigns.

Biomedicine and the Expansion of Antiretroviral Therapy in Nigeria

A central concept I work with in this chapter is 'therapeutic economy', which Vinh-Kim Nguyen defines as 'the totality of therapeutic options in a given location, as well as the rationale underlying the patterns of resort by which these therapies are accessed', and the 'practices, practitioners, and forms of knowledge that sufferers resort to in order to heal affliction' (2005: 126). My concern is how the recent expansion of ART in Nigeria has altered and expanded the therapeutic economy of HIV, how Muslims living with HIV/AIDS and the practitioners who treat them appraise the efficacy of ART, and how the drugs themselves are understood as substances requiring moral evaluation.

Nigeria is an undeniably medically pluralistic society. When Nigerians become ill there are many sources from which they seek healing, including a wide range of 'traditional' healers, spiritual churches, Islamic healers, herbal stores, and street hawkers, in addition to biomedical hospitals, clinics and pharmacies. Patients frequently shop around among different healing options in attempts to find affordable solutions to their problems (Oyebola 1986). In northern Nigeria, as medical historian Ismail Abdalla asserts in his historical ethnography of Hausa medicine, 'even among the educated there are many who see no contradiction in consulting a traditional practitioner in the evening and seeing a Western-trained physician in the morning' (1997: 30).

Biomedicine's arrival in northern Nigeria was recent relative to other therapeutic traditions; prior to the British colonial era it was virtually unknown. The indirect form of colonial rule pursued by the British in the politically powerful Hausa-Fulani emirates that comprise much of today's northern Nigeria curtailed the institutionalization of biomedicine in the region. Seeking to minimize the perception that they were undermining the authority of the emirs, the British administration prohibited Christian missionaries from operating in Muslim areas of northern Nigeria (Wall 1988: 125). This was significant because throughout Africa Christian missions provided the majority of medical care in colonial states (Vaughan 1991: 56). Fewer hospitals and clinics in the Western tradition were established in the north, relative to other parts of Nigeria.

Today the availability of biomedical care remains highly uneven. Rural populations, ostensibly covered by Nigeria's troubled local primary health care facilities, are especially underserved. Despite the fact that oil-rich Nigeria has the second-largest economy in sub-Saharan Africa (after South Africa), government expenditure on healthcare is low. The Nigerian government spends about US$25 per citizen on healthcare annually, ranking Nigeria among the countries with the lowest per-capita spending on healthcare in the world (World Health Organization 2012). Government hospitals and other health facilities are overcrowded and understaffed, often lack drugs, and medical equipment is frequently out of operation. Nigeria's worsening shortages of electricity and municipal water further affect not only hygiene and medical safety, but also compromise Nigerians' faith in their nation's medical system (Last 2004). Wealthy Nigerians commonly seek medical care outside the country.

While biomedical interventions of Western origin have found partial acceptance among northern Nigerian Muslims, in recent years they have at times been met with suspicion and rejection (Last 2005; Renne 2010); this has been particularly true of drugs distributed for free. Such distrust was particularly acute in the case of the polio eradication initiative led by the World Health Organization. In October 2003, Kano's former state governor Ibrahim Shekarau led a boycott of the distribution of the oral polio vaccination based on suspicions that the vaccine contained an anti-fertility agent or was otherwise unsafe (Renne 2010). This mistrust of Western medical interventions among some northern Nigerians has been exacerbated by international conflicts and perceptions of Western aggression in the Muslim world, most notably the 2003 American-led invasion of Iraq. Moreover, such reactions could be understood as one facet of a broader and pervasive resistance to the Westernizing forces of British colonial occupation, and the subsequent threats posed by incorporation into the secular Nigerian state (Barkindo 1993).

Mirroring the government's lacklustre commitment to healthcare more generally has been a weak response to HIV treatment provision. As recently as 2004, only about 50,000 HIV-positive Nigerians were on ART. These 50,000 – those who were lucky enough to be enrolled in the federal government's small pilot ART programme or rich enough to be able to afford the expensive drug regimen themselves – represented less than 3 per cent of the HIV-positive Nigerians who needed ART according to clinical guidelines at the time (Osotimehin 2004). In 2003, seven times as many Nigerians died of AIDS-related illnesses as were on ART (National Population Commission 2003).

Like many sub-Saharan African countries, Nigeria has experienced a rapid scale-up of biomedical HIV/AIDS care since 2004, with new clinics, new laboratories, newly trained and employed medical staff, and newly available ART. Today ART coverage for HIV-positive adults in Nigeria who should be on treatment according to WHO recommendations is 23 per cent[6] (UNAIDS 2010). Given the scale of the country's epidemic this means that over a million Nigerians who should be on ART are still without access. More optimistically, nearly 360,000 Nigerians were on ART by the end of 2010 (National Agency for the Control of AIDS 2011), a more than sevenfold increase in coverage since

[6] The most recent WHO guidelines recommend initiation of ART for all HIV-positive individuals with a CD4 count of ≤350 cells/mm^3 (WHO 2010). The 2006 guidelines recommended ART initiation with a CD4 count of ≤200 cells/mm^3. Thus while treatment in Nigeria and other countries has expanded considerably in recent years, the new recommendations for treatment initiation have meant that a smaller percentage those who should be on treatment actually are, even as absolute numbers on ART have risen.

2004. Hundreds of thousands of people have averted HIV-related illness and death in recent years as a result.

The expansion in ART in Nigeria is largely attributable to a massive influx of international donor funding. In 2008, for instance, less than 8 per cent of the country's total HIV/ AIDS budget came from domestic sources, whereas 48 per cent came from the United States President's Emergency Plan for AIDS Relief (PEPFAR), and 33 per cent came from the United Nations' Global Fund to Fight AIDS, Tuberculosis and Malaria (Resch et al. 2009). As one of 15 PEPFAR 'focus countries,' Nigeria has received over $2.5 billion to date from the United States for HIV/AIDS prevention, treatment and care programmes, with the majority of this money going to ART services and palliative care for HIV-positive people (United States Diplomatic Mission to Nigeria 2012). In 2007, PEPFAR funds supported 83 per cent of all ART provision in Nigeria (Resch et al. 2009), with much of the remainder supported by The Global Fund. In sum, well over 90 per cent of funding for biomedical HIV/AIDS treatment in Nigeria since 2004 has come from outside the country, with about half of all treatment funding coming from the United States.

There has been no large-scale public opposition to the provision of ART in northern Nigeria – and indeed most have warmly welcomed the increased availability of the drugs. Yet some HIV-positive people, as well as practitioners working in Islamic traditions, express misgivings about ART. Some question the interests and profit motives of Western drug companies and governments in distributing ART for free, echoing recent mistrust of Western medical interventions in the region. Others express misgiving about the toxicity and side effects of ART as a chemically manufactured therapy. Still others question the efficacy of ART as a therapy that treats but fails to cure.

Islam and Prophetic Medicine in Northern Nigeria

Islam expanded to what is today northern Nigeria around 1,000 years ago, but came to dominate as a religious and cultural system following the 1804–10 *jihad* led by Usman dan Fodio, which consolidated the area as an Islamic state. The vast majority of northern Nigerian Muslims are Sunni, with the Sufi *Qadriyya* and *Tijaniyya* brotherhoods comprising the greatest proportion of Sunnis for the last 200 years (Paden 2005). Over the last several decades, and particularly in urban centres like Kano, several newer anti-Sufi reformist and Islamist groups have grown in size and influence. These groups have attracted primarily younger adherents who rail against Western influences and aim to bring northern Nigeria into conformity with stricter interpretations of Islamic doctrine – in particular, those found in Saudi Arabia. The most influential among these newer reformist movements has been the Wahhabi-inspired *Jama'atul Izalatul*

Bid'ah Wa'ikhamatul Sunnah (Society for the Removal of Innovation and Reinstatement of Tradition), popularly known as *Izala* for short, or *'yan sunna* (Kane 2003). The *Izala* movement, along with other anti-Sufi Islamist groups (such as Malam Ibrahim al-Zakzaky's primarily Shiite 'Islamic Movement in Nigeria') advocate for literalist interpretations of scripture and the rejection of what they perceive to be un-Islamic – especially American – influences in Nigeria (Paden 2008).

Following Nigeria's return to civilian rule in 1999, and largely in reaction to widespread corruption and government mismanagement, the 12 states that comprise northern Nigeria began formally adopting *sharia*, the Qur'anic codes that stipulate that there be no separation of religious and civil life. In Kano State, implementation of *sharia* courts and criminal codes began in 1999. In 2003, Governor Shekarau greatly expanded *sharia* institutions, establishing a new Sharia Commission, a *hisbah* (vigilante) board, and in 2005 he introduced a wide-ranging programme of 'social reorientation' known as *A Daidaita Sahu* (Straightening the Rows) which aimed at bringing Kano into better alignment with Qur'anic laws and principles (Ostien 2007).

The push for *sharia* in the 12 northern states was indeed a major goal of newer conservative reformist movements (such as the *Izala*) and to an extent it indexed the increasing importance of these groups vis-à-vis the older and more politically entrenched Sufi brotherhoods (O'Brien 2007). However, the institutionalization of *sharia* was not the result of any one sect's efforts; rather, these social realignments found support among a broad cross-section of northern Nigerian Muslims concerned about corruption, the unaccountability of the Nigerian government, and the perceived pernicious slide towards un-Islamic influences (Last 2008). While far from representing the mainstream, the increasingly violent attacks by militant Islamist group *Boko Haram* ('Western Education is Forbidden') against targets including the Nigerian police and government agencies, the United Nations headquarters in Abuja, Christian churches, and beer parlours can be seen as expressions of disenfranchisement and the radical rejection of institutions perceived as un-Islamic.

One aspect of the increasingly Islamic reorientation of northern Nigerian society has been the marked expansion of religious-oriented healing practices. Since the early 2000s classical Islamic modes of healing – with their focuses on the spiritual dimensions of illness, the power of prayer and Qur'anic recitation, and the natural cures proscribed in the Qur'an and the *hadith* (the collected literature on the pronouncements and actions of the Prophet Mohammed) – have increased dramatically in both volume and prominence. Prophetic healing traditions have seen a renaissance throughout the northern states, even though governments have made few formal efforts to back them. As the expansion of ART and biomedical care for people with HIV/AIDS has occurred primarily in Nigeria's cities, so too the expansion of Islamic therapeutic strategies has been most pronounced in metropolitan Kano and other cities – reflecting the tendency of global flows of money and ideas of various origins to concentrate in urban centres (Appadurai 1996).

The Islamic therapeutic strategies most widely adopted in contemporary northern Nigeria lie within a long-established tradition in Islam known as the 'medicine of the Prophet' (*Tibb-ul-Nabbi* in Arabic) dating to the time of the Prophet Muhammad (Wall 1988). Muslim physicians and botanists of the medieval period made significant contributions to knowledge about the effects of plants, drugs, and foods on the human body, building on ancient Greek and Islamic prophetic traditions. By the thirteenth century, Andalusian-Arab botanist Abu al-Abbas al-Nabati introduced the experimental scientific method into this growing corpus of knowledge, and Islamic *materia medica* evolved into the science of pharmacology (Huff 2003).

Abdalla argues that by the time Islam came to northern Nigeria in the late fourteenth or early fifteenth century, Islamic medicine had lost its empirical approach to disease and cures. Rather, it became 'impregnated with religious and para-religious ideas that emphasized the curative property of divination, numerology, and prayer, especially prayer in traditions attributed to the Prophet Muhammad' (1997: 13). As opposed to the more scientific Greco-Islamic medicine developed centuries earlier, 'Islamic medicine among the Hausa [has come] to be understood as nothing other than Prophetic medicine' (Abdalla 1997: 35).

Malamai

Malamai are trained, to various degrees, in Islamic scholarship and Arabic language, although only about half of them teach. Others work in government administration, religious procedure and ritual, medical practice, legal practice, and the formulation of public opinion (Paden 1973: 56). Although only a portion of *malamai* work in the traditions of prophetic medicine, this has become an increasingly vital occupational niche over the past two decades. Compared to the impersonal atmosphere and frequently curt service provided at government health facilities in Nigeria, the 'amicable, intimate, elaborate and often ritualistic approach' of the *malamai* makes Islamic healing a comparatively attractive option to many Nigerian Muslims (Abdalla 1997: 30).

Those who specialize as healers use their knowledge of the Qur'an and other Islamic texts to tackle afflictions both physical and spiritual. The *malam* is considered 'a spiritual leader, an educator, political advisor, judge, secretary, and [medical] practitioner all in one' (Abdalla 1997: 140), who, depending on what scholarly materials are at his disposal and according to his own personal inclinations, 'may function as a counselor, diviner, astrologer, fortune-teller, spiritual adviser, pharmacist, and physician' (Wall 1988: 232). Traditionally, *malamai* have consulted patients from the parlours of their private homes or in mosques. While this home- and mosque-based approach continues today, in recent years many *malamai* have opened more elaborate 'Islamic health centres' replete with fulltime staff, consultation rooms, and Islamic pharmacies.

Malamai base their healing on the depth of their scholarly knowledge of the Qur'an and the mystically charged symbols of Islam and are expected to work within an Islamically orthodox framework (Last 2007: 3). Indeed, because it is considered to be the direct and infallible word of God in Islam, *malamai* tap the Qur'an itself for its perceived curative properties (Wall 1988). As Clifford Geertz argued, the Qur'an 'differs from the other major scriptures of the world in that it contains not reports about God by a prophet or his disciples, but His direct speech, the syllables, words, and sentences of Allah. Like Allah, it is eternal and uncreated' (1976: 1489). One well-known *malam* in Kano referred me to a passage in *Medicine of the Prophet*, a well-known fourteenth century text on prophetic medicine, to explain the centrality of the Qur'an to his healing practice:

> The Qur'an is the complete healing for all illnesses of heart and body and ills of this world and the next. Not everyone is given the qualification or the success to seek healing thereby. When the sick person is able to treat himself with it, and uses it for his illnesses with trust and faith and complete acceptance and certain belief, fulfilling the right conditions, the illness can never resist it. For how could any illness resist the Word of the Lord of Earth and Heaven, whose Word if sent down upon the mountains would shatter them, or upon the earth would flatten it? For whatever illness of heart or body, the Qur'an contains the way pointing to its Remedy, its cause, and protection from it, for whomsoever God grants understanding of His Book. (al-Jawziyya 1998: 250)

People living with HIV and AIDS have consulted *malamai* working in the tradition of prophetic medicine since the disease's emergence in Nigeria in the mid 1980s, decades before the US-led scale-up of ART. Despite the increasing dominance of ART in northern Nigeria's therapeutic economy, HIV-positive people continue to seek care from *malamai*, in addition to or instead of biomedical care. Several anthropologists have argued for greater incorporation of traditional healers into HIV/AIDS care in Africa (e.g., Good 1988; Schoepf 1992; Green 1994). Yet there have been no significant attempts to incorporate practitioners of Islamic or other forms of non-Western medicine into the Nigerian healthcare system. Practitioners working outside the biomedical system have been essentially excluded from the flood of donor money for HIV/AIDS entering the country. While global HIV/AIDS agencies and foreign donors like the U.S. PEPFAR programme have often been keen to enlist faith-based organizations into their efforts, an implicit requirement of this involvement has been that such organizations ideologically support ARV-based treatment regimes over and above any faith-based or 'natural' healing approach.

Early Islamic Materia Medica: Curing with Natural Substances

Prophetic medicine in contemporary northern Nigeria has expanded in several interrelated and at times overlapping directions. Of these, the most ubiquitous have been the thousands of storefront Islamic chemists (pharmacies) that have opened for business over the last decade. Largely unregulated by government and possessing varying degrees of Islamic and medical expertise, these chemists dispense the natural vegetal and mineral *materia medica* proscribed in the Qur'an and *hadith*, among other items.

In Kano, Islamic chemists offer on-the-spot consultations and prescribe natural products indicated in classical Islamic medical exegesis, such as honey, water from the Well of Zamzam in Mecca, *habbatus sauda* (black seed), dates, garlic, olive oil and perfumes. Also frequently available are locally produced remedies indicated for those suffering from witchcraft and spiritual attacks, potions to attract a beloved's affections, and medicines to increase sexual excitement and performance.

The specific items for sale in each chemist's store are subject to some variability, determined both by the size of the operation but more especially the strictness with which a given proprietor adheres to classical Islamic texts. While some chemists carry products not necessarily prescribed by Islam and which are more properly considered of the pre-Islamic Hausa medicine tradition, more religiously conservative operations sell only products and services that they believe to be clearly indicated by Islam. A sign posted at the shop of one *Izala* chemist was indicative of this approach: 'Follow the ways of the Prophet, precisely! Studying the Qur'an and Hadith and applying them is the way to health for Muslims'.[7]

Many northern Nigerian Muslims believe that honey is especially effective for treating a variety of ailments, including HIV. Several HIV-positive people I knew who were on ART said that they always took their drugs with a spoonful of honey, believing that this made the treatment more effective; others expressed the conviction that ART contains honey. Insofar as patients stay faithful to ART, biomedical practitioners rarely discouraged incorporation of honey or other natural *materia medica* into one's daily therapeutic routine, and sometimes tacitly encouraged it. *Malamai* who emphasize treatment with prophetic *materia medica* generally ascribe viral causality to HIV infection and adopt biomedical concepts such as 'viral load' and 'CD4 count'.

[7] In the original Hausa, '*Sunna, Sak! Karatun Al-Qur'an da Hadisi da aiki da shi, shi ne sama lafiya ga Musulmi*'.

Rukiyya: Talking with Jinn

In addition to scripturally based *materia medica*, two other common prophetic strategies are used by *malamai* to treat HIV/AIDS. The first is the increasingly popular practice of *rukiyya*, a form of spirit exorcism: A *malam* recites passages from the Qur'an renowned for their healing powers loudly and repeatedly into the ear of a person believed to be afflicted by *aljannu* (jinn), supernatural creatures mentioned frequently in the Qur'an. Patients typically break down emotionally during *rukiyya* sessions, speaking in the voices of the spirits that have possessed them as the *malam* uses vigorous prayer and even physical violence to pull the spirits (*cire iskoki*) out of the afflicted person's body.

Dr Zaberu began learning to communicate with spiritual beings when he was five years old; he inherited this vocation from his mother. The first time we meet, he tells me: 'You're a man. And just as I'm sitting and talking with you right now, that's how I can sit with jinn and communicate with them. I have treatment for all kinds of jinn.' Black jinn, he explains, are more stubborn and difficult to treat than white ones; sometimes the black ones leave and come back.

Unsurprisingly, *malamai* who specialize in *rukiyya* are more likely to assert that HIV infection is symptomatic of an underlying spiritual affliction than attributing a viral causation. As Dr Zaberu explained, 'Of all people with AIDS,[8] only 30 per cent really have HIV from sexual or blood contact. The other 70 per cent, while they do have HIV, they got it from a jinn.' Before treating a patient for HIV, he sends the afflicted person to a biomedical facility for an HIV antibody test to confirm whether she is positive. If she is, he treats the patient with *rukiyya*, then sends her back for another blood test to confirm that she is now negative. Several *malamai* in Kano claimed that *rukiyya* has the power to cure HIV/AIDS – particularly if the illness is attributed to an underlying affliction by jinn.

While their etiological assumptions may be quite different than those of biomedical practitioners, *malamai* often draw nevertheless on biomedical concepts and processes in their healing practices. *Rukiyya*, for instance, has become institutionalized into clinical format, 'with standardized fees and intake forms that documented the symptoms, treatment, and outcome of each patient's illness' (O'Brien 2001: 225). As this demonstrates, healing strategies may exhibit elements of syncretism, even as underlying presumptions about illness causality remain distinct.

---

[8] He uses the older Hausa term *ƙanjamau* rather than 'HIV' or 'AIDS'. *Kanjamau*, which means simply AIDS in Hausa, comes from the Hausa verb *ƙanjam–*, 'to become thin or emaciated'. Many HIV-positive Hausa speakers take umbrage with the term *ƙanjamau*, finding it stigmatizing and preferring 'HIV' and 'AIDS'.

Rubutun Sha: Imbibing the Word

Literally, 'writing for drinking' in Hausa, *rubutun sha* involves writing verses from the Qur'an with non-toxic ink onto sheets of paper, often thousands of times. These sheets of paper are then washed clean with water and the afflicted person drinks the resulting liquid, literally internalizing the potency of the verse. Like *rukiyya*, *rubutun sha* entails using of verses from the Qur'an to heal. But whereas the body of the afflicted is aurally penetrated by the Qur'an during *rukiyya*, with *rubutun sha* the afflicted literally ingests the power of scripture. The use of Arabic language verses from the Qur'an for medical purposes, whether recited or ingested, are understood as manifestations of prayer, 'an act of piety or devotion aimed at providing succor or comfort for the sick' (Wall 1988: 237). While still popular among some Sufi-oriented healers, *rubutun sha* has been criticized by orthodox reformers as 'innovation' without proper scriptural basis.

Malam Ismaila lives and works in a roadside town 20 kilometres from metropolitan Kano. I come to meet him because a HIV-positive acquaintance from the hospital HIV/AIDS clinic tells me Malam Ismaila administers the cure for HIV. In a room outside the main entrance of his family home, nearly a dozen women in *hijab* are waiting to be seen the day that I visit. In a second room, two male assistants sit on plastic mats in from of dozens of stacks of long white paper on which verses from the Qur'an have been hand-written in golden-brown ink 30 times per sheet. The men collate 18 sheets of hand-inscribed paper at a time, roll them tightly together, and tie these bundles inside thin black plastic bags. These verses, which the *malam* writes for many hours a day, are given to patients on sliding scale based on one's ability to pay.

Malam Ismaila says with a smile that he is obsessed with the Qur'an. Expressing his distrust of biomedicine, he explains that when HIV-positive people come to him for treatment he tells them to stop ART. Citing the Qur'an, he professes that the word of Allah will cure HIV or any other illness – and that it is impossible that it cannot:

> I tell them [HIV-positive people] when they come, 'This one [antiretroviral therapy] is not a cure.' Everyone knows it's not a cure. The drugs they give them in hospital are not a cure. Everyone knows that. So I tell them just to have faith in what I am giving you, because I am giving you medicine from the holy Qur'an, and [with the] holy Qur'an it is inevitable you are going to get cured. Have that faith and forget about the drugs in the hospital. A lot of them have taken the advice I gave them, they have avoided the modern medicine; a lot of them are cured. Those who have started [*rubutun sha*] early have been cured completely.

Malam Ismaila further explains that AIDS is divine punishment for the transgression of conservative sexual morality. From his perspective – a common

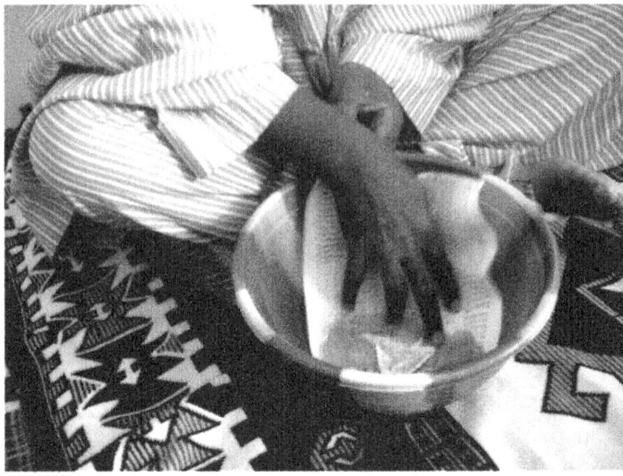

Figure 5.1 *Rubutun sha*: A *malam* washes hand-written verses of the Qur'an in water. An afflicted person will then drink or bathe with the resulting liquid, which is said to cure illnesses – including HIV/AIDS (Source: Jack Tocco)

perspective indeed in Nigeria – human deviance from God's scriptural mandates is the root cause of the epidemic. For Muslims who contend that AIDS came about because of human distance from scriptural mandates and who furthermore believe in the unmediated perfection of the Qur'an, practices such as *rukiyya* and *rubutun sha* are necessarily efficacious forms of therapy. By literally internalizing the Qur'an, the sufferer/sinner overcomes his moral deficiency and is returned to spiritual and physical health.

In summary, the field of Islamic healing in contemporary northern Nigeria encompasses a range of herbal and spiritual approaches centring on the traditions of prophetic medicine and on more heterodox methods such as *rubutun sha*. Promulgated by both Sufi-oriented and anti-Sufi reformers, Islamic medicine is the first resort to care for many northern Nigerian Muslims with a variety of physical and spiritual complaints. The personalized care and more relaxed environment provided by *malamai* contrast with the gruffness and crowding typical of many public biomedical facilities.

Prophetic approaches are sometimes used singly, but they may also be used in combination with each other. For instance, one profitable centre that saw many hundreds of people with HIV in Kano in the years before the expansion of ART sells a treatment that mixes honey, Zamzam water, and *rubutun sha* in measured, pre-bottled doses. They also keep detailed patient records in ledgers that look very much like those associated with a biomedical office, and sent patients for CD4 blood tests to measure their progress. The centre was still in operation when I interviewed its founders in 2010, but had moved to a smaller building in a less prestigious neighbourhood. It was clear that their success had been decimated by the arrival of ART, but they continued to sell their treatments to HIV-positive clients.

Despite the popularity of Islamic healing practices, they are both largely unregulated and largely unsupported by the ministries of health in the northern states. Of the estimated 30,000 Islamic medical centres, Islamic chemists, and other traditional medical practitioners in Kano State, as of 2010 only seven were registered with the Kano State Ministry of Health's Private Health Institutions Registration Unit. On the one hand, if state health ministries support and recognize prophetic and other 'traditional' practitioners, they risk a reproach from the biomedical establishment. If, on the other hand, they more strongly regulate traditionalists – when, for instance, they claim to be able to cure HIV – they risk being branded as anti-Islamic. The compromise that state governments strike, it would seem, is not licensing such practitioners while allowing them to operate.

'Every Disease Has Its Cure'

In many Muslim societies, 'ordinary conversation is laced with Quranic formulae to the point where even the most mundane subjects seem set in a sacred frame' (Geertz 1976: 1491). Muslims in northern Nigeria regularly quote from the Qur'an and *hadith* in everyday discourse to express and affirm guiding principles of social life. This practice is especially common when discussing central concerns, such as life and death, right and wrong, humankind's relation to Allah, and our place in the wider world. In conversations pertaining to health, the most consistently expressed proverb by far is: 'For every disease that God has sent to humankind, He has also sent its remedy'. Attributed to the Prophet Mohammad in several often-quoted *hadith*, this proposition is foundational to Muslim ideas about illness and healing (al-Jawziyya 1998: 9–10). In everyday conversation the proverb is expressed with the more succinct Hausa phrase, '*Kowace cutar da maganinta*' ('Every disease has its cure'). In addition to being a frequent conversational utterance, the proverb is seen in the advertisements and signboards of prophetic medicine practitioners, and even written on the back of some public buses.

The affirmation that Allah sends a cure with every disease is also common in discussions of HIV/AIDS.[9] This sentiment offers hope in the midst of a devastating public health crisis; it also has the potential to unify the Muslim

[9] This has been true for other Muslim communities in Africa too. See for instance Svensson (2009) on Muslims in Kisumu, Kenya.

community's response to the epidemic. From another perspective, however, the proposition that every disease has a cure can be seen as inappropriate and even dangerous when applied to HIV/AIDS. In the dominant biomedical understanding of HIV, the virus presently has no cure. Where highly active antiretroviral therapy (HAART) has been the standard of care since its rollout in 1996 (particularly, that is, in the world's richest countries), HIV infection is now widely considered a manageable, chronic disease. The goal of HAART is not to eliminate the virus, but to suppress it as much as possible, thereby forestalling indefinitely its progression to AIDS. From the biomedical perspective, HIV cure claims have generally been interpreted as the self-serving assertions of denialists and profiteers.

Many *malamai* insist that HIV can be completely cured by faith in the supernatural power of the Qur'an and proper combinations of the *materia medica* prescribed in Islamic texts. The ability to completely cure HIV/AIDS (or, more precisely, to serve Allah's will in manifesting the cure) is avowed in advertisements, radio broadcasts, and other forums where *malamai* discuss the disease. Dr Inusa, with whom I began this chapter, was among the most passionate of the *malamai* I interviewed in articulating his ability to cure HIV, but was far from alone in asserting that Allah reveals the cure to dedicated Islamic scholars. Such assertions constitute a response to the increasing therapeutic hegemony of ART in Nigeria. Taken further, those who profess that HIV/AIDS can be cured by prophetic medicine confirm the omnipotence of Allah and the inferiority of secular (and hence fallibly human) biomedicine.

Without falsifying the proposition that a divine cure for HIV exists, many Muslim patients on ART and the predominantly Muslim biomedical staff who treat them express scepticism about whether Allah has yet to reveal the cure to humans. The growing numbers of HIV-positive Muslims who consume ART, some of whom simultaneously pursue forms of Islamic healing, are therefore positioned somewhere at the intersection of two different cultural-institutional understandings of HIV and its treatment. As Van der Geest and Hardon (2006) point out, 'neo-traditional' drugs for preventing and treating AIDS developed without competition from ART. Whereas health workers advise patients today against neo-traditional treatments out of concern for pharmacological interactions with ART, patients may consider neo-traditional medicines as complementary or even alternative to modern pharmaceuticals.

With the exception of those who claim that ART is inferior to Islamic remedies or too toxic, some *malamai* consider ART to be beneficial, even advising complementary therapy with Islamic treatments. Many patients on ART, and the biomedical staff who care for them, praise ART for the frequently transformative effects these drugs have in the lives of HIV-positive people. But no one I interviewed for my research said they believed ART constitutes a cure.

ART is conceptually distinct from the notion of a cure – which, from the Islamic perspective, is the sole providence of Allah.

On the one hand, Islamic approaches to health emphasize the will of Allah, attending to not only the physical but also to spiritual components of health and disease. Standard biomedical etiology and treatment, on the other hand, focus nearly exclusively on measurable changes to individual bodies, denying the importance or even the existence of spiritual aspects of wellness and illness, and categorically denying the existence of a cure for HIV. How, then, do different people in northern Nigeria talk about ART, cures, and negotiate these two conceptually distinct aspects of the therapeutic economy of HIV?

Isa is in his late twenties, has been HIV-positive for three years, and is a member of a hospital-affiliated support group for people with HIV. While he is enrolled as a patient at a hospital HIV clinic, his doctor has told him that his CD4 cell count is high enough that he does not yet qualify for ART. When I asked him to explain what he thought about HIV treatment, he responded: 'As a Muslim, I agree that God has never made a disease for which He has not also sent its medicine. So even if we don't have the cure [for HIV] now, it's here. We just need to find it, because God has sent it down to us. We just haven't reached the time yet when we can say, here's the medicine; drink it and you're cured.' Here, Isa offers an interpretation of the *hadith* that is common among HIV patients and practitioners operating in the biomedical system: that a cure for HIV exists *somewhere* in the world, but human beings have not yet discovered it. This interpretation does not falsify the *hadith*, which would be considered blasphemous, but proposes instead that revelation of the cure to human beings is forthcoming. In *Medicine of the Prophet*, al-Jawziyya considers a similar interpretation:

> It is also possible that [Muhammad's] actual words were: 'For every disease there is a remedy,' to be taken in a general sense, so as to encompass fatal illnesses and those which no physician can cure. In that case, God the Most Glorious has appointed remedies to cure them but has concealed the knowledge of such remedies from humankind, and has not given man the means to find out. For created beings have no knowledge except that which God has taught them' (1998: 10).

From this perspective, Allah – source of everything in the universe, including human knowledge – has not yet revealed the cure for HIV to people. The cure is, as it were, hidden in our midst.

Ali, another member of the same HIV support group, is a businessman in his mid thirties who fell seriously ill before testing HIV-positive a year before starting on ART. Having spent over 2 million naira (about US$14,000) of his own money trying to cure himself with a variety of herbal treatments, he expressed gratitude to the staff of the hospital HIV clinic – where, he pointed out, the ART was even free. Ali compared his life before and after being on ART:

> I'm not afraid to tell anyone, now, that I have this disease. Before, if you got HIV, you had to hide it because there was no medicine. But I've never been fatter than I am now – I feel strength in my body. Since I've started ART I've never had a headache or malaria. I have a mosquito net, I eat regularly, and I don't mess around with taking my meds at the proper time ...] Before I was enlightened [about HIV], I told you, once someone told me that they would give me a treatment that would cure me – what do they call them, 'native doctors'? I went to Ilorin, I went to Lagos, I went to Kaduna, and I even went out into the bush to seek out a treatment, buy it with my own money, to get healthy and cure myself completely. But now I know it's a lie. People say they have a cure, but they never explain how it works. They say, 'We understand this disease, we know how to eliminate it from someone's body. Just take this treatment once and you'll be cured.' But if you don't mess around with taking your real medicine [that is, ART], you won't have problems.

The costs of treatments provided by practitioners of prophetic medicine vary based on the form and duration of treatment, the practitioner, and the financial situation of the patient. In Nigeria, where the price of most goods and services is negotiated, *malamai* commonly say that they 'show mercy' in pricing their remedies for poorer patients. That being said, it is not uncommon for treatments to cost upwards of the equivalent of US$100 a month for several months – a substantial expense for the great majority of Nigerians. In narrating his therapeutic migration from cure seeking to ART, Ali reflects on his pursuit of a cure as futile and unenlightened. He attributes the major improvements in his health to a strict adherence to his ART and other health promoting habits, such as eating properly and using a mosquito net. He criticizes in no uncertain terms those who claim they can cure HIV on the grounds that they do not explain how these alleged cures work. Like many patients now on ART, Ali's enthusiasm for ARV drugs are associated with the physical, financial, and emotional costs he suffered before he started taking them.

Dauda, an HIV-positive man in his early thirties who is employed as an ART adherence counsellor at a PEPFAR-funded HIV clinic in Kano, expressed similar frustration about those who claim they have a cure, namely because they are not forthcoming about the curative mechanism. When I asked about the difference between the hospital clinic where he worked and a nearby Islamic health centre, he said:

> Some people approve of this [prophetic] type of medicine and some don't. There are differing opinions, and the relationship [between prophetic practitioners and

> biomedical practitioners] isn't always very good. Do you see what I mean? Some [*malamai*] are just doing it to be in the market, to make money. They think that we [at the HIV clinic] are trying to encroach on their business, and they're not happy about it.

Highlighting the economic aspect of the therapeutic economy of HIV, Dauda makes the case that *malamai* working in the prophetic tradition are displeased with biomedical practitioners and their provision of ART because this competition encroaches on their business. He also posits a larger mutual distrust between biomedical and prophetic healers. Dr Inusa responded similarly to Dauda when I asked him about the relationship between prophetic and biomedical practitioners:

> There's a good relationship among those of us who practice Islamic medicine, those who practice traditional medicine. We have a mutual understanding. We even meet together to exchange views and help each other. Every medicine, if it's not Western, it gets called traditional by Westerners [he chuckles]. Westerners don't concern themselves with Islamic medicine. Every medicine that's not Western is 'traditional' to them. So because of that, we [non-biomedical practitioners] unite to help each other out.

Masu maganin gargajiya (traditional healers), the larger category with which many healers working in Islamic prophetic traditions align themselves,[10] consider themselves to be distinct and largely at odds with practitioners of *maganin Turawa* (Western biomedicine). There are several national, state, and local associations in Nigeria for herbalists, traditional doctors, and other non-biomedical practitioners. While *masu maganin gargajiya* are in some ways in competition with each other for patients, and often advertise their practices in a variety of media, they tend to view biomedicine as a much more serious source of competition. *Masu maganin gargajiya* frequently decry their lack of support by the Nigerian government, despite the fact that they are many Nigerians' first resort to care. Dr Inusa's accusation that Westerners lack respect for other healing

---

[10] However, a few prophetic healers also told me in interviews, '*Ni ba mai maganin gargajiya ba ne*' ('I am not a traditional healer'), in order to emphasize the Islamic foundations of their practices and distinguish themselves from herbalists and spiritually based healers who do not adhere as closely, or at all, to Islamic precepts. Hundreds of traditional healers not operating under the rubric of prophetic medicine also exist in Kano; they tend to be found in or near Sabon Gari, Kano's primarily Christian neighbourhood, where many southern Nigerians live and work. While some of these produce and sell herbal 'immune boosters' that are of interest to some people living with HIV, I have never heard these individuals claiming that they can cure HIV.

systems is a frequent refrain among those who work outside the biomedical system. He continued:

> There's a *hadith* that says 'Look for your medicine with Allah. God has never sent a disease for which he has not sent its medicine' It's a *hadith*. And another *hadith* says 'The one who knows the proper cure for something knows it, and the one who doesn't know it doesn't know it.' The one who doesn't know the cure, he shouldn't say it doesn't exist. Rather, he should simply say he doesn't know it. We Muslims don't agree that there's a disease that can't be cured. We don't agree. That's why at this health center we cure our patients. We've even had witnesses come visit and see that the cure is real; they've seen the [blood] test results. You see this gift. Our faith doesn't allow that there is no cure. We give medicine out in the open, and people are cured – praise be to Allah.

Dr Inusa's repeated insistence that he is able to cure HIV is based on what might be considered a literalist exegesis of Islamic texts. According to him, the *hadith* on diseases and their cures imply not only that all diseases are potentially curable, but also that they are necessarily curable now. Addressing critics who doubt the presence of a cure, he rhetorically reframes their scepticism into an agnostic suspension of judgement: How can these critics be so certain that there isn't a known cure? And if they cannot be absolutely certain, shouldn't they say that they are uncertain, rather than saying that there is no known cure? Dr Inusa's insistence that his Islamic centre provides cures for patients with HIV, whereas biomedical facilities provide only non-curative treatments, finds some rhetorical support from another passage from *Medicine of the Prophet* concerning the efficacy of prophetic medicine: 'Religious and Prophetic medicines heal certain illnesses that even the minds of great physicians cannot grasp, and which their science, experiments and analogical deductions cannot reach' (al-Jawziyya 1998: 8).

Another *malam*, who like Dr Inusa was one of the few *malamai* officially registered with the Kano State Ministry of Health's Private Health Institutions Registration Unit, advertised in a popular weekly Hausa-language newspaper, saying that at his centre: 'HIV/AIDS is completely cured [holistically]'[11] Another, advertising in the same newspaper, says perhaps more subtly that 'Every disease has its medicine ... we have medicines [*magani*] for uncontrollable diseases like high blood pressure, AIDS, ulcer, typhoid fever, and the rest.'[12] The Hausa word *magani* is typically translated into English as 'medicine,' but also carries the connotation of 'cure.' Thus, when someone professes to have *magani*

[11] In the original Hausa, '*HIV/AIDS warkewa ake gaba daya* [*holistically*]'.

[12] In the original Hausa, '*Kowace cuta tana da magani ... muna da magungunan gagararrun cututtuka kamar hawan jini, AIDS, gyambon ciki wato ulcer, zazza'bin taifod da sauransu*'.

for an illness, he is at least claiming to have medicine for it – although in Hausa, this is conceptually linked with the concept of a cure.[13]

At any rate, since concepts of 'relief' and 'cure' are often highly subjective, healers have vested interests in defining these terms in ways that are favourable to themselves (Wall 1988). When pressed on how they know whether they have succeeded in curing a patient of his or her HIV infection, some *malamai* will insist that a patient's general physical and emotional improvement evinces the cure. Those who adopt a perspective of HIV as a virus often profess that a substantially improved CD4 cell count is evidence that their treatments have worked – thus adopting the main marker of ART efficacy in Nigeria.[14] Some insist that patients they have cured of HIV subsequently test negative for HIV antibodies, but that the Nigerian government and media suppress news of such HIV-positive to HIV-negative sero-conversions.

Back at the hospital HIV clinic I mentioned to Dauda, the ARV adherence counsellor, that I had been surprised the day before when Dr Inusa told me that he had devised a cure for HIV. To this Dauda responded:

> Yes, there are people who say that they have a cure, and people drink it. Our Islamic belief is that every disease has its cure – except that we might not know it yet. Surely someone will be able to know the cure. But anyone who says they have the cure, it would be better and helpful if he comes out with it, shows it, makes a lot of it, so that we can give it to people to make them well. But if you have the cure and you keep it hidden under your bed – if you only give it to people who pay you a lot of money – hat's not help. If you have the cure, people have to know.

In other words, given the extreme suffering brought about by HIV/AIDS, if someone has truly devised a cure he or she is morally obligated to make it publically available rather than use it for his or her own profit. What is striking about this humanitarian position is that it parallels an argument several *malamai* have joined HIV treatment activists in making against Western drug companies who develop and sell ARV drugs: rather than keeping these treatments metaphorically hidden by intellectual property protections and prices that render them inaccessible to the vast majority of people with HIV, those who manufacture these the treatments have the moral responsibility to make them widely available.

---

13 An HIV-positive man in a support group whom I knew was on ART once asked me: '*Me ya sa har yanzu ba mu da maganin HIV?*' ('Why do we still not have magani for HIV?'). I interpreted him to be asking why there was still no cure for HIV – despite the fact that ART constitutes a form of medicine for the disease.

14 Since it is a much more expensive diagnostic measure than a CD4 cell count, viral load is generally only measured in Nigeria when a patient experiences a substantial drop in their CD4 count despite being on ART.

Dr Salisu, a Muslim biomedical doctor who works at an HIV clinic in Kano, offered this succinct opinion when I asked his opinion of those who profess they have a cure for HIV: 'If they want to treat HIV patients with holy water, honey, and prayer, I don't have a problem with it. But to tell patients that they are cured and should stop taking their ART completely? It's a crime.' Dr Salisu's statement might be interpreted to mean that he believes Islamic treatments offer some net spiritual benefit to HIV-positive patients, or that they at least pose no serious harm to them. He might also be conceding to the realities of practising within the pluralistic therapeutic economy of HIV in northern Nigeria. But by stating that it's criminal to tell patients to stop taking ART, he indexes his doubt about the existence of a known cure.

Such a position finds justification in another *hadith* attributed to the Prophet Muhammad: 'If anyone carries out medical treatment, yet previously he was not known as a medical man, then he takes responsibility' (al-Jawziyya 1998: 105). Al-Jawziyya points out that in this *hadith* the Prophet did not say 'whoever is a physician,' but rather 'whoever practices medicine'; this indicates that the Prophet Muhammad ascribed legitimacy to a range of practitioners, not just established 'medical men.' But, al-Jawziyya (1998: 105) continues: 'When a person carrying out treatment transgresses the limits of his knowledge and expertise and causes harm to the patient, he should be held responsible. One who lays claim to knowledge or practice which he does not have is an impostor.'

When I asked how he responds to those who remain sceptical or suspicious of ART and base the sentiment on Islamic grounds, Dr Salisu said he appeals to the proposition – found not only in Islamic teaching, but rather common to several religious systems – that everything good is God's blessing:

> I tell them that both Muslims and non-Muslims are created by God; Westerners – that is Europeans and Americans, developed societies – are created by God, just like we are. And God's mercy can come through both Muslims and non-Muslims. Just like we receive medication and treatment for other ailments apart from HIV through the Western society, just like we receive good food, better than ours, just like we import vehicles and use planes produced by Western society to go for pilgrimage. So it's a blessing from God almighty, but it's coming through his creations who have different culture and religion than ours. You can't say that Western society is not the creation of the Almighty. So, the same way, if we have a disease, whether global or restricted to our society, the treatment or the cure may eventually come through any of God's creations, or any of God's doing, whether in the Western society or here. And I used to tell them that having treatment for HIV which suppresses the virus and makes someone to live well and longer is also a mercy of God, coming through Western scientists. Ok? We learn from what you [Western] people develop and transfer that mercy of God to our people. And you

can't deny the impact of other interventions by Westerners in our health system. Would they [people critical of ART] then say that it's not the mercy of God?

Conclusion

In 2009 Nigeria's largest single Islamic organization, the Nigerian Supreme Council for Islamic Affairs (NSCIA), released a national Islamic policy on HIV/AIDS in an effort to unify the Muslim response to HIV/AIDS in Nigeria. In the policy's forward (NSCIA 2009: iv), His Eminence Muhammad Sa'ad Abubakar III, the Sultan of Sokoto and President-General of the Council, writes: 'The Policy is based on the Teachings of The Glorious Qur'an and the Traditions of the Holy Prophet (SAW)[15]' – a statement that is repeated several times throughout the 31-page document. Indeed, every page of the policy includes passages from the Qur'an.

Furthermore, the policy asserts that Muslims 'are committed to ensuring that persons infected or affected by HIV/AIDS including orphans and vulnerable children receive appropriate treatment, care and support in line with the National Guidelines for treatment of HIV and AIDS in adults and adolescents as well as the National Guidelines for paediatric HIV and AIDS treatment and care. To achieve this, access to quality healthcare and referral systems shall be encouraged with focus on ART, palliative care and establishment of support groups' (NSCIA 2009: 15). By emphasizing ART, NSCIA aligns itself with the national treatment guidelines established by the National Agency for the Control of AIDS (NACA), which itself follows UNAIDS's biomedical focus on ART as the currently accepted treatment for HIV. No mention is made in the policy of the existence of a cure for HIV, or of treating HIV/AIDS with natural substances, or of spiritual causes of HIV infection.

The policy states that Nigeria's Islamic HIV/AIDS policy 'shall be based on the injunctions of the Glorious Qur'an and Sunnah of the Prophet (SAW)' (NSCIA 2009: 6), without further stating that the Qur'an *itself* be the primary medicinal agent (as in the practices of *rukiyya* and *rubutun sha*). In its assertion of a unified Muslim position that is closely aligned with mainstream biomedical approaches to treating HIV/AIDS, the policy makes no mention of a range of common practices and perspectives on the disease among northern Nigerian Muslims who find their inspiration not from the policies of programs like UNAIDS or PEPFAR, but from classic Islamic texts.

Aside from being Islamic, what prophetic treatment practices share is a deep history not associated with ART. From the perspective of nonbelievers,

[15] 'SAW' is an abbreviation for the Arabic phrase *Sallallahi Alaihi Wasallam* (Peace be upon him), and commonly follows mention of the Prophet Mohammad in Islamic texts.

Islamic prophetic medicine may seem supernatural and unconnected to scientific reasoning. For many people in northern Nigeria, however, the curative mechanism of ART is similarly shrouded in the unknown. And while some patients found little contradiction in consulting both biomedical and prophetic care for their treatments, the practitioners themselves were much more likely to have ill will towards the other system and its practitioners. This was particularly true to the extent that it was felt the other system disrespected one's own, harmed one's business, or put patients at risk.

In research on the polio eradication initiative in northern Nigeria, Renne (2010) demonstrates that there is no monolithic Islamic view on the value, effectiveness, and safety of the polio vaccine. Rather, parents' decisions about whether or not to have their children vaccinated against polio or other childhood diseases depends on education and social class, as well as particular understandings of the Qur'an and *hadith*. Becker (2009) found similarly that Tanzanian Muslims' attitudes towards AIDS and ART are less predetermined by restrictive religious notions than they are influenced by the political process and different kinds of knowledge, reminding that Islam (like all religions) is lived in socially, politically, and culturally specific contexts. In a similar vein, I have argued that a multiplicity of perceptions and values are expressed about ART and other HIV treatments in northern Nigeria. Despite the surety of language in the *National Islamic Policy on HIV/AIDS*, there is far from any consensus among Nigerian Muslims on HIV treatments in light of Islamic beliefs about healing and treatment efficacy. Recent moves by NSCIA to emphasize ART as the singular appropriate treatment for HIV and AIDS reflect how religious organizations often align themselves with broader secular, national and international donor policies about HIV treatment.

ART remains the provenance of biomedical doctors, while practitioners working in Islamic traditions have no authority and in most instances little interest in distributing the drugs. Furthermore, many *malamai* practising prophetic medicine stake their professional reputations, not to mention their faith, on their ability to cure patients of their ills. Naturally, this logic is extended to treating HIV/AIDS. ART therefore highlights the disconnect between how nationally and internationally positioned Islamic organizations assert a unified 'Islamic perspective' on HIV/AIDS, and how many healers working in Islamic traditions in Nigeria talk about and treat the disease. Abdalla's (1997: 88) insight that 'the Hausa people in general [have] shifted back and forth from one medical system to the other in order to maximize their own interest in the continuously changing socioeconomic conditions of Hausaland' finds particular salience in the recent history of HIV/AIDS care in northern Nigeria. Given the rapidly expanded availability of ART since the mid 2000s, there has been a marked movement towards biomedical clinic-based care for cases of HIV/AIDS in those parts of northern Nigeria where international donor funding has made these therapies available. Concurrently, and following the larger socio-political reorientation towards conservative Islam, healing as a whole in northern Nigeria has shifted towards classical Islamic approaches.

As a therapeutic practice that treats but cannot completely cure, ART thus complicates popularly held assumptions about disease and medicine in northern Nigerian Muslim society. I have suggested that one's position within the recently ARV-centred therapeutic economy of HIV in northern Nigeria – and one's perceived net gain or loss in terms of social reputation, economic benefit, and health outcome – influences both how one perceives ART and how one interprets widely known Islamic scriptures on disease and healing.

References

Abdalla, I.H. 1997. *Islam, Medicine, and Practitioners in Northern Nigeria*. Lewiston, NY: Edwin Mellen Press.

al-Jawziyya, I.Q. 1998. *Medicine of the Prophet*. Translated by Penelope Johnstone. Cambridge: Islamic Texts Society.

Appadurai, A. 1996. *Modernity At Large: Cultural Dimensions of Globalization*. Minneapolis, MN: University of Minnesota Press.

Barkindo, B.M. 1993. Growing Islamism in Kano City since 1970: Causes, form and implication, in *Muslim Identity and Social Change in Sub-Saharan Africa*, edited by L. Brenner. Bloomington, IN: Indiana University Press, 91–105.

Becker, F. 2009. Competing explanations and treatment choices: Muslims, AIDS and ARVs in Tanzania, in *AIDS and Religious Practice in Africa*, edited by F. Becker and P.W. Geissler. Leiden: Brill, 155–87.

Farmer, P. 2001. *Infections and Inequalities: The Modern Plagues*. Berkeley, CA: University of California Press.

Federal Republic of Nigeria 2012. *Global AIDS Response Progress Report 2012*. [Online]. Available at: http://www.unaids.org/en/dataanalysis/monitoring countryprogress/progressreports/2012countries/ce_NG_Narrative_Report[1].pdf [accessed: 3 February 2013].

Geertz, C. 1976. Art as a cultural system. *MLN*, 91(6), 1473–99.

Good, C. 1988. Traditional healers and AIDS management, in *AIDS in Africa: The Social and Policy Impact*, edited by N. Miller and R. Rockwell. Lewiston, NY: Edwin Mellon Press, 97–113.

Gray, P. 2004. HIV and Islam: Is HIV prevalence lower among Muslims? *Social Science and Medicine*, 58(9), 1751–56.

Green, E. 1994. *AIDS and STDs in Africa: Bridging the Gap between Traditional Healing and Modern Medicine*. Boulder, CO: Westview Press.

Hasnain, M. 2005. Cultural approach to HIV/AIDS harm reduction in Muslim countries. *Harm Reduction Journal*, 2 (23), doi: 10.1186/1477-7517-2-23.
Huff, T. 2003. *The Rise of Early Modern Science: Islam, China, and the West*. Cambridge: Cambridge University Press.
Kane, O. 2003. *Muslim Modernity in Postcolonial Nigeria: A Study of the Society for the Removal of Innovation and Reinstatement of Tradition*. Leiden: Brill.
Last, M. 2004. Hausa, in *Encyclopedia of Medical Anthropology: Health and Illness in the World's Cultures*, edited by C.R. Ember and M. Ember. New York: Kluwer Academic/Plenum Publishers, 718–29.
Last, M. 2005. Religion and healing in Hausaland, in *Christianity and Social Change in Africa: Essays in Honor of J.D.Y. Peel*, edited by T. Falola. Durham, NC: Carolina Academic Press, 549–62.
Last, M. 2007. The importance of knowing about not knowing, in *On Knowing and Not Knowing in the Anthropology of Medicine*, edited by R. Littlewood. Walnut Creek, CA: Left Coast Press, 1–17.
Last, M. 2008. The search for security in Muslim northern Nigeria. *Africa*, 78(1), 41–63.
National Agency for the Control of AIDS 2011. *Fact Sheet 2011: Antiretroviral Therapy (ART) in Nigeria*. [Online]. Available at: http://naca.gov.ng/content/view/417/lang,en/#art_dec_2010 [accessed: 3 February 2013].
National Population Commission [Nigeria] 2003. *Nigeria Demographic and Health Survey*. Calverton, MD: ORC Macro.
Nguyen, V.-K. 2005. Antiretroviral globalism, bio politics, and therapeutic citizenship, in *Global Assemblages: Technology, Politics, and Ethics as Anthropological Problems*, edited by A. Ong and S.J. Collier. Malden, MA: Blackwell Publishing, 124–44.
Nigerian Supreme Council for Islamic Affairs 2009. *National Islamic Policy on HIV/AIDS*. Abuja: NSCIA.
O'Brien, S. 2001. Spirit discipline: Gender, Islam, and hierarchies of treatment in postcolonial northern Nigeria. *Interventions*, 3(2), 222–41.
O'Brien, S. 2007. La Charia contestée: démocratie, débat et diversité musulmane dans les 'états charia' du Nigeria. *Politique Africaine*, 106(June), 46–68.
Osotimehin, B. 2004. HIV/AIDS in Nigeria today. Paper to the 4th National Conference on HIV/AIDS, Abuja, Nigeria, 2–5 May 2004.
Ostien, P. 2007. *Sharia Implementation in Northern Nigeria 1999–2006: A Sourcebook*. Ibadan: Spectrum Books.
Oyebola, D.D.O. 1986. National medical policies in Nigeria, in *The Professionalisation of African Medicine*, edited by M. Last and G.L. Chavunduka. Manchester: Manchester University Press, 221–36.
Paden, J.N. 2005. *Muslim Civic Cultures and Conflict Resolution: The Challenge of Democratic Federalism in Nigeria*. Washington, DC: Brookings Institution Press.

Paden, J.N. 2008. *Faith and Politics in Nigeria: Nigeria as a Pivotal State in the Muslim World*. Washington, DC: United States Institute of Peace Press.

Renne, E.P. 2010. *The Politics of Polio in Northern Nigeria*. Bloomington, IN: Indiana University Press.

Resch, S., Wang, H., Ogungbemi M.K. and Kombe, G. 2009. *Sustainability Analysis of HIV/AIDS Services in Nigeria*. Bethesda: Health Systems 20/20 Project/Abt Associates.

Rhine, K. 2009. Support groups, marriage, and the management of ambiguity among HIV-positive women in Northern Nigeria. *Anthropological Quarterly*, 82(2), 369–400.

Schoepf, B. 1992. AIDS, sex and condoms: African healers and the reinvention of tradition in Zaire. *Medical Anthropology*, 14, 225–42.

Svensson, J. 2009. 'Muslims have instructions': HIV/AIDS, modernity, and Islamic religious education in Kisumu, Kenya, in *AIDS and Religious Practice in Africa*, edited by F. Becker and P.W. Geissler. Leiden: Brill, 189–219.

UNAIDS 2010. *Report on the Global AIDS Epidemic 2010*. Geneva: UNAIDS. [Online]. Available at: http://www.unaids.org/documents/20101123_GlobalReport_em.pdf [accessed: 3 February 2013].

United States Diplomatic Mission to Nigeria 2012. *U.S. President's Emergency Plan for AIDS Relief (PEPFAR)*. Abuja: Embassy of the United States of America. [Online]. Available at: http://nigeria.usembassy.gov/pepfar.html [accessed: 3 February 2013].

Van der Geest, S. and Hardon A. 2006. Social and cultural efficacies of medicines: Complications for antiretroviral therapy. *Journal of Ethnobiology and Ethnomedicine*, 2(48), doi: 10.1186/1746-4269-2-48.

Vaughan, M. 1991. *Curing Their Ills: Colonial Power and African Illness*. Cambridge: Polity Press.

Wall, L. 1988. *Hausa Medicine: Illness and Well-Being in a West African Culture*. Durham, NC: Duke University Press.

World Health Organization 2010. *Antiretroviral Therapy for HIV Infection in Adults and Adolescents: Recommendations for a Public Health Approach*. [Online]. Available at: http://whqlibdoc.who.int/publications/2010/9789241599764_eng.pdf [accessed: 3 February 2013].

World Health Organization 2012. *Global Health Observatory Data Repository: Health financing, health expenditure per capita*. [Online]. Available at: http://apps.who.int/ghodata/?vid=1901 [accessed. 3 February 2013].

Chapter 6
'Silent Nights, Anointing Days': Post-HIV Test Religious Experiences in Ghana[1]

Benjamin Kobina Kwansa

Introduction

The majority of the people infected with HIV that I interviewed during my fieldwork in Ghana between 2007 and 2011 recalled that they found out about their positive status when they went to a hospital with a 'normal' illness and, just like any other patient, went through the rudiments of registering in the Outpatients Department (OPD). They explained that they then went to the nurse to have their vital signs (blood pressure, temperature, weight and height) measured and then joined the (usually long) queue to see the doctor. Some of them had to see the doctor several times before their persistent condition warranted an HIV test. Others were asked to have the test at their first appointment with the doctor. Abiba,[2] a 32-year-old Muslim woman with four children, narrated:

> The doctor told me that I needed to do some more tests ... so he could find out exactly what was wrong with me. This time, he asked me to go to that room to see Mr Owusu [the counsellor in one of the hospitals]. Well, at first I didn't think anything about it ... about this disease, so I went with the help of my mother. When we got there, Mr Owusu asked my mother to wait outside because he wanted to talk to me alone. It was then that he asked whether I knew why I was asked to come to him. When I replied in the negative, he told me that they wanted to check whether I had some of the worms that have recently been around (*emmoa yi a aba yi bi*).[3] I missed a heartbeat when he said that. Why would they

---

1 An earlier version of this chapter appeared in the *African Journal of AIDS Research* (AJAR) 9/4 (2010), in a special section on religion and antiretroviral therapy. Permission to reprint – in part or in whole – from that publication was kindly granted by AJAR.

2 All the names used here are pseudonyms.

3 The literal translation of the phrase commonly used to disclose test results – èmmoa *no bi* èwò *wo mogya mu* – connotes [small] animals, but the people I interviewed usually referred to it as 'worms'. The understanding was that because of the delicate nature of issues surrounding HIV due to the levels of stigma associated with it, counsellors preferred to

> have to test me for this? I hadn't messed up. And I am also not one who will meddle in the affairs of others, for them to want to hurt me. Why would anyone think about killing me? Mr Owusu, however, spoke to me at length and advised me to be calm. He then told me that I wasn't going to die if I listened to him and did whatever he and the doctors told me to do. Maybe you won't be positive, he said. At that point, all that he was telling me was falling on deaf ears. I was just thinking about the consequences of a possible positive result. My mother would die if she heard about it ... how about my father; he didn't even want to see my face at that time. He would just kick me out of his house. I didn't have any choice, so they did the test and I was positive, as expected.

Unlike the case of Abiba who was informed about the test before it was conducted, analyses of the life stories of people who had been to Komfo Anokye Teaching Hospital (KATH) and St. Patrick's Hospital (SPH), the two ART facilities in Kumasi and Offinso, respectively, used in this study, showed that every so often the clients claimed to have been told about the test when their positive test results were about to be disclosed during post-test counselling (see below). This was usually the case for pregnant women since HIV tests are 'provider-initiated' on the maternity wards unless one opts out.

I return to this issue involving Abiba later and how she pursued spiritual therapy to ward off those who might be trying to harm her but, suffice to say here, several scholars have shown how serious illnesses in Ghana, usually those with an inexplicable diagnosis, prognosis and treatment, are attributed to the supernatural (Wyllie 1983; Awusabo-Asare and Anarfi 1997; Radstake 2000). The term 'spiritual' is used in this chapter not necessarily in the context of associating oneself with any religious order, denomination or particular doctrine, but to highlight how people make meanings out of and act on their relationships with the supernatural. Although religion can provide a strong base for a person's spirituality, being spiritual in this context does not necessarily mean one is religious. In other words, a person could believe that supernatural powers underline a particular situation and may use supernatural means to understand, tap and even alter the situation. This person may, however, not subscribe to a particular set of beliefs and practices, as pertaining to a specific religious doctrine, denomination or order. One's spirituality can therefore affect one's decisions in life, such as health-seeking behaviour, when and how they plant their fields, and whether or not they participate in risky but potentially beneficial social action (Ver Beek 2000; Dei 2002). Spiritual therapy is thus used here to show how people living with HIV and their families and close associates make meanings

---

use the much softer 'worms in the blood', which is oftentimes ambiguous and arouses less shock than when the word HIV is used. In this chapter, I use 'worms' instead of the literal translation of '[small] animals'.

out of and subscribe to magico-religious concepts, acts and symbolism in their bid to find relief and/or a solution to their specific (health) predicament.

Animals feature prominently in the customs, religions and folklore of human societies worldwide, being held in high esteem in some societies as untouchable gods or spirits and totems, and in others as evil, deadly and despicable creatures with magical, almost supernatural attributes (Attuquayefio 2004). Attuquayefio notes how it is thought in Ghana that animals (especially snakes) can be 'sent' as agents of the devil to bite the enemies of people who might have been offended by the actions of such people. Witches are especially likely to use animals and insects, such as snakes, spiders, owls and other birds as agents. In such cases, the victim may then have a serious illness with abnormal symptoms and one that is difficult to cure and will lead to his/her death. As Abiba's case highlights, 'having worms that can only be detected by a blood test', which is unusual for a 'normal' worm, makes a case for ascription of the cause to the supernatural. Like many of the people with HIV that I interacted with, she spent 'silent nights' of soul-searching to find the causative possibilities – 'I haven't messed up. And I am also not one who will meddle in the affairs of others, for them to want to hurt me. Why would anyone think about killing me?' A number of HIV-positive persons have searched for spiritual therapy ('anointing days' with mainly prophet-healing Pentecostal and charismatic churches) after such soul-searching.

Spiritual therapy is significant in HIV discourses in Ghana because of the problem of stigma and its effect on health-seeking behaviour and access to healthcare facilities. The objective of the scale-up of Voluntary Counselling and Testing (VCT) and ART services supported under the WHO's '3 by 5' treatment initiative was partly to address this problem. This was based on the assumption that, as more people got tested and knew their status, the probability of understanding the conditions of people living with HIV (PLHIV) becomes higher, thereby decreasing stigma towards affected people. This notwithstanding, the level of HIV stigma continues to be high in Ghana (Kwansa 2013; Radstake 2000; Awusabo-Asare 1995). People infected with HIV thus adopt strategies to keep their status secret (Kwansa 2013). Accessing counselling, testing and treatment poses an even greater challenge for many. As Kwansa (2010) shows, spiritual therapy is a pragmatic way of avoiding stigma which is surrounding HIV, and still allowing patients to access medical help.

This chapter describes the experiences that people infected with HIV have with counselling and testing. Significantly, it shows how ambiguities, such as using the 'worm' metaphor as a way of disclosing test results, leads clients to use spiritual therapy to establish meaning and cope with their predicament while preventing future consequences. The worm metaphor may not in itself have led people to spiritual therapy, but it is the ambiguities in its usage – whether it is a 'normal' (for example intestinal parasite) or an 'abnormal worm' (for example witchcraft) or a combination of the two that necessitated and ensured its pursuance even after spiritual therapy. It also shows that having access to antiretroviral treatment, which suppresses the human immunodeficiency virus as far as possible, does not exclude a search for spiritual therapy. Significantly, this chapter highlights the infected people's compromises, reorientation and conversion, and the cost to not only their social lives but also financially too, as they pursue spiritual therapy.

Methods and Setting

The project that this chapter is based on was conducted in communities served by the KATH in Kumasi and SPH in Maase Offinso respectively. Kumasi, Ghana's second-largest city, has a long and proud history as the centre of the Ashanti Kingdom and is the capital of the Ashanti Region. Officially, Kumasi has a population of around 700,000 but most estimates put it at just over a million. Maase Offinso is quite a small town where SPH serves a community of about 100,000 and others in its 60 km or so catchment area. I explored the hospital clients' points of view regarding VCT and ART, and the way these services were offered through medical channels. Uncovering social and cultural perceptions about HIV-related blame, shame and stigma were central in the research. The project combined qualitative and quantitative methods, taking a multidisciplinary approach with a multi-stakeholder perspective to compare and contrast the interests and views of the different actors in the management of HIV and AIDS. The study examined the issue of VCT and ART uptake from two other perspectives: (i) health professionals who offer VCT and ART (Dapaah 2012); and (ii) district, national and international policy makers. Data was collected from August 2007 to July 2008, November 2009 to January 2010 and from June to August 2011. As a project researcher, I conducted ethnographic fieldwork using a combination of observations, in-depth interviews, focus-group discussions and case studies to elicit data from 49 clients from the two health institutions being studied. Living among these HIV-positive people and their close relatives and friends, I spent time listening, asking questions and observing their everyday lives. I also worked with them when the situation allowed, such as in stone quarries and at selling points. I attended church services with them too, and accompanied them on errands for 'spiritual breakthrough' as well as to social gatherings, such as funerals. I found that how HIV test results are disclosed to people contributes significantly to the individuals' pursuit and use of spiritual therapies.

Counselling and Testing in Ghana

As in most countries, VCT is the main entry point for accessing ART services in Ghana. HIV counselling and testing began with a pilot study in June 2003 at Agomenya and Atua government hospitals in the Eastern Region. Other sites followed in December 2003 and February 2004 in the two tertiary teaching hospitals in Ghana: Korle-bu in Accra and KATH in Kumasi. As of 2009, there were 3,222 sites offering VCT services to the country's population of over 20 million people. About 200,000 people in the Ashanti Region have undergone VCT at approximately 466 sites that offer these services since February 2004 (NACP/GHS 2010). From my observations, the majority of those who went for counselling and testing at the two hospitals seemed to be general patients at the hospitals because these services were mainly initiated by the doctors there. The majority of the testing done at the hospitals was not voluntary. The clients, mainly locals from the communities served by the hospitals, were between 18 and 50 years of age and belonged to the middle to lowest wealth quartiles. There were twice as many women as men receiving counselling. Although counselling is a relatively new concept and has only been around in the healthcare system in Ghana for about two decades, all the clients at the facility were expected to go through a standard procedure, namely pre-test counselling, the test itself and then post-test counselling.

Pre-test Counselling

Pre-test counselling helps the client to decide whether s/he wants to have the HIV antibody test. Those who had used the service explained that the counsellor probed why the client had decided to come for counselling, exploring his/her personal history of marriage, sexual behaviour, general health problems, and their knowledge of HIV/AIDS. Some members of the focus-group discussion indicated that the counsellor explained the test procedure and how one could interpret the results. The counsellors then talked about the positive or negative results of the test and how to stay as healthy as possible for as long as possible. Although pre-test counselling is aimed at allowing the client to make an informed decision as to whether to take the test or not, most of the respondents who went through pre-test counselling said they felt the counsellors did not present them with any options. Melissa a 25-year-old banker and a member of the focus group explained:

> as if their only focus is to get you to test, your feelings and emotions come second. They make it seem like you don't have an option. You definitely have to do the test, otherwise they [the counsellors] may think that you are bad.

Oppong (a systems analyst in his early thirties and a member of the group) said:

> The counsellors focus too much on the effects of a positive result and that will definitely make you shake. I was asked what impact I thought a positive or indeterminate result would have on my life and how I was going to react to that. I had not given all these [points] the slightest thought, so my heart started beating fast. If fright could cause one to be infected, I knew I was already positive!
>
> They even asked me whom I would disclose the information to if I got a positive result, and that really sunk me. I couldn't tell anybody. I knew I was not positive that's why I went in for the test. Do you think if I had the least suspicion of not being negative I would go in for the test?

Most of the infected people who took the text voluntarily did not remember exactly what they were told during their pre-test counselling. They cited reactions such as fright, shock and thoughts of the effects of a possible positive result as preoccupying their minds when they realized that they were going to have an HIV test. These cases of the HIV-positive persons and of the young professionals could be interpreted to mean that those who had pre-test counselling did not find the service to be very useful. However, 26-year-old Kojo, who was a member of the focus-group discussion, insisted that counselling before testing was necessary and that he had learnt 'so much' from the counsellor.

> I learnt that a negative result does not necessarily mean that you don't have any HIV antibodies as it should be confirmed some months later [if you had engaged in a risky venture]. Neither does a positive result show that you are positive since you may need another test to confirm it. In addition, though I knew medicines were available for a positive result, I didn't know much about it – where to get them, how long you would have to take it, whether there were different types, and even the problems associated with taking the medicines, [among others].

Though some of those infected also said that they thought the pre-test counselling was useful, they had difficulty enumerating the benefits they had derived from it.

The Test

For those who took the test voluntarily and those who were tested on the initiative of their health institution, a sample of their blood was drawn for the test. Since HIV testing became available in Ghana, most of the facilities have used the ELISA HIV antibody test, which was used on some of the respondents who used the ART facility in KATH. From their narratives, it appears that two main problems were associated with this service. Firstly, due to the lengthy period of waiting for the test result, many people refused to collect their results, especially in cases where they suspected that they were being asked to do a HIV test. Maakua, a 40-year-old woman who had lost her husband and the younger of her two daughters to AIDS, recalled that after her husband died she was also asked to go for a test by his family because they got to know about it before his death.

> I worked with my husband in another town. His family was very rich and we [she and her husband] received substantial support from them. When my husband became very ill some few years ago, his uncle took him to several places for medical help until they finally got to 'Gee' [Komfo Anokye] where he was diagnosed as being HIV-positive.
>
> Probably because he thought no amount of money and/or medicines would help cure his nephew, the uncle immediately stopped all payments for his treatment and so he was subsequently discharged and came home to die. As if this was not enough, he summoned all the family and announced my husband's plight. They subsequently took me back to 'Gee' to check my status so they could help me if I was also positive. I refused to go in for the results, though it made no difference because the entire community had already heard the news. My husband's family then threw my children and me out of their house and subjected us to public humiliation and disgrace. It became worse when my second daughter died some months later also after a persistent illness. My first daughter also followed with the same persistent illness and soon it was my turn. That was when I went back for the test and found out I had this thing and started treatment with my daughter.

People who take the test and have to wait for days for the results, as in the case with ELISA, can have a change of heart about it. On the other hand however, it presented people like Oppong [a member of the FGD] and Maakua, who felt coerced into taking the test, with a second chance to decide about whether they wanted the test result or not. Indeed, some respondents who did not go for their test results, started considering spiritual therapy in the hope that their results would be negative. HIV tests that do not give an on the spot result, run into problems globally. The Centre for Disease Control in the US, for instance, reported that out of the approximately 2.1 million HIV tests that are conducted annually in publicly funded counselling, testing, and referral (CTR) programmes, in 2000 30 per cent of persons who tested positive and 39 per cent of persons who tested HIV negative did not return to pick up their test results (CDC 2000). At the time of writing, there are no statistics available for retention rates for counselling sessions for ELISA testing, although the problem has been dealt with by using the rapid test.

Hardon et al. (2011) show how African AIDS programmes, especially those in East Africa, have changed dramatically from being client-initiated counselling and testing (as found in VCT) to being provider-initiated testing and counselling

(PITC). In the latter case where less emphasis is put on counselling, health providers recommend and test clients unless the patient declines this service (WHO/UNAIDS 2007). In our research settings in Ghana, the rapid HIV test was used in most of the hospitals, private clinics, private laboratories and during sensitization campaigns due to the obvious advantages it has regarding the period of waiting for test results. It tended to limit however, the extent of client involvement in the decision about whether to test or not, since the whole process could be done within 20 minutes, by which time the client might have had to make a life-long decision, especially in the case of diagnostic testing. Those who wanted to know their status themselves without being referred by a doctor, used private facilities. As my observations showed, in some of the private laboratories in the Ashanti Region, it seemed that counselling (both pre- and post-test) was rarely offered. One technician in a private laboratory explained that there were two main groups that access the HIV testing service in their laboratory. He explained:

> The first are the cases referred from the hospital [that do not have a counselling and testing session]. For this group we [the technicians] prefer to assume that they already know about the test that is being conducted. If they don't know, then we are not responsible for breaking the news. The majority of the cases are clients who initiate the test themselves [either because of their own perception of personal risk, a demand by a church as a pre-requisite for marriage, for a work-related reason such as joining the military, or to travel outside of the country – to the US or China (until recently) for example]. In these cases too, clients know what they are coming in for and therefore do not need counselling.

Generally, although the private laboratories were found not to have the right staff to offer counselling services, many people preferred these instead of the hospitals. This was because 'they were fast', 'there are no queues', 'they do what you ask them to do, and not what they think you should do or what they want you to do', and, importantly, 'they do not condemn you', according to informants.

Post-Test Counselling

Post-test counselling was, according to the HIV-positive persons I interviewed, an occasion when the client was again made to express his/her feelings about the possible result and any expected reaction. After the test results came out, the counsellor made them available to the clients. Those who went in voluntarily could see the outcome by just looking at the kit because they were shown how to interpret the results of the rapid test. However, clients who had a diagnostic test and who did not know that the test was being conducted, were taken through some of the issues that should have been discussed at the pre-test counselling stage, before the results were delivered. Esther, who is an unmarried trader in her late twenties, explained that although she did not know that an HIV test had been conducted, when the counsellor started talking about managing physical and mental issues, better social relations and safe-sex practices, she feared the worse. It was still a surprise though, when she was finally told that 'you have some of the worms in your blood' (èmmoa *no bi* èwò *wo mogya mu*).

When the client is informed about the result of the test, whether it is negative or positive, the various options available to the client are discussed. Counselling in the case of negative results was found to be used to educate clients (again) on HIV prevention, and those with problematic high-risk behaviour are referred to specialized organizations, such as the Planned Parenthood Association of Ghana (PPAG), for 'treatment'. For clients with a positive result, the counselling session was used to educate them on issues including partner notification and for referral for medical and psychosocial support and care. The facilities were expected to offer follow-up services to clients to enable them utilize existing care and support services, including access to ART and home-based care services.

For those who test positive, the post-test counselling is a time for soul-searching and to decide on one's next course of action. Mama Panyin, a 44-year-old divorcee who sells processed food, expressed her feelings after the test:

> For me, after the results were announced, I didn't remember anything that the counsellor said again. I started feeling dizzy. I was confused. I knew that was it ... I am done.

Some of the clients had issues with how their positive results were explained to them during post-test counselling. In almost all the cases investigated, the PLHIV said they were told that 'worms or small animals were in the blood/system' (èmmoa èwò *me mogya mu* or èmmoa èwò *me mu*), as was the case with Esther and Abiba. This was probably the best way for counsellors to communicate the situation to the person infected, as HIV/AIDS has no specific name in the local language. The logic is that the virus is a small animal that gets into the blood and then works its way out. In everyday conversations, other terms such as an 'extreme form of gonorrhoea' (*babaso nwènfo*), 'that sickness' (*saa yareè no*) and 'a sickness whose name cannot be mentioned' (*yareè a yènbò din*) were used to identify the virus.

It was probably because these phrases aroused negative sentiments, especially for people who were unwell, that they were not used during post-test counselling. The counsellors thus preferred the much softer 'worms', which is more ambiguous and arouses less shock by way of reaction to the news. Others, however, explained that such ambiguities as to whether it is 'this worm or that worm' lingered on in their minds, and so they did not take on board all that was said during the post-test counselling. Some persons teased fellow patients for buying medicines literally to de-worm after they were given their results. It was only when they were referred to the ART clinic for care and support that they realized the magnitude of these 'worms'. It is this ambiguity that offers the client the leeway to access other forms of therapy, other than that provided at hospitals. This is because even before some clients had found out about their 'worms', they had moved between self-therapy, folk medicine, biomedicine and spiritual therapy in an attempt to remedy their worsening health. However, the majority of the people in the study considered spiritual therapy only after they had received their test results. Although they had resorted to spiritual therapy for various reasons before, this time – after their soul-searching – it was mainly because they associated their ailment with the supernatural.

Disease Aetiology and the Search by PLHIVs for Spiritual Therapy

It is not unusual in Ghana to attribute spiritual causation to serious disorders like HIV and AIDS (Wyllie 1983). Awusabo-Asare and Anarfi (1997) found that PLHIV who visited traditional healers did so because they related their infection to spiritual causes, mainly witchcraft and curses. The worm analogy, therefore, fitted the link to the spiritual. As is evident in Abiba's case and is reminiscent of the majority of cases investigated, the subtlety of the worm in disclosure gives clients a reason to link their ailment to the supernatural, usually witchcraft. The majority, unsurprisingly, claimed that they were victims and had not been infected through casual sex or promiscuity, which were the dominant perceptions of being the causes of HIV infection in the communities studied. To buttress their point, these HIV-positive individuals cited malevolent people and powers as the main means of becoming infected (cf. Radstake 2000). Some of the expressions the PLHIV I met used were: *yè tò maame* (it was bought for me); *èyè dua bò'* (it's a curse) and *omo ayème* (they've messed me up). Kaakyere, who was in his mid thirties, recounted that *aboa bèka woa èfiri wontuma mu* (an insect that will bite you will definitely come from your own clothes):

> My family members are bad. Can you believe I am the only surviving male in my entire [extended] family? Look! Look at what they are doing to me [pointing to himself regrettably]! I married quite early because I didn't want to play around. Now look! I'm not any different from those who played around. They think they've gotten me now. But *Insha Allah* [God permitting], it won't happen. You see ... I'm regaining my strength again.

It is interesting how the metaphors of the insect and the worms used during counselling relate to something that has more than a physical cause. Although, the insect Kaakyere refers to is more about the closeness of the person causing the harm, the effects of HIV infection, which included physical pain leading to exhausted, weak, thin and atrophic bodies, made room for the spiritual linkage. Such seemingly inexplicable conditions only fit the supernatural in view of the fact that 'it is beyond human comprehension'. Other informants in the study linked the effects to curses from deities for unfulfilled vows or to rivals casting spells. Many people cited cases of witchcraft. Thus, no matter the weight of biomedical proof of the virus, many of the PLHIV thought that their predicament had an aspect of spiritual causation. Egya (a 65-year-old informant and a former director at the university who was managing his infection together with diabetes and high blood pressure) said: 'Nothing happens in a vacuum, there must be a reason for it happening to me at this particular point in time ... why me at this time?'. During my research, however, a few people with HIV gave reasons ruling out the supernatural by citing their previous high-risk sexual encounters, accidents during surgery at the hospital, and spousal infidelity. Interviewing counsellors and other healthcare professionals fell outside the purview of this aspect of the project[4] and so it was not clear why counsellors continued to use the worm metaphor when it was obvious that it aroused linkages with the supernatural. Informal conversations with a counsellor (who works outside the study areas) showed that if there was a choice between mentioning HIV and AIDS during post-test counselling and having clients make a scene due to fear, guilt and shame and using the worms and causing ambiguities that may still have them pursue antiretroviral therapy (and spiritual therapy too), the latter was more morally acceptable. It therefore became a win-win situation, where counsellors did not have to feel uncomfortable in presenting the results, and the clients also did not feel shame and guilt as a result of infection.

Some people who correctly noted that there is no known cure for HIV also asserted that they believed it is a spiritual illness, and thus a reason for seeking spiritual therapy. Explanations given by some PLHIV were: 'It is no ordinary illness'; 'Even the white man has not been able to find a solution'; and 'It is a prophecy that has come to pass, so there is nothing that can be done about it'. In the latter case, 31-year-old Kay, who claimed to have turned to Christ a year after being put on ART, claimed that:

> God told the Israelites if you diligently heed to the voice of the Lord, your God, and do what is right in His sight ... then He will put none of the diseases on you, which He has brought on the Egyptians who are constantly doing abominable things. It is only He [God] who will bring a cure when He has forgiven them their sins.

[4] The perspective of nurses, counsellors and doctors can also be found in Dapaah (2012) although he does not show why counsellors mention 'worms' and 'small animals' in post-test counselling.

In relation to this, some leaders of Pentecostal and charismatic churches[5] and traditional healers claimed to have a cure for HIV. Such pronouncements have been common in Ghana, with the most famous being that of the late Nana Kofi Drobo, who gained international prominence after publicly claiming to have the cure for HIV.[6] In the narratives of PLHIV, it was not uncommon to hear about a healer being 'very powerful'. These were largely healers who claimed to have already healed people or who could heal those with HIV. Similar claims have been heard in other countries. In Uganda, for instance, health workers have expressed concern over the growing number of HIV-positive teenagers who abandon their HIV treatment after turning to spiritual therapy, mainly in Pentecostal churches.[7] Thus, the biomedical option that allows people living with the virus appealed less than the belief that a person can be healed and restored to their prior state of health through spiritual therapy.

The alternative offered by spiritual therapy – that HIV infection, the 'worms' or AIDS illness is curable – seemed in tune with many of the informants' personal realities. As traditional healers are usually familiar with their clients' cultural traditions, fears and wishes, some utilize such knowledge in their curative practices, sometimes as a form of psychotherapy with strong elements of suggestion in their healing practices (Twumasi 1972; Kayombo et al. 2005). In addition, procedures surrounding spiritual therapy, which can involve divination, sorcery or clairvoyance, are used to diagnose, treat or cure, and further protect against some sicknesses. This gives meaning to the complaint of illness and hence the remedy given is embraced dutifully because of the faith

---

5 Though several works have focused on HIV and AIDS and issues of stigmatization, religion and spiritual therapy in Ghana, specifically healing campaigns by Pentecostal and charismatic churches (PCC), very few have detailed the spiritual lives of PLHIV; see Wyllie (1983), Gifford (1994, 2004), Meyer (1998), van Dijk (1997, 1999), Radstake (2000), Takyi (2003) and Asamoah-Gyadu (2004, 2005). These Pentecostal charismatic and revival missions may be referred to as spiritual churches in generic terms and although they have different backgrounds and characteristics, they all claim healing as a main objective in spreading the good news of Christ.

6 The story appeared in the *People's Daily Graphic*, 26 August 1992. Cited in Crentsil (2007: 150).

7 An online report at http://allafrica.com/stories/201010140054. html claims that in Uganda: 'Over the years, growing trends of adolescents and caregivers have withdrawn from treatment with a belief of having been cured of HIV/AIDS in church', according to the comment of a counsellor coordinator at Baylor College of Medicine Children's Foundation. The report cites 'a 2007 study by Makerere University's Infectious Disease Institute ... found that 1.2 per cent of 558 respondents undergoing HIV treatment discontinued therapy because they believed they had been spiritually healed. A total of four out of six restarted therapy, but three required much more expensive second-line salvage therapy.'

that the client finds in the system (cf. Crentsil 2005). An informant named Frank attested to the fact that:

> If the healer is able to tell me so much of my secrets and draw connections from situations I hadn't even imagined, why wouldn't I believe him if he says my colleague bought this sickness for me in order to take my position? I believe it, and the signs are there for all to see ... However, the prognosis by biomedicine cannot tell exactly how I got infected, what happened, the exact time the infection came, who brought it ... and they give medicines that cannot even cure but only manage it.

Frank attended a Pentecostal church about 20 km from his home but did not belong to any religious denomination. It was his search for a cure for HIV that led him to follow a fellow sufferer to the church.

Significantly, many of the clients I met viewed spiritual therapy as a survival and coping strategy. They did not feel socially accepted and were blamed for their predicament. They thus resorted to the Supreme Being since, according to some of them, he is 'the helper of the helpless', 'only He understands man's innermost secrets' and *òno na obedi m'asem ama me* [he can vindicate me]. An undying hope that there may be a cure for HIV one day made them hold on to such beliefs. More than this, the hope that they may save their souls from eternal damnation, even if they cannot enjoy the last days of their earthly lives because of the disease, was enough motivation for them to seek spiritual therapy (cf. Dilger 2007).

What the informants thought was the origin of their situation correlated with their health-seeking behaviours (Janzen 1978; Kleinman 1980; Awusabo-Asare and Anarfi 1997). My examination of some of the people's life stories showed that their initial state after knowing about the 'worms in the blood' was frequently one of re-examination. They spent countless 'silent nights' in soul-searching and considering options to overcome such a worrying condition. This led some to think that they were suffering from *èfiè yareè* (illness from home), *sumsum yareè* (spiritual illnesses) or *duabó* (a curse), which demanded a different type of diagnosis and healing, and thus 'was not meant [only] for the hospital'. A number went on various expeditions (which Abiba referred to as 'anointing sessions') to heal and cure them. Spiritual therapy was thus very common among the majority of the PLHIV I met during my research in the area, although its magnitude and intensity were largely related to what they believed was the possible source of their HIV infection. Those who were convinced that the cause of their HIV infection was not physical were more likely to devote time and resources to finding a form of spiritual therapy, mainly Christian and/or traditional and/or Islamic.

The Search for Spiritual Therapy

Plummer et al. (2006) noted in a study in Tanzania how many people consulted both traditional and medical facilities when faced with HIV infection or AIDS. The main motivation was that traditional healers were accessible, affordable and culturally acceptable (Kayombo et al. 2005). Wyllie (1983) described how among spirit-guided healers in Winneba, a coastal town in Ghana, most claimed their diagnostic and remedial actions were informed and guided by spirit entities, with whom they stood in a special relationship as a medium or earthly representative. These traditional healers typically claim that Western scientific medicine may be effective in dealing with naturally caused illnesses but that only traditional healers' 'special, spiritually informed knowledge and expertise' can help in the treatment of illnesses caused by spiritual agents. It is this knowledge and expertise that leads them to diagnose PLHIV concerns (such as worms that can only be detected in a blood test) and give prescriptions that are in tune with the belief and realities of clients. The belief that antiretroviral medicines may be effective in dealing with the naturally caused aspects of the predicament but that only spiritual therapy can deal with the spiritual causes explains why many continued using spiritual therapy after being enrolling on ART.

A variety of medical practices occur within the medical set-up in Ghana. These include the activities of herbalists, bonesetters, traditional midwives, Muslim scholars like *mallams* and *marabouts*, possession priests (like *trònua* among the Ewe, *akomfo* among the Akan), *Tigare* and *Mami Wata* shrines, and a variety of Christian healers and prophets. However, the different methods are not neutral vis-à-vis one another (Krause 2006). In the Ashanti cosmology, there are no fewer than 18 powerful gods who regulate the daily activities of people although some are more powerful than others. However, gods from Cote d'Ivoire, especially the river god *Bobo*, who was often mentioned, are particularly feared for their punishments (Ashitey 1988; Agadzi 1989; Anarfi 1995; Decosas et al.1995; Radstake 2000). People curse and are cursed for using these gods. Others appeal to these gods because of personal issues, such as financial problems, a visa to travel, needing intelligence in education, protection against evil spirits, the undoing of a spell or for healing. Adherents cut across all spheres of life, regardless of wealth, education or religion. The PLHIV I interviewed mentioned that they appeal to this range of traditional healers for help when they feel at a loss for other options. This includes even those who were previously not adherents. Pentecostal and charismatic churches were also consulted. They claim to heal sufferings that are not easily cured by biomedicine, including mental disorders, infertility, impotence, epilepsy, witchery, and life-threatening health problems such as cancer, strokes and HIV/AIDS. Not all churches boast this divine gift of being able to ward off and exorcize the dangerous powers that cause these ailments but it is very common among the

PCCs, which thus increases the numbers of people who throng to their premises for spiritual help (Gifford 1994; de Witte 2003; Meyer 2004). The informants seldom mentioned Islamic healing practices, though the activities of *mallams*[8] had some prominence. Apart from their ability to heal spiritually, those who visited *mallams* explained that the latter had a special gift of giving charms and amulets to clients to ward off evil spirits based on Quranic verses. This appealed to them because, as Ahoofe puts it, 'those who got me infected would stop at nothing to finish me; so as I seek treatment, it is better for me to protect myself from future harm'. Ahoofe, who is in her late twenties, travelled about 40 km to the ART centre every month and frequented the services of a *mallam*, also far from her home in the Ashanti Region.

The usual pattern followed was to confer on various options (traditional healers, spiritual churches, *mallam*) until the PLHIV arrived at one or more that they hoped would ensure improvement in their health. Feierman (1981) shows how in north-eastern Tanzania, people try different therapeutic options to establish and advance the process of diagnosing an illness by treating it to see whether the condition improves. If it improves, the person continues therapy or moves on to other alternatives. Most of those who I met in my study had followed (or were following) several regimes, although they were also on ART. They were quite pragmatic in their choices, and remained with an option as long as their needs were being met. Using a particular option did not necessarily correlate with the profession of faith or belief. When they found one that met their needs better, they moved on. Due to the numerous options in terms of spiritual therapy, many people negotiated between the various systems. However, these negotiations frequently resulted in the PLHIV compromising some strict religious doctrine or practice, and at times led them to join new ones. Accordingly, there is often a crossing of religious and denominational boundaries in people's search for therapy.

HIV infection and the search for a cure made those infected take decisions that would otherwise have been considered contradictory. Often, adherents to a particular option are not free to join or combine it with others because of the strong adverse relationship between them, sometimes resulting in tensions and animosity. For instance, Pentecostal churches may strongly discourage traditional healers and shrines (as well as the *mallam*). What is interesting here is how infected people negotiate these tensions between (temporary) commitments to a certain faith and ideological prescriptions of a specific denomination as they take steps that they deem to be pragmatic in finding solutions to their predicament (see Kwansa 2010).

---

8 *Mallam* is usually a term for Islamic scholars but is commonly used to refer to adherents who practise folk medicine in Ghana.

The people in my study devoted a lot of time to prayer for the forgiveness of sins and commitment of themselves into God's care. Observations at the two ART facilities and at meetings of the various associations of PLHIV showed that a great deal of time was spent singing songs of 'praise and worship' and 'sharing of the Word' before the day's main agenda commenced. Although these services were Christian in nature and not all the members at the clinics and in the associations were Christians, there were no complaints. All the members spoke fondly of these words of encouragement that they hear monthly. Abiba, who belongs to the Hope for the Best Association, said she takes great delight in listening to the words of advice and encouragement. Though a Muslim, she travelled from another region where she lived to attend the meeting. She indicated that the words of encouragement are 'very helpful and keeps [her] going through the month', and that makes her long for meeting days. In another case, Mama Sofo, a women's leader in a Protestant church, not only secretly enrolled at an ART facility far from her village but also went to 'a very powerful pastor' to be prayed for.

At the stage of compromise, many of the people I met tended to combine their previously held faith with that of the newer one. Even though they might have been very lax in the past, they could still seem to be compromising. Some people appeared to justify their new faith by being very committed to its activities. For them, and as Abiba mentioned above, 'A little from here and a little from there will keep us going'.

In the course of the study, however, I observed that some people had a total religious reorientation and converted wholly to a new faith. In their quest for spiritual therapy, some lost their previously held faith either because the new one addressed their needs better or because the old and the new did not go together. In cases of the former, a place that a client initially intended to visit only for prayers later became their main place of worship when s/he envisaged a better chance of healing in the new place:

Others were found to have manoeuvred between religions, especially in cases where the old faith and the new one could not coexist. For example, Kaakyere, a staunch Pentecostal, went to a traditional shrine for help when alternatives seemed to have failed. He explained that once he became thin and emaciated, his pitiable sight had led his relatives to convince him to seek help from the shrine. He was given a ring as a sign of the covenant between himself and the god of the shrine. The relationship would be abrogated once Kaakyere returned the favour by going back to the shrine to thank the god for help after he felt better. He was not told to pay a specified sum but instead he promised to send some money, drinks and two fowls. Even though he was initially sceptical and unwilling to go, he noticed some drastic improvement after he made the visit. He later found out his HIV-positive status when he went to the ART centre and has been on ARVs ever since. Four years later, he was still unable to go to church.

The various advantages that adherents claimed for the need to limit the destructive functions of the 'worms in the blood' notwithstanding, religion was another context in which PLHIV were stigmatized when their HIV status became suspect (Takyi 2003; Crentsil 2007). Since 2005, the Ghana AIDS Commission (GAC), which regulates all activities on HIV/AIDS in the country, has been collaborating with the major religious bodies (the Christian Council of Ghana and the Council of Pentecostal and Charismatic Churches) to fight stigma and discrimination of PLHIV. Some churches had departments and agencies responsible for lending care and support. Popular advertisements on this collaboration were aired on television and shown on billboards, with some portraying the leadership of the Christian Council of Ghana, the chief imam and the leaders of other Muslim groupings embracing people identified as PLHIV. They conveyed messages such as 'Don't fight the people, fight AIDS'; 'Who are you to judge?'; 'Jesus didn't judge, why should you?'; 'Judging is not Christ-like' and 'Reach out, show compassion to PLHIV'. Yet in reality, these groups also contributed to the discrimination of PLHIV (Kwansa 2010).

In addition, it was common for some of these healers, mainly Pentecostal pastors, to set up camps for their clients.[9] Some HIV-positive persons spoke to me about their experiences in these prayer camps where there were very poor housing, sanitation and dietary conditions. Visits to camps in the study area confirmed that clients were made to undergo several days of fasting and prayer. Consequently, some people stopped taking their ARVs, while others took their pills without food. On one occasion, after I made several futile visits to 22-year-old Ewurama's house, I found her in a prayer camp, visibly dehydrated, starving and unkempt. She died after six months at the camp. The ramifications have been that people very often return to an ART facility in worse shape than before attending a prayer camp. At the camps, clients are denied rest and quiet because the causative agent (disease demons) must be allowed no peace. The demons are at times 'smoked out' by smells and fumigation. And if the evil spirits are strong enough to endure these hardships, they must be lured elsewhere, such as to take up abode in an inanimate object (Twumasi 1972). In some cases, PLHIV were severely lashed with canes in a bid to drive out demons from people's bodies. Others were made to carry heavy goods on their heads and run for a certain distance, in the belief that the evil spirits would be 'let loose' during the course of the run. Clearly, these and many more practices would compound the infected person's health problems. The search for spiritual therapy therefore did not necessarily guarantee better health conditions. Indeed, the majority of the infected people had spent their savings on transport, charms, amulets and concoctions used in healing rituals in an attempt to find healing and a cure.

---

9 See also Van Dijk (1997).

ART brings financial burdens too. The anti-retrovirals cost GHS 5 per month and are not covered by the national insurance scheme. Additional costs are involved too, including transport, other hospital expenditures and medicines (such as folders, hospital cards, laboratory tests, anti-retrovirals and other medicines prescribed), and food for their demanding appetite as a result of the antiretroviral medicines (Kwansa 2013). However, the costs of spiritual therapy are found to be often more expensive than those of ART.

Conclusion

While counselling in the overall healthcare system in Ghana is relatively new, it is no different from what pertains in other African countries (Ego and Moran 1993; Lamptey and Coates 1994). However, counselling in most parts of Sub-Saharan Africa has generally been in the form of advice from 'experts' to patients and their relatives (Awusabo-Asare 1995). This advice is to a large extent taken as a given. And so, when counsellors inform clients that they have 'worms in the blood', some people decide to take this literally and look elsewhere than the hospital to treat this extraordinary condition. The nights of contemplation and days of expedition often lead them to the services of *dunsifoò*, *asòfoò*, *akòmfoò* and *mallams*.

People who are HIV-positive search for spiritual therapy but this does not necessarily begin after discovering their HIV status, although, as this chapter has shown, a belief in the spiritual causation of HIV infection, coupled with a need to heal holistically, has led most of the PLHIV studied to some form of spiritual therapy. This has mainly been pursued not just to find a cure, but also to locate the real cause of the infection and avert future (or further) attacks. It is this aspect of spiritual therapy that the PLHIV described as 'holistic' since it addressed many of their lingering questions such as 'why me', 'why this time' and 'who caused it' in the pursuit of healing the body of physical illness and the soul of spiritual sickness.

Significantly, the case material suggests that the use of spiritual therapy to manage HIV infection may not be very different from how it is used to manage other afflictions deemed to have a spiritual cause. However, pertinent to cases of HIV where levels of stigma are very high, spiritual therapy seems to be one of the limited options available to HIV-positive persons. In this sense, spiritual therapy offers an opportunity to escape the social blaming (stigmatization) that comes with being infected with HIV. Seeking spiritual therapy can thus work as a coping strategy by shifting the 'blame' or responsibility onto others (for example malicious people or powers), either perceived or real.

Interestingly, a lot of spiritual therapists in the Ashanti Region have laid claim to having a cure for HIV. Likewise, some Pentecostal pastors were noted for being powerful and having the ability to cure HIV infection. For this reason, PLHIV who were desperate to relieve themselves of their current predicament have sought their services. Often, the 'authority of God' and the power of biomedicine were used to complement each other. PLHIV rationalized this by saying that 'God heals and the doctors get money for it'. Given that people spend more money on God than on ART, this assertion cannot be true. Indeed, while the activities of the medicine men and spiritualists in Ghana are not regulated (leaving room for some to prey on the genuine spiritual beliefs or unguarded ignorance of clients), some clients are left in worse conditions, as is the case of many of the people infected with HIV attending prayer camps. In fact, the healers were found to 'get more money' in their healing bid than the doctors, since ART is a relatively inexpensive option. The research found that some providers of spiritual therapy, having good knowledge of the epidemiology of HIV/AIDS, have used it to perpetuate the infected person's spiritual needs. In a client's pursuit of holistic treatment therefore, their services may seem indispensable.

Research in medical pluralism in Ghana, and elsewhere in Africa, has shown that the health-seeking behaviour of people more often follows proximate, seemingly pragmatic decisions than decisions guided by the principles of a medical system (Twumasi 1979; Mullings 1984; Fink 1987; Krause 2006, 2007). Earlier researches have shown that an important element in people's search for healing and well-being is the crossing of denominational and religious boundaries through compromises, reorientation and, sometimes, conversion (see Kwansa 2010). This state of uncertainty is intrinsically tied to the maintenance of hope, whereby clients claim they will do whatever it takes to restore their health and status. In effect, although some PLHIV mentioned that experiences with spiritual therapy had strengthened their spiritual beliefs, the search for spiritual therapy can be seen as a pragmatic approach to a 'hopeful end', and not necessarily a profession of faith or a belief in only traditional healings or cures.

References

Agadzi, V.K. 1989. *AIDS: The African Perspective of the Killer Disease*. Accra: Ghana Universities Press.

Anarfi, J.K. 1995. Female migration and prostitution in West Africa: The case of Ghanaian women in Cote d'Ivoire. *Studies in Sexual Health No. 1*. Accra: Deutsche Gesellschaft fuer Technische Zusammenarbeit (GTZ), Regional AIDS Programme for West and Central Africa.

Asamoah-Gyadu, K.J. 2004. *African Charismatics: Current Developments within Independent Indigenous Pentecostalism in Ghana*. Leiden: Brill Academic Publishers.

Asamoah-Gyadu, K.J. 2005. Anointing through the screen: Neo-Pentecostalism and televised Christianity. *Ghana Studies in World Christianity*, 11, 9–28.

Ashitey, G.A. 1988. *Disease Control in Ghana*. Accra: Ghana Universities Press.

Attuquayefio, D.K. 2004. The snakes of Ghana: Myth, science and reality. *Ghana Journal of Science*, 44, 73–86.

Awusabo-Asare, K. 1995. HIV/AIDS education and counselling: Experiences from Ghana. *Health Transition Review*, 5 (Supplement), 229–36.

Awusabo-Asare, K. and Anarfi, J.K. 1997. Health-seeking behaviours of persons with HIV/AIDS in Ghana. *Health Transition Review*, 7, 243–56.

Centres for Disease Control and Prevention 2000. HIV and AIDS cases reported through December 2000. *HIV/AIDS Surveillance Report: Year-end Edition*, 12, 2.

Crentsil, P. 2005. A dark world: Supernaturalism and illness among the Akan of Ghana. *Suomen Anthropologi*, 30(1), 53–71.

Crentsil, P. 2007. Death, Ancestors and HIV/AIDS among the Akan of Ghana. PhD thesis, Faculty of Social Science, University of Helsinki.

Dapaah, J.M. 2012. *HIV/AIDS Treatment in Two Ghanaian Hospitals: Experiences of Patients, Nurses and Doctors*. Leiden: African Studies Centre.

De Witte, M. 2003. Altar media's 'Living Word': Televised charismatic Christianity in Ghana. *Journal of Religion in Africa*, 33(2), 172–202.

Decosas, J., Kane, F., Anarfi, J.K., Sodji, K.D.R. and Wagner, H.U. 1995. Migration and AIDS. *The Lancet*, 346 (8978), 826–8.

Dei, G.J.S. 2002. Learning culture, spirituality and local knowledge: Implications for African schooling. *International Review of Education*, 48(5), 335–60.

Dilger, H. 2007. Healing the wounds of modernity: Salvation, community and care in a neo-Pentecostal church in Dar es Salaam, Tanzania. *Journal of Religion in Africa*, 37, 59–83.

Ego, M.L. and Moran, M. 1993. HIV/AIDS counselling program: A rural Ghana experience, in *Sexual Networking and HIV/AIDS in West Africa*, edited by J.C. Caldwell et al. Supplement to *Health Transition Review 3*. Canberra: Australian National University, 85–92.

Feierman, S. 1981. Therapy as a system-in-action in Northeastern Tanzania. *Social Science and Medicine*, 15(B), 353–60.

Fink, H.E. 1987. *Religion, Disease and Healing in Ghana*. Munich: Trickster Wissenschaft.

Gifford, P. 1994. Ghana's charismatic churches. *Journal of Religion in Africa*, 24(3), 241–65.

Hardon, A., Kageha, E., Kinsman, J., Kyaddondo, D., Wanyenze, D. and Obermeyer, C.M. 2011. Dynamics of care, situations of choice: HIV tests in times of ART. *Medical Anthropology*, 30(2), 183–201.

Janzen, J.M. 1978. *The Quest for Therapy: Medical Pluralism in Lower Zaire*. Berkeley, CA: University of California Press.

Kayombo, E.J., Mbwambo, Z.H. and Massila, M. 2005. Role of traditional healers in psychosocial support in caring for the orphans: A case of Dar-es Salaam City, Tanzania. *Journal of Ethnobiology and Ethnomedicine*, 1, 3.

Kleinman, A. 1980. *Patients and Healers in the Context of Culture*. Berkeley, CA: University of California Press.

Krause, K. 2006. The double face of subjectivity: A case study in a psychiatric hospital, Ghana, in *Multiple Medical Realities: Patients and Healers in Biomedical, Alternative and Traditional Medicine*, edited by H. Johannessen and I. Lázár. New York and Oxford: Berghahn Books, 54–71.

Krause, K. 2007. Science treats, but only God can heal: Medical pluralism between religion and the secular in Ghana, in *Religion and its Other: Secular and Sacral Concepts and Practices in Interaction*, edited by H. Bock, J. Feuchter and M. Knecht. Frankfurt am Main: Campus, 185–98.

Kwansa, B.K. 2010. Complex negotiations: 'Spiritual' therapy and living with HIV in Ghana. *African Journal of AIDS Research*, 9(4), 449–58.

Kwansa, B.K. 2013. *Safety in the Midst of Stigma: Experiencing HIV/AIDS in Two Ghanaian Communities*. Leiden: African Studies Centre.

Lamptey, P.R. and Coates, T.J. 1994. Community-based interventions in Africa, in *AIDS in Africa*, edited by M. Essex, S. Mboup, P.J. Kanki, R.G. Marlink and S.D. Tlou. New York: Raven Press, 513–31.

Meyer, B. 1998. 'Make a complete break with the past': Memory and post-colonial modernity in Ghanaian Pentecostalist discourse. *Journal of Religion in Africa*, 27(3), 316–49.

Meyer, B. 2004. 'Praise the Lord': Popular cinema and Pentecostalite style in Ghana's new public sphere. *American Ethnologist*, 31(1), 92–110.

Mullings, L. 1984. *Therapy, Ideology and Social Change: Mental Healing in Urban Ghana*. Berkeley, CA: University of California Press.

NACP/GHS 2010. *2009 HIV Sentinel Survey Report*. Accra, Ghana.

Plummer, M.L., Mshana, G., Wamoyi, J., Shigongo, Z.S., Hayes, R.J., Ross, D.A. and Wight, D. 2006. 'The man who believed he had AIDS was cured': AIDS and sexually transmitted infection treatment-seeking behaviour in rural Mwanza, Tanzania. *AIDS Care*, 18(5), 460–66.

Radstake, M. 2000. *Secrecy and Ambiguity: Home Care for People Living with HIV/AIDS in Ghana*. Leiden: Africa Studies Centre.

Takyi, B.K. 2003. Religion and women's health in Ghana: insights into HIV/AIDS preventive and protective behaviour. *Social Science and Medicine*, 56, 1221–34.

Twumasi, P.A. 1972. Ashanti traditional medicine. *Transition*, 41, 50–63.

Twumasi, P.A. 1979. A social history of the Ghanaian pluralistic medical system. *Social Science and Medicine*, 13(4), 349–56.

Van Dijk, R. 1997. From camp to encompassment: Discourses of trans-subjectivity in the Ghanaian Pentecostal diaspora. *Journal of Religion in Africa*, 27(2), 135–59.

Van Dijk, R. 1999. The Pentecostal gift: Ghanaian charismatic churches and the moral innocence of the global economy, in *Modernity on a Shoestring*, edited by R. Fardon, W. van Binsbergen and R. van Dijk. London and Leiden: SOAS/ASC/Anthony Rowe, 71–91.

Ver Beek, K.A. 2000. Spirituality: A development taboo. *Development in Practice*, 10(1), 31–43.

World Health Organisation/UNAIDS. 2007. *Guidance on Provider-Initiated HIV Testing and Counselling in Health Facilities*. Geneva: WHO.

Wyllie, R.W. 1983. Ghanaian spiritual and traditional healers' explanation of illness: A preliminary survey. *Journal of Religion in Africa*, 14(1), 46–57.

Chapter 7

The Blood of Jesus and CD4 counts: Dreaming, Developing and Navigating Therapeutic Options for Curing HIV/AIDS in Tanzania

Dominik Mattes

Introduction

It was not long before the lady sitting next to me on the plane inquired about my opinion concerning 'Babu'. It was early May 2011, I was about to start my second field stay in Tanzania, and I had already heard about this 'miracle healer' dispensing a herbal concoction to thousands of sick people in the village of Samunge (Loliondo Division) in the remote Sonjo plains close to the Kenyan border. Before I could answer, the lady readily explained that she was originally from Dar es Salaam but had worked as a nurse in Europe for decades. She expressed her doubts about the hygienic conditions of Babu's medicinal cups, which she suspected were not thoroughly cleaned after each use and could thus spread infections among already weakened patients. After issuing further doubts about the concoction from a scientific point of view, however, she slowly argued her way towards its potential efficacy. The long-lasting skin disease of her sister's neighbour, for instance, had supposedly been cured through Babu's medicine. 'His skin looks beautiful now!' her sister had rejoiced on the phone. Elaborating on her own indecisiveness, the lady finally concluded that she had to see for herself: 'Seeing is believing!'

This lady's ambiguity is emblematic of the state of the Tanzanian public at the time, which was engaged in a multilayered and intense debate about scientificity and efficacy, faith, medical and religious authority, governmental, civic and media responsibility, and economic and political development, which had been sparked by Babu's 'magic cup'.

Drawing on in-depth interviews with patients on antiretroviral treatment (ART) and an exhaustive collection of articles in daily newspapers, this chapter documents the complex entanglements between ART and local and national discourses of 'healing' in Tanzania. To this purpose, I will first elaborate on the extraordinary phenomenon of 'Babu wa Loliondo' (Kiswahili: the Grandfather of Loliondo), who started providing a 'miracle cure' for HIV/AIDS in August 2010, and not only attracted millions of people from Tanzania and abroad but also incited a highly informative public controversy revolving around scientific and religious understandings of healing. The political connotations and social context of this phenomenon are first analysed in comparison to a similar African prophetic movement, followed by an exploration of the epistemological crossroads between science and religion through the perspectives, concepts and practices of people living with HIV/AIDS in Tanga[1] who flexibly and pragmatically navigated between both spheres. An outline of the studies that have to date addressed the intersection between treatment for HIV/AIDS and religious practice will serve as the point of departure.

ART in Articulation with Religious Concepts of Healing

The interrelations between HIV/AIDS and religious practice have recently gained heightened attention. Most of the existing studies, however, refer to the era before the large scale roll-out of ART in Africa or do not specifically address the interrelation between ART and religion. Yet in times of ART, the embedding of HIV/AIDS within religious conceptual frameworks is of significant analytical importance. The complete biomedicalization of people's ideas about HIV/AIDS, suffering and death, in correspondence with the expanding availability of ART, is hardly ever the case. 'Indigenous ritual and Qur'anic (as well as Biblical) language have a force that biomedical explanations and recommendations cannot match' (Becker 2009a: 161). The ethnographic research upon which this chapter is based revealed scepticism towards the biomedical truths propagated at Care and Treatment Centers in urban Tanzania (see Mattes 2011). Despite their often positive experiences with antiretroviral medicines (ARVs), many patients kept looking for alternative remedies. Their concept of 'healing' could not be narrowed down to rising CD4 counts and increased body weight.

Among the few studies on the mutual impact of expanding ART and religious practice in Africa, the formation of patients' new subjectivities and 'responsible selfhood' figures prominently (Burchardt 2009; Nguyen 2009). But there are also critical voices that call for a careful examination of the socio-political contexts of such processes, in order not to constrain the argument of self-formation to the

[1] Fifteen months of fieldwork were conducted in Tanga, a city on the Tanzanian Swahili coast with approximately 250,000 inhabitants. The study explored the incorporation of ART into the fabric of everyday life and social interrelations of people living with HIV/AIDS, their families, medical staff, traditional medical practitioners, religious leaders, and local government authorities.

individuals' 'encounter with illness, counseling and subsequent rediscovery of their religion' (Becker 2009b: 6).

Other studies examine the integration of ART into Muslim thinking and practices in Nigeria. Balogun (2010) presents a theological discussion of the legitimization of ART in relation to Islamic rules as deduced from the Quran; Tocco (2010: 14) demonstrates that there exists 'a multiplicity of perspectives and values attached to these technologies, rather than a singular way in which all Muslims perceive them in light of Islamic beliefs about healing and treatment efficacy'.

Regarding Christian theological understandings of ART there are two studies of interest. Kalipeni et al. (2009: 5) examine 'the Church in Southern Africa' as a '"double edged sword" when it comes to combating the HIV/AIDS epidemic', referring to the churches' large contribution to the care of people living with HIV/AIDS on the one hand, and their position towards condom use that compromises prevention efforts on the other.[2] By citing two influential clergymen's answers to the same questions about the use of ART, Kalipeni and colleagues demonstrate significantly opposing attitudes towards ART across varying Christian denominations. In his study on the understanding of life, death and healing in Botswana, Togarasei (2010: 433) calls for a new theology 'that accommodates ARVs in the realm of God' – a 'theology of ARVs' based on the principles of 'the sanctity of life' and the notion 'that scientific discoveries that enhance human life should be seen as God sanctioned'.

These studies suggest that the concept of healing is constituted differently in relation to socio-political, cultural and theological contexts, and that ART is unlikely to detach the concept from these wider contexts. In fact, it has been observed that even a few years into the large scale roll-out of ART in sub-Saharan Africa, 'bodies and people were not disciplined by the available biomedical treatment regimes in the ways envisaged (or at least hoped for) by national and international policymakers as well as local healthcare providers' (Dilger et al. 2010: 380). The Loliondo phenomenon serves as a vivid example of this observation.

'Relief for the Troubled Mankind': The 'Wonder of Loliondo'

When the first articles on Babu appeared in early March 2011, the sick had already been flocking to Samunge in their thousands to see Ambilikile Mwasapile. The 76-year-old retired pastor of the Evangelical Lutheran Church

[2] In consideration of the panoply of Christian denominations in Africa it has to be mentioned that accordingly there exist vastly differing stances towards condom use across but also within different Christian communities (see e.g., Rasing 2007).

of Tanzania (ELCT) had had a dream in which God had shown him how to prepare a concoction from a particular tree's roots to cure major chronic diseases such as HIV/AIDS, cancer, diabetes and hypertension. In the dream, Mwasapile was also instructed that the medicine should be delivered exclusively by him at the modest cost of 500 Tanzanian Shillings (Tsh) per cup – the price of a regular cup of tea.

Mwasapile initially provided his medicine to a few fellow villagers. Some indeed felt their afflictions improving and the word spread like bush fire. By March 2011, people were arriving from all parts of Tanzania, their vehicles queuing for kilometres on the rough dirt roads crossing the Ngorongoro Conservation Area. More and more people were attracted by the testimonials of relatives and friends who had supposedly been cured of all kinds of diseases. Biblically inspired narratives of the lame walking and the blind seeing circulated. The first testimonial of a 30-year-old HIV-positive widow living in Samunge featured in a newspaper in mid March. Since drinking 'God's miracle cure for the ailing nation' (*The Citizen*, 13 March 2011), the woman, who had been on ART for several years, claimed that her CD4 levels had started rising until, to the amazement of her clinicians, she had tested HIV-negative (*Mwananchi*, 14 March 2011). This story fuelled people's hopes and increased the influx to the village – and the infrastructural chaos this created in the entire region. At the height of its popularity, approximately 6,000 people were provided with the cup on a daily basis. Disastrous hygienic conditions, insufficient accommodation and excessive prices for food and drinking water endangered the survival of the severely sick who had been removed from hospitals by relatives and had already struggled with the exhausting journey.

Minister of Health and Social Welfare Dr Haji Mponda issued his first statement on 10 March, prohibiting further distribution of the medicine until the hygienic conditions were addressed, Mwasapile had 'registered his services in line with laid down procedures', and an expert task force had assured that the medicine was safe for human consumption (*The Guardian*, 10 March 2011). Bishop Laizer of the Evangelical Lutheran Church reacted with a rebuke. 'It is not right to halt the service, which has spiritual elements and it is also not right to take such action without involving stakeholders who are *wananchi* [citizens]', he reprimanded, and requested that the government actively support Mwasapile's services for the benefit of the citizens. On the following day, Minister of State Mr William Lukuvi mitigated the Health Minister's directive, saying that 'the government cannot interfere with religious beliefs because it is not in its policy to do so' (*Daily News*, 11 March 2011). He rather intended to 'ensure peace and security for the 6,000 patients already camped in the area to get the medicine before allowing more people in' and 'to improve the environment by engaging more health workers, first aid teams and ambulances to make life in the otherwise surrounding bush area become habitable'.

The dispensing of Mwasapile's medicine was never officially stopped. More and more high-level politicians, including the former Prime Minister, several current ministers, regional commissioners, and parliamentarians, arrived in Samunge in order to have their share. Several parliamentarians organized free transportation for their constituents as a sign of their generosity and care and made sure to inform the press over the millions of Shillings they invested. They even offered helicopter flights to Samunge to affluent potential voters who could afford the 1,000 USD fare. One Member of Parliament, Beatrice Shelukindo, 'the first high profile opinion leader in the country to come out in the open testifying the potency of the "miracle drug"' (*Guardian on Sunday*, 13 March 2011), encouraged all Tanzanians to 'fully exploit the golden chance'. Claiming that relatives of hers had been cured of cancer, HIV/AIDS, and diabetes, she reasoned that 'not everything is politics', that this was a matter of 'divine power', and – alluding to the government's notice of ongoing scientific research on the concoction – that 'God is unresearchable' (ibid.).

Two logics of efficacy were entangled in Babu's concoction: scientifically verifiable *materia medica* in the form of medicinal plant extracts on the one side, and faith in God and his servant Mwasapile on the other. This rendered the 'magic cup' a polysemantic symbol that provided ample contact surface for both proponents and critics of natural science and religiously informed concepts of illness and healing. While some traditional healers[3] were scandalized that Mwasapile had not been obliged to register according to Tanzania's *Traditional and Alternative Medicines Act* (United Republic of Tanzania 2002) – a procedure whose breach could be heavily fined (*Mwananchi*, 26 March 2011) – Mwasapile himself insisted that he was no traditional healer in the first place. He had no expert knowledge of medicinal plants but simply functioned as an instrument of God; the efficacy of his medicine rested solely in unconditional belief in the healing powers of the Almighty (see *Mtanzania*, 17 May 2011). '[T]his medicine ... has the power of the blood of Jesus Christ, the son of God, so even if the bugs [viruses] are still there, they will not be able to fight with the blood of Jesus', he explained (*An-Nuur* 3–9 June 2011a).[4]

---

[3] The terms 'traditional healers' and 'traditional medicine' bracket together a wide variety of medical practices and imply equally heterogeneous – sometimes politically instrumentalized – assumptions of what 'the traditional' designates. 'Traditional healers' in Tanga engage in diverse therapeutic practices such as herbalism, divination, spirit exorcism, and Quranic healing. The official registration as a 'practitioner of traditional or alternative medicine' includes the payment of registration fees, the presentation of testimonials of the applicant's healing competence, and the provision of 'a written statement from the local government authority within which he is practising' (United Republic or Tanzania 2002: 12). Satisfaction of these requirements grants a certificate valid for three years.

[4] All quotes from interviews or newspaper articles have been translated from Kiswahili to English by myself.

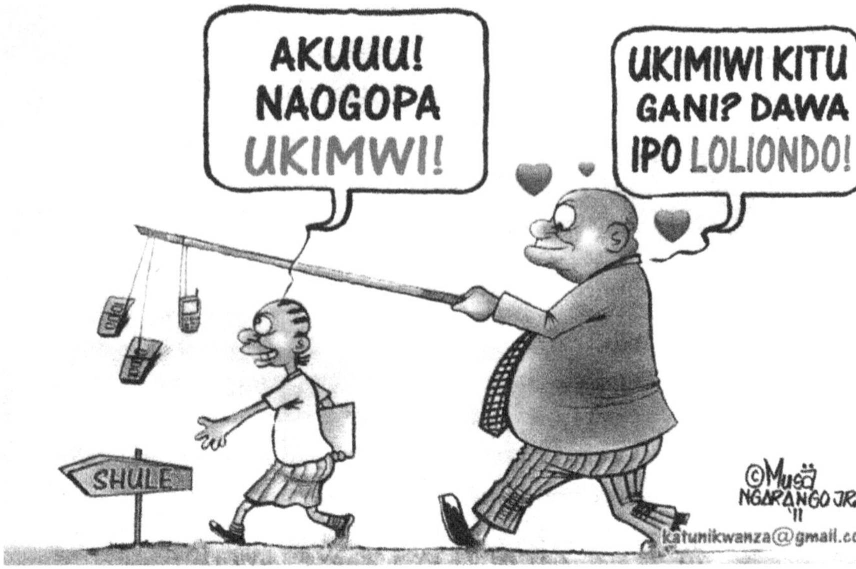
AKUUU! NAOGOPA UKIMWI!
UKIMIWI KITU GANI? DAWA IPO LOLIONDO!
SHULE
©Musa NGARANGO JR. '11
katunikwanza@gmail.com

Figure 7.1 'I am afraid of AIDS!' – 'AIDS, what's that? There's medicine in Loliondo! (Source: Musa Ngarango, *Tanzania Daima*, 6 May 2011)

More than Mwasapile himself, who displayed rather modest behaviour, it was his circle of close confidants who, with their public sermons, started a process of mystifying him. The crowds were repeatedly reminded of the holiness of the pastor's compounds and urged to refrain from sinful and antisocial behaviour (see e.g., *An-Nuur* 3–9 June 2011b). Only in two situations Mwasapile himself added a slightly moralizing twist to his healing practice. Once he admonished high-level society members to wait for their turn as anyone else, otherwise the medicines would not prove effective for them (*Nipashe*, 21 March 2011). On another occasion he emphasized that his medicine should not be mistaken for a vaccine against HIV/AIDS and other diseases; thereby reacting to reports of middle-aged men who after taking the concoction thought themselves safe to indulge in unprotected sexual activities (Figure 7.1).

Mwasapile claimed that God had told him to start treating the nation's orphans and inmates, whereupon he requested the government to support the organization of respective initiatives (*Nipashe*, 7 May 2011). On other occasions God had issued concrete instructions concerning the price of the medicine and had finally allowed Mwasapile to accept donations by the cured, which he had vigorously refused before (*An-Nuur*, 3–9 June 2011b). Mwasapile also refused to have his medicine processed into pills – a recommendation made by an expert delegation from the World Health Organization – arguing that God had not agreed to that (*Mwananchi*, 1 May 2011).

The Tanzanian Christian community was divided concerning Mwasapile's alleged close ties with God. While some leaders encouraged their church members 'that it was alright Biblically for them to drink the Loliondo medicine' (*Daily News*, 11 March 2011), other – predominantly Pentecostal – leaders issued warnings against engaging in Babu's 'satanic work'. Bishop Kakobe, founder of the Full Gospel Bible Fellowship Church and himself actively engaged in individual and collective faith healing ceremonies (see Dilger 2007), sharply attacked Mwasapile for applying the 'power of darkness', precluding the possibility that God would collaborate with somebody who was not 'saved'.[5]

Muslim leaders issued hardly any comments in public. The Sheikh of Samunge's Muslim community, however, considered Mwasapile to be a charlatan. The inhabitants of the Sonjo Plains had been using the *mugariga* plant long before Mwasapile's revelations, he explained. Without denying the plant's therapeutic potency, he clarified that it could not cure diseases like HIV/AIDS or diabetes. He rather assumed that expanding the influence of Christianity among 'irreligious' locals was Mwasapile's real intention (see *An-Nuur*, 1–7 July 2011).

Obviously, these publicly staged disputes had no significant effect on the pilgrims' faith in the miracle potion. By mid May, Mwasapile was reported to have dispensed some 3 million cups (*Tanzania Daima*, 9 May 2011). The massive influx of patients effected an immense boost of entrepreneurship in Samunge and along the main entryways leading to the village. Government authorities issued obligatory licenses (5,000–10,000 Tsh, *c.* US$3–6) for every car heading towards Samunge. Countless safari companies in Arusha, the closest large city to Samunge (400 km away) and the main starting point for the touristic circuits in the national parks of northern Tanzania, adjusted their portfolios. Return tickets to Samunge were sold for up to 150,000 Tsh, a sum equivalent to three or four months' salary for the poorer pilgrims. Restaurants, tea stalls, small shops, tent hotels, and sanitary services all sprang up along the routes, providing their owners with considerable income. Even large companies jumped at the chance of capitalizing on Babu's popularity. Major mobile communication companies expanded their coverage to Loliondo and gave Mwasapile cell phones as gifts. A solar energy enterprise bestowed him with a medal for his 'selfless service' and with a donation of technological equipment worth some 4 million Tsh brought light to the enlightened (*Habari Leo*, 11 May 2011).

The government authorities struggled to contain the chaotic situation in and on the way to Loliondo. Upon Babu's request, Prime Minister Pinda called for the

[5] The idea of being 'saved' or 'born again' through the complete commitment of one's life to Jesus and a break with any 'sinful' practices of one's 'old' life is a central element of Pentecostal thought and practice (cf. Dilger 2005: 254).

public not to set out for Loliondo for seven days and further cars were prohibited from continuing their journey. This caused considerable protest among travellers who were stuck on the roads and held the authorities responsible for casualties among the waiting sick. At this point in time there were about 24,000 people queuing for Babu's cup. On the other hand, the government tried to ameliorate the situation by ordering the authorities of Ngorongoro District to install water pipes at Mwasapile's house, set up tents and toilets for the waiting, improve the conditions of the roads and the local dispensary, and provide sufficient space for burying the dead (*Nipashe*, 29 March 2011).

Scientific Claims and Religious Appeals

After Health Minister Mponda's ineffective orders to halt Babu's services, the next official statement was issued by Arusha's Regional Medical Officer, who stressed that 'so far nobody suffering from HIV/AIDS has been clinically proven to be healed from the alleged miracle cure' (*Daily News*, 18 March 2011). At the same time, however, he conceded that the potion might indeed be effective in the treatment of diabetes.

In contrast to his initially sceptical position, a few weeks after ordering the prohibition of Mwasapile's service, Mponda stepped into the breach *for* him. Since Mwasapile attracted equally high numbers of pilgrims among Kenyan and Tanzanian citizens, Kenyan Public Health Minister Beth Mugo had vigorously requested that he be immediately arrested and stopped from misleading the public. Mponda, however, dismissed this suggestion as 'unfair', saying that his Kenyan colleague 'had no sufficient evidence to prove her statement', and rather referred to ongoing scientific research about the safety of Babu's medicine for human consumption (*The Guardian*, 28 March 2011).

On the following day first respective results were published. Two researchers from the National Institute for Medical Research (NIMR) and the Muhimbili University of Health and Allied Sciences in Dar es Salaam had identified Babu's miraculous tree as *Canissa Spinarum*, which is commonly used for therapeutic purposes and as a nutritional supplement by various Tanzanian pastoralist ethnic groups (Malebo and Mbwambo 2011: 10f.). Drawing on a meta-analysis on the plant's chemical properties, the researchers concluded that Babu's cup was fit for human consumption and may in fact have therapeutic (antiepileptic, anti-inflammatory, cardiotonic, antioxidant, and antiviral) effects (ibid.: 11ff.). However, they strongly recommended further investigation 'on optimum dosage, dosing schedule and duration of treatment per ailment' (ibid.: 21). On the basis of this report, Mponda and a representative of the Tanzania Food and Drugs Authority publicly stated that the consumption of Babu's medicine was not harmful. Nevertheless, they also made clear that its actual levels of efficacy were still being investigated and that the results could not be expected any time soon (*Nipashe*, 29 March 2011).

Meanwhile, the Commission of Science and Technology (COSTECH) had begun verifying the possibility of patenting Babu's concoction, and to this purpose had tried to establish the medicine's unique characteristics (*The Guardian*, 1 April 2011). The possibility that – contrary to the NIMR report – Babu's medicine could contain an undiscovered active ingredient was equally considered in a report of the Tanzania Medicinal Plant Foundation, which claimed to have verified that the concoction either consisted of a combination of *Canissa Spinarum* and another plant, or was made from a completely different plant altogether (*The Citizen*, 19 April 2011). The concoction's efficacy was further investigated by researchers of the NIMR, COSTECH, and WHO, who explained that they were involved in the close observation of 200 persons who had drunk Babu's potion, and that trials with diabetic laboratory rats were being conducted (*Mwananchi*, 30 April 2011).

The absence of scientific evaluation of precisely what effects Mwasapile's medicine had on diverse physical afflictions seemed not to have any effect on the mass of Loliondo pilgrims. Incomplete and misleading media reporting further fuelled the run for the miracle cure. 'Experts: Babu's cup is fantastic protection', headlined *Habari Leo* (6 May 2011), citing the results of the preliminary NIMR report, while the *Business Week* (13–19 May 2011) quoted a representative of the Tanzanian Medicinal Plant Foundation who said that 'though not all, people are getting cured of HIV and other incurable diseases after getting Loliondo treatment'.

While on the one hand the governmental position was informed by scientific rationality, the actions and statements of some politicians illustrated an incongruous stance and a general reservation about interfering in matters of faith. Although announcing the intention to take strict disciplinary measures against any type of self-proclaimed healer advertising cures for chronic diseases similar to Mwasapile's (*Majira*, 26 May 2011) – and indeed several copycats were barred from dispensing their herbal brews –, Deputy Minister of Health Dr Lucy Nkya explained that the government was not able to intervene in Mwasapile's case 'because his work involves faith' (*Daily News*, 1 July 2011). Reports of members of the political elite drinking Babu's cup did not stop.

Mwasapile's impact on the treatment itineraries of people living with HIV/AIDS was quite tangible. 'I repeat again, those suffering from HIV/AIDS need just one cup of my medicine and they don't have to continue taking hospital medication', read his most explicit statement in this respect (*Daily News*, 29 June 2011). Indeed, many patients throughout the country and abroad gratefully acknowledged his encouraging instructions and stopped taking ARVs after supposedly being cured. The numbers of patients who did not return for their drug refills were reported to increase at varying treatment centres.

As time elapsed, however, testimonials of people who had waited in vain for their miracle cure increased. Infuriated relatives of those who had succumbed to the relapses of their afflictions raised their voices. 'Medically verifiable stories of cures are totally absent in the media. Whose interests are being served, only the profiteers'?' asked a columnist with regard to the government officials and entrepreneurs for whom the mass of pilgrims constituted a lucrative source of income (*Guardian on Sunday*, 29 June 2011). By mid July the 'Mseto[6] of faith' had lost much of its credibility and the increasing death reports exerted significant impact. The number of cars passing through Samunge each day had decreased to 100–50 and Samunge's 'new economy' started collapsing (*Mtanzania*, 13 July 2011).

In late July, first threats of taking Mwasapile to court were made by Rev. Christopher Mtikila, the highly controversial leader of the anti-Islamic nationalist Tanzania Democratic Party, who claimed to act on behalf of deceased Loliondo pilgrims. He also intended to call those politicians to account who had publicly taken Babu's cup and thus fuelled the run to Loliondo (*Sani*, 20–22 July 2011). In August, the chair of the Tanzania Network of the Organizations for People Living with HIV/AIDS (TANOPHA) issued similar threats (*Ukweli na Uwazi*, 16–22 August 2011), and the Vice President of the Medical Association of Tanzania (MAT) once more emphasized the danger of discontinuing biomedical therapies after taking Mwasapile's medicine and called for the government to communicate this in an unmistakable manner (*Nipashe*, 25 August 2011). Reacting to this and previous fierce critique of the government's passive stance towards Babu's medicine, Health Minister Mponda called for patience until the scientific evaluations of the cup's efficacy yielded results (*Nipashe*, 31 August 2011), and Mwasapile continued dispensing his medicine without hindrance. The tuberculosis ward at a nearby hospital was closed in September due to the lack of new admissions. Mwasapile took this as proof of God's healing powers and a further legitimization to continue his services: 'I don't cure people, but the Almighty God does it. It is illogical to blame the one who brings relief to the troubled mankind' (*The Citizen*, 17 September 2011).

Ambilikile Mwasapile: An Uncharismatic Semi-Prophet? A Socio-Political Interpretation

In order to explain the enormous momentum of the 'Wonder of Loliondo', I suggest examining the phenomenon in the context of prophetic movements in Africa, particularly in comparison to a similar case in Malawi where in the

---

[6] 'Mseto' is an acronym for a common artemisinin based antimalarial pharmaceutical drug.

early 1990s one Billy Chisupe equally attracted hundreds of thousands with an herbal cure for HIV/AIDS. In some articles Mwasapile was addressed as *nabii*, an Akkadian term of the Old Testament designating 'one who is either called by God or announces the message of God' (Johnson and Anderson 1995: 8), which found its way into Kiswahili through Arabic influence. 'The prophet was conscious of the fact that the revelation he received came from God and that it had not originated from his own consciousness', explains Oosthuizen, referring to the prophets of the Old Testament (1992: 3). In this literal sense, it seems appropriate to designate Mwasapile as a prophet. As has been argued in a considerable body of historical literature, however, the crucial aspect of what makes a prophet is his/her role as a leader in times of ecological, social, or political crisis, and as an instigator of social change in the sense of Wallace's 'revitalization' (1956) and Weber's 'charismatic authority' (1974). Throughout the nineteenth and twentieth centuries, African prophetic movements have emerged as a response to destructive external influences in the form of colonial conquest and associated epidemics as well as to a community's or society's perceived inner moral decay, all three phenomena often being closely interconnected (see Ranger 1992). Johnson and Anderson (1995: 19) extend the definition of 'prophet' correspondingly:

> The utterances of prophets need not always be directly predictive: they will also encompass commentary upon the past, and may be interpreted as offering guidance on the regulation of social and political practice in the present. This more pervasive relation sustaining the moral community places the prophet in a social context that is much broader than mere reaction to crisis: the prophet is also a barometer of social and political behaviour.

The case of Billy Chisupe has been largely interpreted along these lines (Probst 1995; Schoffeleers 1999). As with Mwasapile he had revelational dreams, although in his case it was not God but his grandfather and an unknown man who showed him a plant that could cure HIV/AIDS. After his story had been broadcast on a national radio channel, thousands started pouring into his remote village demanding his concoction, known as *mchape*, which was dispensed for free. The naming of the concoction was reminiscent of the witch cleansing movement that swept Malawi in the 1930s, which was also referred to by the name *mchape*. The mass influx to Chisupe's village caused infrastructural chaos similar to the situation in Loliondo, and the Malawian government equally struggled to counter Chisupe's attractiveness with scientific evidence of his concoction's inefficacy (see Probst 1995: 121). Unlike Mwasapile, however, Chisupe refused to have his medicine scientifically investigated, arguing that the Malawian government and the Western 'AIDS establishment' would not acknowledge the positive results anyway (see Schoffeleers 1999: 416). All this happened at a time of 'all-pervasive … crisis caused concretely by the AIDS pandemic, a severe famine caused by a succession of poor rainy seasons, a drastic devaluation of the Malawian Kwacha and, more generally, a widely shared disappointment in the way things had been developing after the elections of 1994' (ibid.: 411). Chisupe responded to this multilayered crisis by providing a cure that the government and scientific community had not been able to come up with in association with explicitly articulated social and political protest. This induced Probst (1995: 121) to interpret the phenomenon as 'a kind of revitalisation … of the old moral patterns, with the new problem of AIDS being substituted for the old problem of witchcraft' and to reflect 'that just as the old *mchape* was a local comment on the effects of the colonial intervention and the global economic recession, the recent *mchape* was a new and timely comment on just another feature of "modernity's malcontents" (Comaroff and Comaroff 1993), this time in the form of AIDS …' The second *mchape* cult was considered a 'counter-institution' to 'the hegemony of the post-Banda state' (Probst 1995: 125), with Chisupe as its leader bestowed with personal charisma implying 'a break with the established order', similar to the description by Ter Haar (1992: 239) of the Zambian Catholic Archbishop Milingo, whose healing ministry attracted large numbers of followers as well as the disapproval of the Catholic establishment in the 1970s.

There are striking similarities between the Wonder of Loliondo and Chisupe's *mchape* '95 cult. The political and socioeconomic situation in Tanzania is widely perceived to be in a state of multilevel crisis, especially by the poor and low educated without formal employment or any form of social security. Disappointment is often expressed by Tanzanians who on a daily basis are confronted with large scale corruption cases among the country's political, business, and religious leadership, as well as the government's inability to provide the most basic conditions for 'development' such as a stable power supply. The complaint of 'those up there' not caring about 'us down here' was a persistent comment on the seemingly ruthless national elite.

Negative experiences with the public health care infrastructure were equally frustrating. Although in a city like Tanga hospitals and health centres were in reach, the staff of the overcrowded facilities was often insufficiently trained and basic medical equipment and medicines had to be purchased in private pharmacies. Searching for treatment for relatively minor physical afflictions could become a painstaking odyssey through health facilities and pharmacies with an uncertain outcome, and could easily consume a family's entire financial reserves. In the light of such experiences, associating the Wonder of Loliondo with the desolate situation of the national health care delivery seemed natural:

> Some say the Loliondo rush is an indication of a failed health system, which over the fifty-year independence period hasn't responded to the health demands

> of millions of people in the country. With an under-funded budget, Tanzania's healthcare system has in some cases become a 'death trap', condemning some people to death, not because they are severely sick, but as a consequence of poor medical services. (*Guardian on Sunday*, 27 March 2011)

There was, in short, a 'serious crisis of expectation' similar to the one in Malawi during the early 1990s where 'people had become disillusioned with politics and everything that had to do with the common good' (Schoffeleers 1999: 410). At this moment, Mwasapile emerged as an almost Messianic figure. 'To offer healing is to offer hope. And hope is that state wherein we know that some kind of response or change or reconciliation or transformation is possible' (Bednarowski 2005: 195). Mwasapile offered hope to the entire 'ailing nation' (*The Citizen*, 13 March 2011), and a connection was made to Tanzania's highly venerated 'father of the nation' Julius Nyerere, respectfully called *mwalimu* (teacher), who 50 years earlier had redeemed the country from the ailment of colonial subjugation:

> The number of women and newly born dying in delivery is among the highest in the world, and real reform is rejected in all quarters of political society, and many are preparing to destroy the peace in the country if certain preconditions of policy are not met. The Loliondo priest looks eerily like the late Mwalimu, his name Ambilikile is close to Mwalimu's teasing name of 'Haambiliki', the potion he administers is the restoration of the Arusha Declaration[7] that many wish for'. (*The Guardian*, 26 March 2011)

The entanglement of longings for both spiritual and political leadership became even more apparent in an article, which referred to Mwasapile as the 'Grandfather of the nation' and emphasized the concept of 'being saved' commonly used by Pentecostal Christians (*Tanzania Daima*, 11 March 2011).

Just as Chisupe's cult was read along the lines of historic protest movements against colonialism, the Loliondo narrative carried an anti-imperialist undertone conceptualizing Mwasapile and his miracle cure as a challenge to neocolonial capitalist exploitation in the form of the western HIV/AIDS industry alleged to capitalize on the African AIDS sufferer (*The African*, 11 May 2011).

While these readings of the Wonder of Loliondo suggest a remarkable similarity with the movement of *mchape* '95, there is a significant difference between the two. Chisupe formulated fierce critique against the political establishment and actively co-constructed his role as a leader in the process of Malawian society's moral renewal. Mwasapile, by contrast, was a 'soft-

---

[7] In the 'Arusha Declaration' of 1967, Julius Nyerere laid out his socialist vision for Tanzania.

spoken, economically modest, socially humble, publicity-shy Loliondo senior citizen who has shot to virtual international stardom, obviously against his will' (*Guardian on Sunday*, 13 March 2011). Apart from his warning that his concoction should not be mistaken for an invitation to engage in 'immoral sexual behaviour' and his socially levelling appeal to the 'rich and mighty' to queue like anyone else, Mwasapile neither issued any judgements on the society's moral state, nor expressed his protest against its fraudulent leadership or his interest in political power. He repeatedly emphasized his own ordinariness and reminded the crowds to praise God instead of himself (see e.g., *Mtanzania*, 13 July 2011). Rather than positioning himself contra the state 'as the cult's 'ritual other'' (Baumann in Probst 1995: 118) he personally welcomed every politician to Samunge, and even politely posed in pictures wearing the VODACOM or AIRTEL t-shirts he was given by these multinationals that epitomize more than anything else 'neo-imperialistic' capitalism.

Due to his political reticence and modest appearance Mwasapile was possibly perceived as not powerful enough to incite a politically motivated protest movement and was thus spared more from governmental regulation and interference than Chisupe in Malawi. Rather than being a prophet in his own right, Mwasapile seemed to have become a projection surface for the disillusioned masses watching out for one.

Another remarkable point is the enormous economic boost that Mwasapile brought to an entire region far off Tanzania's economic hubs. The masses of pilgrims constituted a considerable source of income for private entrepreneurs along the pilgrimage routes. They also flushed enormous amounts of money into the registers of government authorities, who through taxing all incoming cars and helicopters made millions of Shillings over the months, inducing local villagers' protest that – as so often – nothing of these revenues trickled down to those who actually had to cope with the ecological and social damage caused by the pilgrims' stampede. By the end of March 2011, Mwasapile himself was reported to have made some 50 million Tsh, of which the ELCT and Mwasapile's assistants were given 20m each, and Mwasapile remained with 10 million Tsh (*Nipashe*, 31 March 2011).

Patients on the Quest for Redemption

The Loliondo phenomenon undeniably sparked a fierce discussion between the proponents of biomedical science and those defending a religiously informed concept of faith healing. In practice, however, these factions were not so discrete. The government's ambivalence, the considerable number of high-level politicians queuing up for the cup, and the masses of pilgrims for whom scientific evidence was unimportant, suggested that large parts of the population running through all social strata did not adhere exclusively to biomedical logic but considered the *possibility* of there being a cure for their ailments beyond insulin, ARVs, and antihypertensive pills. While the widespread acceptance of religious healing power in the form of Mwasapile's cup was statistically proven common among the Tanzanian citizenry,[8] in-depth interviews I conducted with HIV-positive persons in Tanga brought to the fore how differing etiological concepts and therapeutic pathways were combined, negotiated, and contrasted in highly individualized ways. While it was rather difficult to find patients who were willing to talk openly about their experiences with Babu's medicine because they knew that they had acted against the strict rules of their biomedical treatment regime, the following exemplary vignettes depict these individualized conceptualizations and negotiations.

How to Measure Faith? – Jemima Zephania

Jemima[9] was working as a teacher, 48 years old, and had two sons of 10 and 19 years. When all three of them had been tested HIV-positive a few years ago, her husband accused her of 'having brought this disease' and drove them all out of his house. When I got to know them, Jemima and her sons lived in a house on the outskirts of Tanga with two tenants from whom they concealed their illness. If the tenants were at home when it was time to take their medication, they all slipped secretly into Jemima's bedroom where they quickly took their pills. Jemima had suffered from various side effects when she began taking ARVs in 2010 and still complained about disproportionate accumulations of body fat even though 'she did exercise as usual'. Her sons, by contrast, did not fare badly with the medicines. At least they were not sick all the time as they had been before starting ART.

Although Jemima had witnessed considerable health improvements after initiating ART, she continued to search for something better. Taking ARVs every day, she complained, 'is something that exhausts you ... Another time ... the children forget if they don't pay attention. So if all of a sudden you see medicine that cures completely, it would be better.' Her two sisters actively supported her search for a cure and informed her about every possible remedy they came across. Jemima had already tried several products, but felt very uncertain and almost haunted:

8 According to a survey by *Synovate*, a multinational market research company, 59 per cent of the Tanzanians surveyed believed in Mwasapile's medicine, and 78 per cent of those who had taken the cup self-reported to be cured of their afflictions (see *The Citizen*, 4 August 2011).

9 All names in this chapter are pseudonyms.

> We are confused, to tell the truth ... When you have a problem, [the doctors] tell you, you can't be cured right away. So [there's treatment] here and there, here and there. When you're told '*here* is very good medicine' – all right, you swallow it. And then '*there* is very good medicine' ... So I took it but I don't know about its quality, because I am not a doctor.

Her biggest problem was the lack of financial resources. Once her sister had informed her about a promising compound from South Africa, but the price of 500,000 Tsh[10] for a single dose far exceeded her means. Jemima would neither have been able to afford the journey to Loliondo had her sister not insisted and paid her and her sons' bus tickets. They all drank Babu's medicine, but even this time Jemima remained sceptical:

> This more expert like thing [ARVs] and faith are two different things. It's not like I was running towards the side of faith. I haven't seen anyone who said 'I stopped taking the medicine [ARVs] and I was cured,' [so] I'm not in a hurry. I'm going slowly. First we asked Babu: 'Should we continue taking ARVs?' And he said: 'If your faith is strong, leave it! But if your faith is not strong, continue taking your medicines, because my medicine works slowly.' So when I heard this, I did not stop and my children are still given their medicine.

Jemima wondered if her religious integrity would suffice for a manifestation of a cure:

> Maybe it is possible. But I personally don't have too much confidence. Because I am a human being and maybe I have failed God in many ways that I don't even know of. And I don't even know why I got this problem in the first place ... Maybe God is trying me saying 'You have failed me' and he wants to bring me back this way, I don't understand ... I don't believe that you can leave the medicines aside directly and God will cure you. It's true, He's helping me to be cured, but I don't know the amount of mistakes I have committed on His account. So, there is faith and I also believe that there is [scientific] expertise (*utaalamu*). I haven't decided yet which direction I should take.

Ultimately, she considered that biomedical judgement should have the last word regarding her therapy. Unless the doctors at the treatment centre where she and her sons were enrolled told her to stop taking ARVs she would not do so, she claimed. However, she did not put much effort into pursuing a biomedical evaluation of the efficacy of Babu's concoction. Several months after she and her

---

[10] At the time of the interview (19 August 2011) this was equivalent to approximately 300 US$ or two-and-a-half times Jemima's monthly salary as a primary school teacher.

sons had taken the medicine, none of them had undergone a new HIV test. Jemima apparently preferred to continue living with her doubts – but also with hope for the unexpected to come true in the future.

You Need to Fish with Two Things! – Samuel Mbago

In 2008, 46-year-old Samuel was admitted to the hospital with cerebral malaria. Fortunately, he recovered, but from then on was semi-paralyzed and had to begin taking ARVs since an HIV test conducted during his hospitalization had turned out positive. When he first started taking the drugs he remembered being tired all the time, and his legs feeling so numb and heavy that he could barely walk. Slowly these negative effects had vanished to some extent.

Three years later, in spring 2011, his younger brother learned of Mwasapile's healing activities. He proposed for Samuel to go there and contributed 70,000 Tsh (*c.* US$42) for the travel expenses. Samuel himself had already heard several stories of sick people being cured and readily embarked on the journey that would take him six days and cost around 350,000 Tsh. In Samunge, Samuel managed to shake hands with Babu. 'If you've drunk this cup of mine you'll already be cured', Mwasapile assured him. Even if the 'bugs' were still visible, they had been reduced for sure, and Babu's medicine was still at work, Samuel hopefully concluded. 'Once you've taken the cup, this medicine does its work all the way'.

In our conversation, he reported feeling a lot better since he had drunk the medicine – and since he had stopped taking his ARVs. At the time of the interview, he had already interrupted his therapy for three months. He regularly talked to one of Mwasapile's assistants via telephone. 'If your progress is good, that's it, just go on like that, don't use your medicines [ARVs]', he had told Samuel during their last conversation. Samuel seemed to ascribe his improvement in equal measure to Babu's concoction and to the disruption of his biomedical therapy. After starting ART his health had also improved to a certain extent, he admitted. 'But right now I'm improving a lot more than at the beginning ... Since I stopped taking [ARVs] I feel a certain lightness.' Nonetheless, he was still in a 'wait-and-see mode' and by no means averse to continuing his biomedical therapy should his improvements be limited:

> I got faith from going to Babu's. He told me not to stop believing. So I thought by myself 'wait and let the [antiretroviral] medicines rest for a little bit until you see how *these* things [improvement through Babu's medicine] are developing.' If there will be no changes, I'll return to exactly where I've been before and I'll continue taking [ARVs]. You have to try everything ... but if you don't have faith you can't be healed ... Faith comes before medicine. If you have faith, this medicine will also help you ... You need to fish with two things, faith and medicine.

Similar to Jemima, Samuel could not tell where the fish would bite. After a few weeks he intended to undergo an HIV test in order 'to know what to do'. 'If the "bugs" are all gone I'll thank God. If they're still there I'll go back to the hospital and continue with the drugs. I'll know that Babu's medicine will have decreased [the "bugs"'] strength but that it didn't cure completely.' Samuel knew about the risks of developing resistant virus strains when interrupting ART, but even the constant insistence of a Home Based Care worker could not motivate him to resume therapy earlier.

Samuel's opinion about other healers claiming to cure HIV/AIDS affirmed the voices of those who strongly criticized the government for not informing its citizens properly about the Loliondo cure:

> These others are liars, liars, liars. But I see that Babu is still there until today and the government supports him. If Babu was a liar, the government wouldn't care about him. Instead it organizes a good procedure, good resting places, good transportation, permits ... Until today they keep putting good regulations in place for him.

Calculations, Pragmatism, and Hope

Jemima and Samuel were grateful for being able to undergo ART but at the same time their accounts underlined how ARVs effected new hardships in their lives. Severe and persistent side effects had to be coped with and could provoke treatment fatigue throughout the course of the lifelong therapy. Experiences of stigma and the consequent creation of secrecy surrounding one's sero status also complicated the therapy.[11] Life with ARVs was by no means a life without HIV, and Jemima and Samuel's quest for a cure – their desire to 'try out everything' – raises the question of how much 'redemption' there actually is in 'the redemptive moment' (Dilger et al. 2010: 377) induced by the growing availability of ART in developing countries.

In both Jemima and Samuel's cases, a set of close relatives actively contributed to their quests for a cure with material and immaterial sources and assisted with calculating the probabilities of a prospective remedy 'being real' (cf. Doran 2007). Yet, while they helped to estimate Mwasapile's spiritual legitimacy, the evaluation of Jemima and Samuel's own spiritual aptness was left to themselves. These calculations and estimations left ample space for uncertainty, which was experienced as deeply demoralizing doubt in one moment and overwhelming

[11] For a more detailed account of the difficulties of living on ARVs in contexts of extreme economic scarcity and the struggle to maintain one's moral standing in the world, see Mattes (2012).

confidence in the next. In both cases, however, the efficacy of the Wonder of Loliondo was undoubtedly thought to be a matter of faith. In fact, Jemima did not even mention the herbal brew in her reflections on a possible cure, and for Samuel having faith was the indispensable condition for the medicine's efficacy. Despite this obvious attribution of therapeutic power to faith rather than to the concoction, Mwasapile in his role as a healer or godly medium seemed to be of minor relevance. While Samuel at least once mentioned him to be 'a man of God', Jemima did not refer to any of Babu's personal characteristics or statements that would point to the importance of topics such as moral reorientation or an expiation of sins. Her speculations about religious integrity were not triggered by a 'moralizing prophet' but were the result of her own reflections. Moreover, Jemima's account resembled those of others who had received the cup without even getting out of their car, and who then immediately embarked on their return trip. God's healing power, condensed in the cup, had become a commodity and had become largely detached from the exigencies of inner catharsis or from the prioritization of profound commitment to Jesus as issued by the leaders of Pentecostal healing churches (cf. Van Dijk 2009). Bishop Kakobe's anxiety about losing followers to this commoditized, more easily accessible form of faith healing may not have been entirely groundless.

Finally, similar to the health seeking behaviour of HIV-positive people in Ghana, who transgress denominational borders in their quest for a cure in a pluralistic therapeutic economy, Jemima and Samuel's accounts clearly demonstrate that 'uncertainty is intrinsically tied up with the maintenance of hope, wherein clients claim they will do whatever it takes to restore their health and status' (Kwansa 2010: 456). It is not only denominational but also epistemological borders that are transgressed in ways that are at times highly pragmatic and often flexible.

Conclusion

The exponential expansion of ART can indeed be seen as a 'redemptive moment' after years of depriving HIV/AIDS sufferers in developing countries of effective treatment. However, many affected by HIV/AIDS still have to cope with stigmatization and severe economic scarcity, and despite their undeniable therapeutic power ARVs also cause a considerable array of side effects, pose new burdens through their lifelong intake, and ultimately fail to satisfy patients' most profound longing for a complete cure.

Even in times of ART, the biomedically declared incurability of HIV/AIDS leaves ample space for a polyphonic concert of healing promises from religious and traditional healers, and patients readily embark on the search for a cure in other terrains than the biomedical. The impact of an expected or subjectively experienced cure is most striking when patients interrupt their biomedical therapies and it is hardly imaginable that these cases will cease as long as science cannot provide a complete cure.

As was demonstrated, government interference, regulation, and standardization of traditional medicine were restricted to the area where healers' epistemologies coincided with the biomedical, and HIV research was exclusively understood as a search for effective *materia medica*. Moreover, the government's 'mixed messaging' (cf. Doran 2007: 404) in the context of the Loliondo phenomenon made evident that even though the official discourse of governmental bodies may be the separation of scientifically verifiable *materia medica* from their religious contexts of meaning and the personal powers of healing figures (cf. Langwick 2011: 80), their individual personnel may nevertheless resort to these same 'non-scientific' healing methods in the search for relief from their afflictions. Epistemological divides, in this case, remain restricted to theory. Economic aspects may equally influence decisions regarding governmental interference in the sphere of traditional or religious healing, in addition to calculations about the extent to which a prominent healer figure poses a threat to governmental authority.

For most people living with HIV/AIDS, the complex entanglements of varying actors' interests in the quest for a cure are as untransparent as their strategies to secure therapeutic authority. Scientific evidence of certain healing practices is often not available, while for many it is also not fully comprehensible or simply not relevant. Patients' health seeking behaviour may thus be informed by mainly pragmatic calculations but could also be a search for meaning and more profound redemption in a situation of permanent – not only medical – crisis. Healers and prophets – be they self or externally constructed – will remain important figures and avenues for troubled persons in these troubled times. It remains to be seen how (if at all) their role will change if and when a definite biomedical cure for HIV/AIDS becomes available, a development that will hopefully do away with at least one major misfortune of people living with HIV/AIDS in Tanga and other parts of the world.

References

Balogun, A. 2010. Islamic perspectives on HIV/AIDS and antiretroviral treatment: The case of Nigeria. *African Journal of AIDS Research*, 9(4), 459–66.

Becker, F. 2009a. Competing explanations and treatment choices: Muslims, AIDS and ARVs in Tanzania, in *AIDS and Religious Practice in Africa*, edited by F. Becker and P.W. Geissler. Leiden and Boston, MA: Brill, 155–89.

Becker F. 2009b. Ethical self-fashioning and living with ARVs: Open questions. Paper to the Conference: 'Prolonging life, challenging religion' of the International Research Network Religion and HIV/AIDS in Africa, Lusaka, Zambia, 15–17 April 2009.

Bednarowski, M. 2005. 'Our work is change for the sake of justice': Hope community, Minneapolis, Minnesota, in *Religion and Healing in America*, edited by L. Barnes and S. Sered. Oxford: Oxford University Press, 195–215.

Burchardt, M. 2009. Subjects of counseling: Religion, HIV/AIDS and the management of everyday life in South Africa, in *AIDS and Religious Practice in Africa*, edited by F. Becker and P.W. Geissler. Leiden and Boston, MA: Brill, 333–58.

Comaroff, J. and Comaroff, J. 1993. *Modernity and its Malcontents*. Chicago, IL: University of Chicago Press.

Dilger, H. 2005. *Leben mit AIDS. Krankheit, Tod und soziale Beziehungen in Afrika*. Frankfurt a.M.: Campus.

Dilger, H. 2007. Healing the wounds of modernity: Community, salvation and care in a Neo-pentecostal church in Dar es Salaam, Tanzania. *Journal of Religion in Africa*, 37(1), 59–83.

Dilger, H., Burchardt, M. and van Dijk, R. 2010. Introduction. The redemptive moment: HIV treatment and the production of new religious spaces. *African Journal of AIDS Research*, 9(4), 373–83.

Doran, M. 2007. Reconstructing *Mchape* '95: AIDS, Billy Chisupe, and the politics of persuasion. *Journal of Eastern African Studies*, 1(3), 397–416.

Johnson, D. and Anderson, D. (eds) 1995. *Revealing Prophets: Prophecy in Eastern African History*. London: James Currey.

Kalipeni, E., Muula, A. and Liwewe, O. 2009. HIV and religion in Africa: The politics of treatment and prevention in a changing religious landscape. Paper to the Conference: 'Prolonging life, challenging religion' of the International Research Network Religion and HIV/AIDS in Africa, Lusaka, Zambia, 15–17 April 2009.

Kwansa, B. 2010. Complex negotiations: 'Spiritual' therapy and living with HIV in Ghana. *African Journal of AIDS Research*, 9(4), 449–58.

Langwick, S. 2011. *Bodies, Politics, and African Healing: The Matter of Maladies in Tanzania*. Bloomington, IN: Indiana University Press.

Malebo, H. and Mbwambo Z. 2011. *Technical Report on Miracle Cure Prescribed by Rev. Ambilikile Mwasupile in Samunge village, Loliondo, Arusha*. Dar es Salaam: National Institute for Medical Research.

Mattes, D. 2011. 'We are just supposed to be quiet': The production of adherence to Antiretroviral treatment in urban Tanzania. *Medical Anthropology*, 30(2), 158–82.

Mattes, D. 2012. 'I am also a human being!': antiretroviral treatment in local moral worlds. *Anthropology and Medicine*, 19(1), 75–84.

Nguyen, V.-K. 2009. Therapeutic evangelism: Confessional technologies, antiretrovirals and biospiritual transformation in the fight against AIDS in West Africa, in *AIDS and Religious Practice in Africa*, edited by F. Becker and P.W. Geissler. Leiden and Boston, MA: Brill, 359–78.
Oosthuizen, G. 1992. *The Healer-Prophet in Afro-Christian Churches*. Leiden: Brill.
Probst, P. 1995. *Mchape* '95, or, the sudden fame of Billy Goodson Chisupe: Healing, social memory, and the enigma of the public sphere in post-Banda Malawi. *Africa*, 69(1), 108–38.
Ranger, T. 1992. Plagues of beasts and men: Prophetic responses to epidemics in eastern and southern Africa, in *Epidemics and Ideas: Essays on the Historical Perception of Pestilence*, edited by T. Ranger and P. Slack. Cambridge: Cambridge University Press, 241–68.
Rasing, T. 2007. The role of Christianity in the context of HIV/AIDS: Dealing with HIV/AIDS in Pentecostal and mainstream churches in Zambia. *Word and Context*, 6, 33–50.
Schoffeleers, M. 1999. The AIDS pandemic, the prophet Billy Chisupe, and the democratization process in Malawi. *Journal of Religion in Africa*, 29(4), 406–41.
Ter Haar, G. 1992. *Spirit of Africa: The Healing Ministry of Archbishop Milingo of Zambia*. Trenton, NJ: Africa World Press.
Tocco, J. 2010. 'Every disease has its cure': Faith and HIV therapies in Islamic northern Nigeria. *African Journal of AIDS Research*, 9(4), 385–95.
Togarasei, L. 2010. Christian theology of life, death and healing in an era of antiretroviral therapy: Reflections on the responses of some Botswana churches. *African Journal of AIDS Research*, 9(4), 429–35.
United Republic of Tanzania 2002. *The Traditional and Alternative Medicines Act*. Dar es Salaam.
Van Dijk, R. 2009. Gloves in times of AIDS: Pentecostalism, hair, and social distancing in Botswana, in *AIDS and Religious Practice in Africa*, edited by F. Becker and P.W. Geissler. Leiden and Boston, MA: Brill, 283–306.
Wallace, A. 1956. Revitalization movements. *American Anthropologist*, New Series, 58(2), 264–81.
Weber, M. 1974. *On Charisma and Institution Building: Selected Papers*, edited by S.N. Eisenstadt. Chicago, IL: University of Chicago Press.

Newspaper Articles

An-Nuur
2011 Siku ilipoingia Samunge kwa Babu, 3–9 June a.
2011 Uso kwa uso na Babu Loliondo, 3–9 June b.
2011 Wachungaji Loliondo kwa Babu wacharuka, 1–7 July.

Business Week
2011 HIV/AIDS cure: Where is the truth? (by Yakobe Chiwambo), 13–19 May.

Daily News
2011 'Magic cure' seekers controlled, 11 March.
2011 Medics doubt efficacy of Loliondo herb on HIV, 18 March.
2011 No child yet? Go to 'Babu' (by Marc Nkwame), 20 June.
2011 Loliondo miracle herb still investigated, 1 July.

Guardian on Sunday
2011 How thousands will initially consult the Loliondo cleric, then go to early grave (by Any Jozen), 13 March.
2011 Tricky balancing between secular medicine, divine healing… (by Wilson Kaigarula), 13 March.
2011 This is a golden chance – Shelukindo (by Rodgers Luhwago), 13 March.
2011 The magic man, the tree and a cup of life (by Richard Mgamba), 27 March.
2011 Loliondo's new billionaires (by Jack Mikaili), 27 March.
2011 Samunge is not it … But there are many reasons to promote a lie (by Pat Patten), 29 June.

Habari Leo
2011 Wataalamu: Kikombe cha 'Babu' ni kinga bomba (by Gloria Tesha), 6 May.
2011 Babu wa Loliondo apewa cheti maalumu (by John Mhala), 11 May.

Majira
2011 Waganga wa jadi wanaojitangaza hawana uwezo wa kutibu (by Lilian Justice), 26 May.

Mwananchi
2011 Daktari: Mgonjwa Loliondo amepona UKIMWI, 14 March.
2011 Serikali kutoa tamko ya tiba la Loliondo leo, 26 March.
2011 Hospitali nne kuchunguza dawa ya Babu (by Mussa Juma and Claude Mshana), 30 April.
2011 Mchungaji Mwasapila apinga dawa yake iwe ya vidonge (by Mussa Juma), 1 May.
2011 Waliofariki Samunge wafikia 92 (by Mussa Juma and Moses Mashalah), 14 May.

Mtanzania
2011 'Babu' Loliondo arusha kombora (by Eliya Mbonea), 16 May.
2011 Babu akana kuwa sangoma (by Eliya Mbonea), 17 May.
2011 Wafanyabiashara wakimbia Samunge (by Eliya Mbonea), 13 July.

Nipashe
2011 Babu asitisha tiba Loliondo, 21 March.
2011 TFDA yasafisha dawa ya Babu, 29 March.
2011 Mamilioni aliyokusania Babu Loliondo yatajwa, 31 March.
2011 Babu aitaka serikali kujiandaa kupokea wageni wengi toka nje (by Asraji Mvungi), 7 May.
2011 Madaktari: Tiba ya Babu imeleta maafa Cosmas Mlekani, (by Cosmas Mlekani), 25 August.
2011 Serikali kutolea tamko rasmi dawa ya Babu wa Loliondo (by Richard Makore), 31 August 2011.

Nyakati
2011 Kulola sasa adai Babu katumwa na jinni (by Alex Mwachali), 3–9 June.

Sani
2011 Mtikila kumburuza Babu wa Loliondo mahakamani, 20–22 July.

Tanzania Daima
2011 Babu wa taifa waokoe watanzania wanaumwa (by Christopher Nyenyembe)
2011 Milioni 3 wanywa kikombe Loliondo (by David Frank), 9 May.

The African
2011 Needed: Protection to Pastor Ambilikile (by Gazpar Hiza), 11 May.

The Citizen
2011 Woman who set off the rush for the 'drink' (by Tom Mosoba), 13 March.
2011 Foundation says Mwasapila has not been saying the truth (by Frederick Katulanda), 19 April.
2011 Survey: 59pc of Tanzanians believe in Mwasapila 'cure', 4 August.
2011 Hospital closes tuberculosis ward for lack of patients, 17 September.

The Guardian
2011 'Miracle cure' herbalist's services halted, 10 March.
2011 Loliondo cup: Pact with God or the devil? (by Ani Jozen), 26 March.

2011 Retired pastor suspends services to new patients (by Lusekelo Philemon), 28 March.

2011 COSTECH: Trademark for 'Babu' cure on the way (by Lydia Shekighenda), 1 April.

2011 Government's silence over 'Babu's cure' worries stakeholders (by Lydia Shekighenda), 21 April.

Ukweli na Uwazi

2011 Babu kortini (by Makongoro Going), 16–22 August 2011

PART III
Emergent Organizational Forms in Times of ART

Chapter 8

Societal Dynamics, State Relations, and International Connections: Influences on Ghanaian and Zambian Church Mobilization in AIDS Treatment[1]

Amy S. Patterson

Introduction

In recent years, donors, scholars, and civil society activists have paid greater attention to the role of churches in the response to HIV and AIDS (Marshall and van Saanen 2007). This chapter compares Ghanaian and Zambian church mobilization on HIV/AIDS, with a focus on access to anti-retroviral treatment (ART). In 2009, Zambia's HIV rate was 14 per cent and Ghana's was 1.9 per cent. Even with its relatively low HIV rate, only about 40 per cent of HIV-positive Ghanaians who needed ART were accessing it in 2009, compared to almost 70 per cent of Zambians (UNAIDS 2010a; Ministry of Health, National AIDS Council, and UNAIDS 2011). Despite this situation, church and civil society demands for ART provision in Ghana have been much more muted than in Zambia. Using societal, state, and international-level explanations, this chapter analyses why interest in HIV/AIDS had declined in Ghana by the mid 2000s, but had strengthened in Zambia, and why church involvement in ART access has been less apparent in Ghana than Zambia. The article then takes the Zambia case one step further to investigate what effect HIV and AIDS activities have had on Zambian churches since 2005.

This chapter examines the church responses to AIDS at two historical junctures. The first is the period between roughly 2003 and 2010 when ART became widely available in many African countries. While not all Africans who needed ART medication could access it in 2010, the number of Africans with access had increased at least tenfold from 2002. In that year, only 2 per cent of

[1] An earlier version of this chapter appeared in the *African Journal of AIDS Research* (AJAR) 9/4 (2010), in a special section on religion and antiretroviral therapy. Permission to reprint – in part or in whole – from that publication was kindly granted by AJAR.

Africans who needed ART could obtain the life-saving medications; by 2008, the figure was 44 per cent (Africa Health Dialogue 2010). Most of the chapter deals with this period. The Ghana case shows how churches grappled with the new emphasis placed on biomedical solutions to AIDS instead of behavioural or moral messages. The second historical juncture encompasses the routinization of ART treatment, and the chapter's final section on church HIV/AIDS activities on Zambia in 2011 is situated within that period. During this time, churches have worked to administer ART programmes, urge patient adherence, and maintain continued financial commitment among donors and African governments.

Churches as Political Actors

I treat churches as institutions, or structures with resources, members, rules, histories, leaders, procedures for making decisions, and formal and informal norms (North 1990: 3). Church efforts on HIV/AIDS are political, because they shape formal and informal decision-making on resource allocation and they influence acceptance of particular values. Churches use various sources of power, from tangible assets like constituencies, expertise, and material resources, to intangible sources such as moral authority and symbols. Because African political life is 'inextricably bound up with religious belief,' (Jenkins 2007: 162) and because churches may sidestep formal government processes through alliances with external actors such as donors, they can implicitly shape political decisions (Ellis and ter Haar 1998).

This work is divided into six parts. I first explain my methodology. Next, I provide background on each country's HIV/ AIDS efforts. Third, I examine differences in church involvement on HIV/AIDS and ART. The fourth section analyses how societal, state, and international factors help elucidate church HIV/AIDS activities. Fifth, the chapter investigates the long-term effects of Zambian HIV/AIDS activities for church legitimacy, church-donor relations, and church-state power. The conclusion raises questions for future research.

Methodology

I incorporate the comparative case study methodology to investigate the factors that shape church activities on HIV and AIDS. Highlighting variations between the country cases challenges the conventional wisdom that churches act either as obstacles or unsung heroes in the HIV/AIDS response (Dilger 2007). While my approach of examining churches within a particular state context may risk 'seeing like a state' and leaving out cross-national movements or subaltern voices

(Scott 1998), it also facilitates analysis of church-state dynamics within certain political and historical contexts.

I chose Zambia and Ghana for this study because they have very different HIV rates, a fact that allows me to investigate how the larger disease environment may affect church HIV/AIDS activities. Also, although the populations of both are majority Christian, the size of these majorities differs: roughly 82 per cent of Zambians and 55 per cent of Ghanaians are Christian (Barrett, Kurian, and Johnson 2001). This factor may affect the nature of church involvement on HIV/AIDS. Third, the countries differ in the ultimate outcome I am trying to explain: church HIV/AIDS mobilization on ART access.

The countries also are similar, a fact that limits alternative explanations for church HIV/AIDS mobilization. Poverty affects both countries (UNDP 2008a; UNDP 2008b).[2] Both experienced democratic transitions during the 1990s, although freedom of expression, rule of law, and competitive elections are more extensive in Ghana than Zambia (Freedom House 2008a, Freedom House 2008b). Both have diverse Christian populations, including mainline Protestants, Catholics, Pentecostals, and African Initiated Churches (AICs) (Lumbe 2008; Gifford 2004: 25–7).

Data for this work come from news articles, government documents, donor reports, and over 100 semi-structured interviews conducted in Accra in 2008 and in Lusaka in 2007 and 2011. I chose interviewees based on their affiliation with AIDS organizations that I identified through newspaper articles and reports. While I focused on churches, I also interviewed secular AIDS activists, government representatives, and bilateral and multilateral donor officials in order to situate church activities in a broader context. I acknowledge that the work does not include analysis of the activities of AICs. Interviewees were predominantly from Catholic, mainline Protestant, and Pentecostal churches. While some AICs are involved with HIV and AIDS, most activities tended to revolve around the old mission churches and the new urban Pentecostal churches.

Interviewees were asked about the factors that shaped church mobilization, church-state relations, societal perceptions of the disease, and church-donor relations. Interviews in Zambia in 2011 also asked about long-range programme development and church interest in HIV and AIDS. Because I wanted interviewees to share honest opinions about this politically and theologically sensitive topic, I assured them of anonymity in publications. To ensure accuracy, I verified facts through other interviews, news articles, and reports.

---

2 In 2005, 68 per cent of Zambians lived below the poverty line, while 39.5 per cent of Ghanaians did (UNDP 2008a; UNDP 2008b).

National Efforts to Address HIV and AIDS

Although the first AIDS cases appeared in the two countries at roughly the same time (1984 in Zambia and 1986 in Ghana), the countries have differed in their approaches to the disease. The first difference is each country's focal point in the HIV/AIDS response. Ghana has concentrated on AIDS awareness through media campaigns that inform people about HIV prevention. In 2008, when the Ghana research was completed, Ghana emphasized HIV testing. In 2009, only 6.8 per cent of Ghanaian females and 4.1 per cent of males had been tested, compared to 15.4 per cent of Zambians (UNAIDS 2010a; UNAIDS 2010b). In contrast, Zambia's higher HIV rate has led it to focus on HIV prevention, care, support, ART access, and improved health-care capacity (Makwiza et al. 2006; UNAIDS 2010a). Churches have been extremely involved in these actions in Zambia, unlike in Ghana.

A second difference is each country's approach to ART access. In 2004, the Zambian government declared AIDS to be a national emergency, an action that enabled it to begin providing free ART in 2005. In 2006, the Zambian government removed user fees at all private and public health facilities to increase ART uptake (Moszynski 2006). In 2002, Ghana used US Agency for International Development (USAID) funds to introduce ART into select health-care centres. While the number of sites with ART increased to over 100 in 2008, many of these clinics, such as the Fevers Unit at Accra's Korle Bu Hospital, segregate ART programmes (*Daily Graphic*, 18 November 2008; AIDS NGO leader, 14 October 2008, Accra). Unlike in Zambia, as of 2009, ART in Ghana was not completely free; patients paid roughly 5 GHC per month for treatment, while the National Health Insurance Programme covered the remaining costs (AIDS NGO leader, 30 November 2008, Accra; UNAIDS 2010a). In both Ghana and Zambia HIV testing and prevention-of-mother-to-child transmission programmes are free (UNAIDS 2010a; UNAIDS 2010b).

Third, social mobilization for treatment has been less political in Ghana than Zambia. Ghana's treatment movement began in 2002 when the Ghana AIDS Treatment Access Group demanded that Coca Cola Bottling Company provide free ART to its HIV-positive workers. While the campaign gained publicity, many Ghanaians perceived it to be confrontational. More recently, newer groups such as Youth Activists Against AIDS and the National Association of People Living with HIV/AIDS have emerged to urge treatment literacy, although their demands for free ART have been limited and their criticisms of government, muted (multilateral donor, 8 October 2008, Accra). Churches have not participated in these efforts. Instead they have worked alongside the Ghana AIDS Network, an umbrella organization which has accessed donor and government funds and rarely has challenged government policies (Haven and Patterson 2007).

In contrast, the Network of Zambian People Living with HIV/AIDS, a group founded in 1996 to provide support for HIV-positive people, organized mass marches and helped place ART access on Zambia's political agenda (*IPS Inter Press Service*, 13 November 2003). Since 2006, the group has demanded that the government provide high quality ART programmes in public clinics (*Kaiser Daily HIV/AIDS Report*, 17 February 2006). But as in Ghana, the Zambian treatment movement has become increasingly fragmented, particularly after the Treatment Action Literacy Campaign formed in 2005. As a result, and because some of the biggest service providers in Zambia are faith-based, organizations of people living with HIV have been somewhat side lined in AIDS policymaking (government official, 14 August 2007, Lusaka; AIDS NGO official, 17 August 2007, Lusaka; multilateral donor, 23 February 2011, Lusaka).

A fourth difference between the countries lies in the structure of external funding for HIV and AIDS. By structure I mean *where* money comes from, *who* receives it, its *magnitude*, and *changes* in funding over time. As of 2009, 84 per cent of Ghana's AIDS funding and 85 per cent of Zambia's came from external sources (UNAIDS 2008b; UNAIDS 2008e; UNAIDS 2010a). A look at the two biggest HIV/AIDS money sources – the Global Fund to Fight AIDS, Tuberculosis and Malaria (Global Fund) and the US President's Emergency Plan for AIDS Relief (PEPFAR) – reveals additional country differences. Zambia gets money from a wider variety of donors, including PEPFAR. In contrast, most of Ghana's money for HIV/AIDS comes from the Global Fund and bilateral donors, though in 2010 the country did receive $13 million from PEPFAR (Global Health Facts 2011).

Another difference is in who the recipients of this incoming money are. In terms of Global Fund grants, the Ministry of Health has received approximately $42 million of the $61 million Ghana has gotten (Global Fund 2011a). In contrast, two non-state actors in Zambia – the Churches Health Association of Zambia and the Zambia National AIDS Network – and one international organization – the United Nations Development Programme – have received sizeable sums from the Global Fund. Between 2004 and 2011, these grants amounted to roughly $119.7 million to the Churches Health Association of Zambia, $62.9 million to the Zambia National AIDS Network, and $81 million to the United Nations Development Programme. In contrast, Zambia's Ministry of Health received $40 million (Global Fund 2011b).

The magnitude of these donations differs between the countries. Between 2004 and 2010 Zambia received over $1.34 billion from PEPFAR and $332 million from the Global Fund, while Ghana received roughly $61 million from the Global Fund (PEPFAR 2007, 2008, 2009a, 2009b; Global Health 2011; Global Fund 2011a, 2011b). These numbers meant that in 2006 alone (the last year of data), Zambia spent roughly $260 million on HIV/AIDS; in comparison, Ghana spent $38 million in 2007 (UNAIDS 2010a; UNAIDS 2010b).

Over time, funding has changed in each country. Zambia's amounts increased between 2003 and 2010, mostly because of the surge in PEPFAR money from $70 million in 2004 to $277 million in 2010. While Ghana in 2011 has more funding for AIDS than in 2003, it has experienced recent declines in assistance, particularly between 2007 and 2008. USAID funding to Ghana has vacillated, from $20 million in 2002, to $6.8 million in 2008, to $14 million for 2010 (USAID 2008; USAID 2010).

Church Involvement on HIV/AIDS and ART Access

The differences in each country's HIV/AIDS efforts are echoed in the contrasting ways churches have approached the disease. I compare these efforts in terms of their frames, timing, continuity, engagement with ART, and participation in state policy making institutions.

Ghanaian churches tended to frame HIV and AIDS in terms of moral messages, particularly calls for youth to abstain from pre-marital sex (church AIDS worker, 29 August 2008, Accra). One pastor said that on HIV/AIDS, 'there is no compromise on immorality' (pastor, 12 November 2008, Accra). Support for condoms among church leaders from all denominations was limited (pastor, 27 August 2008, Accra; government official, 8 October 2008, Accra). This morality focus has meant limited attention to support and care programmes for people living with HIV in churches.

In Zambia, pastors wanted youth to abstain from pre-marital sex and they preached marital faithfulness, but some acknowledged that hunger and unemployment drove people to make risky sexual choices (Fikansa 2009; Kelly 2007). By 2007, the national church umbrella organizations – the Council of Churches in Zambia (mainline Protestants), the Evangelical Fellowship of Zambia (primarily Pentecostals), and the Zambia Episcopal Conference (Catholics) – called for a response that framed HIV and AIDS as resulting from underdevelopment and poverty, not solely from 'immoral choices' (church AIDS worker, 15 August 2007, Lusaka; FBO leader, 14 August 2007, Lusaka).

In terms of timing, Ghanaian churches developed an early high level, public advocacy HIV/AIDS campaign in 2000. Low HIV awareness drove the Christian Council of Ghana (the country's oldest and largest Protestant ecumenical body), Catholic bishops, Muslim leaders, and the Ghana AIDS Network to design the 'Compassion Campaign' to educate the public and address stigma, particularly in the religious community (church AIDS worker, 24 September 2008, Accra; church AIDS worker, 2 December 2008, Kumasi). With funding from USAID, the campaign first organized workshops for high-level Christian and Muslim religious leaders. The campaign then held training sessions with 3 000 clergy and lay leaders, and it embarked on a media campaign that urged the public to show compassion toward people living with HIV/AIDS (Compassion Campaign 2002). The Compassion Campaign officially ended in 2003, when USAID began to channel money into other programmes. One study credited the campaign for the decline in negative attitudes about people living with HIV and AIDS between 2001 and 2003 (Boulay, Tweedie, and Fiagbey 2008).

Zambian churches did not engage in a similar early, public AIDS campaign, despite providing care and support to their sick members. As early as 1995, the Zambian government called for churches to do more for HIV education and stigma reduction (*Deutsche Presse-Agentur*, 25 November 1995). Two years after Ghana began its efforts, Zambian Catholic bishops first issued a public letter that challenged the government to address AIDS (*Post* [Zambia], 8 November 2002). In 2005, the country's three ecumenical bodies set up a task force to respond to HIV and AIDS (*Times of Zambia*, 13 October 2005). Churches also pressured the government to remove television ads on condoms which church leaders thought were sexually explicit (church AIDS worker, 13 August 2007, Lusaka). However, these early actions tended to be episodic and reactive, unlike Ghana's coordinated Compassion Campaign. Because Zambian churches were overwhelmed with the high demand for care and support, they had less time for public advocacy (Mukuka and Slonim-Nevo 2006; church pastor, 20 August 2007, Lusaka).

When we examine continuity in church AIDS efforts, Ghanaian church interest has declined since the Compassion Campaign. Recent efforts include local-level HIV education and stigma reduction programmes by the Christian Council and the establishment of voluntary counselling and testing (VCT) centres at urban neo-Pentecostal churches. Several church and secular interviewees criticized church inaction in Ghana. Some point out that churches are unwilling to develop and fund care and support programmes (church AIDS worker, 24 September 2008, Accra). Others believe that the churches do not want to do more than promote compassion, because increased involvement on HIV and AIDS would align churches with people who were infected through 'immoral behaviour' (multilateral donor, 8 October 2008, Accra). Church leaders complain that congregants are 'tired of hearing about AIDS' (church AIDS worker, 29 August 2008, Accra). And perhaps most telling, by 2008, many central figures in the Compassion Campaign no longer worked on HIV/AIDS in Ghana. Some left because of 'burn out,' and others, because they thought AIDS was no longer a dynamic and urgent issue (church AIDS worker, 10 November 2008, Accra).

In contrast, church involvement with AIDS has increased in Zambia. Churches have designed new HIV prevention efforts and developed ART treatment projects, and church home-based care programmes have grown exponentially (UNAIDS 2008c: 66). Some of the larger, urban churches, such as Bread of Life, Northmead Assemblies of God, and Chreso Ministries have developed ART clinics and designed income-generating activities for people with HIV. While churches have 'come quite late' to the advocacy role, they have begun to speak out more on the disease at both the national and local levels (Zambian FBO official, 24 October 2007, Grand Rapids, Michigan).

Zambian and Ghanaian churches differ in their involvement with ART. As of 2008, Ghanaian church advocacy for ART availability was muted. Church inactivity both reflects and causes the limited politicization of treatment in Ghana. Even though some church-related hospitals and clinics provide ART (*Public Agenda*, 10 December, 2007), the level of church support for treatment is unclear. On one hand, Ghanaian churches have signed global ecumenical statements on the need for Africans to have wider access to medicines (*East African Standard*, 12 June 2004). On the other hand, as of 2008, Ghana's national-level ecumenical bodies and its major church health association (Churches Health Association of Ghana) eHeahad not joined the Ecumenical Pharmaceutical Network (EPN), a pan-African church movement to increase availability of medicines. Ghanaian church leaders no doubt resemble other African pastors, who often have little information on ART and in surveys demonstrate some suspicion of ART programmes (EPN 2004, EPN 2008).

In contrast, the three Zambian church mega-organizations and the Churches Health Association of Zambia publicly appealed to the government to provide free ART (*Times of Zambia*, 21 February 2005, *Times of Zambia*, 24 August 2005). In 2006, the Churches Health Association of Zambia worked with bilateral donors, who provided evidence that user fees were hampering ART uptake, to push for the elimination of these fees (bilateral donor, 15 August 2007, Lusaka; FBO leader, 16 August 2007, Lusaka). Since then, church leaders have called for greater food security for people on ART and increased ART access in rural areas (Fikansa 2009). By 2011, church leaders advocated for continuous donor and government attention to and funding for ART (pastor, 17 February 2011, Lusaka).

Finally, the countries' churches differ in their representation and power in each country's two major HIV/AIDS policy institutions: (1) the national AIDS councils; and (2) the Global Fund-mandated Country Coordinating Mechanisms. Since 2003, Ghana's five church umbrella organizations – the Christian Council, Catholic Secretariat, Pentecostal Council, Council for Independent Churches, and Traditional Healers' Association – have had representation on the Ghana AIDS Commission Steering Committee, which makes day-to-day policy decisions (government official, 10 October 2008, Accra). Despite widespread representation, it appears that Ghanaian churches act as relatively weak veto players and not policy instigators on the Ghana AIDS Commission. They have had limited effect when they have sought to change some AIDS policies, particularly on condoms (government official, 10 October 2008, Accra).

In Zambia, church representation on the National HIV/AIDS/STI/TB Council (National AIDS Council) is more contentious and less representative, but more effective than it is in Ghana (church AIDS worker, 15 August 2007, Lusaka; FBO worker, 14 August 2007, Lusaka). Churches with active HIV/AIDS programmes, the Zambian Interfaith Networking Group on HIV/AIDS, and the Churches Health Association of Zambia have official representation on the National AIDS Council. However, the three national ecumenical bodies do not have representation, except through Churches Health Association of Zambia. Since 2008, the chairman of the National AIDS Council has been the charismatic Bishop Joshua Banda, senior pastor at the 2,000-member Northmead Assemblies of God Church in Lusaka. Interviewees confirmed that church leaders and the Churches Health Association of Zambia play a large role in consultation on government AIDS policy making (bilateral donor, 15 August 2007, Lusaka; FBO worker, 14 August 2007, Lusaka).

A second policy institution is the Country Coordinating Mechanism, or the decision-making entity which applies for and oversees Global Fund grants. The churches are represented on these national-level committees through their health-care associations, the Churches Health Association of Ghana and the Churches Health Association of Zambia. Governments in both countries pay the salaries of health workers at clinics and hospitals associated with these health organizations, which provide 42 per cent of Ghana's total health care and 30 per cent of Zambia's (WHO 2005; CHAG 2005; UNAIDS 2008c).

The Churches Health Association of Zambia and the Churches Health Association of Ghana differ in their influence in HIV/AIDS decision-making. As a principal recipient of Global Fund money, the Churches Health Association of Zambia can control the HIV/AIDS resources that go to denominations, congregations, and faith-based organizations. Because the Churches Health Association of Zambia can set health priorities through its funding decisions, the government listens to it in decision-making (FBO official, 16 August 2007, Lusaka; bilateral donor, 15 August 2007, Lusaka). On the other hand, the Churches Health Association of Ghana is not a principal recipient of Global Fund money and must rely on allocations from the Ministry of Health and the Ghana AIDS Commission, a fact which limits its autonomy and influence.

Why These Differences?

To elucidate the factors that explain these different patterns in church AIDS involvement in the two countries, I focus on societal, state, and international levels. This multi-level analytical tool recognizes the complex and interconnected variables that shape outcomes.

The Societal Level of Analysis

The consequences of AIDS stigma, each country's religious composition, and the nature of civil society partly explain church action on AIDS and ART access in each country. Defined as discriminatory actions toward the HIV-positive person, stigma may lead to public shaming, ostracism, and denial of services such as health care, housing, or employment. For the HIV-positive person, these actions (or fear of them) may cause psychological stress, loss of identity, self-blame, secrecy about sero-status, and reluctance to seek ART (Mwinituo and Mill 2006; Nyblade et al. 2003). Stigma may cause HIV-positive church members to leave their Christian fellowship and HIV-negative members to deny fellowship or communion to the infected person.

While the AIDS stigma affects both countries, its impact on church AIDS activities in Ghana is more pernicious. Ghanaians commented that both self-stigma and external stigma are very high, partly because of cultural understandings which label sexually transmitted diseases as disgraceful. Many Ghanaians stress that spiritual forces punish those who are promiscuous (Asamoah-Gyadu 2005). Stigma leads to widespread secrecy and fear about AIDS; caregivers often hide their HIV-positive patients (Mwinituo and Mill 2006), and many Ghanaians refuse to be tested for HIV. As a result, even with increased availability of ART, AIDS deaths in Ghana increased between 2001 and 2007 (UNAIDS 2008a).

Research demonstrates that stigma tends to be higher in communities with low HIV prevalence (Zukoski and Thorburn 2009). Ghana's low prevalence means most people never encounter someone with AIDS (Afrobarometer 2004). The decline in Ghana's HIV prevalence from 3.3 per cent in 2003 to 1.9 per cent in 2007 also made citizens complacent because they thought the country had successfully combated HIV and AIDS (multilateral donor, 8 October 2008, Accra; UNAIDS 2008a). The increase to 2.9 per cent in 2009 did not seem to increase concern about HIV infection among the general population (UNAIDS 2010a). Because other conditions such as malaria, diarrheal disease, maternal mortality, heart disease, and cancer have a large impact on Ghana, some health and church officials complained that HIV and AIDS had already gotten more attention than it warrants (church AIDS worker, 10 November 2008, Accra; pastor, 27 August 2008, Accra; *Daily Graphic*, 23 October 2008; *Ghanaian Times*, 13 October 2008; *Daily Graphic*, 6 November 2008).

Fear and stigma may have pushed Ghanaian churches to act early on HIV/AIDS and to justify compassion to HIV-positive people, 'so that they won't wilfully infect other people' (church AIDS worker, 2 September 2008, Accra). Stigma and the low prevalence also have meant church-sponsored care programmes for HIV-positive congregants are rare, a situation which reinforces stigma since church members do not gain personal exposure to people with the disease. Stigma and complacency hampered church public discussion of HIV and AIDS and mobilization on ART access (pastor, 2 December 2008, Kumasi).

In contrast, groups such as the Network of Zambian People Living with HIV/AIDS combat AIDS discrimination and self-stigma (AIDS NGO, 20 August 2007, Lusaka). Churches also have helped to challenge stigma (Nyblade et al. 2003). Pentecostal mega-churches, such as Bread of Life International and the Northmead Assemblies of God started AIDS support groups and programmes (church AIDS worker, 14 August 2007, Lusaka; pastor, 14 August 2007, Lusaka; Ndhlovu 2007).[3] Because the HIV rate in Zambia has remained relatively steady, AIDS continues to be an issue that concerns many citizens and directly affects families (church AIDS worker, 11 March 2011, Lusaka; Afrobarometer 2004).[4]

As stigma has declined in Zambia, churches have expanded their HIV/AIDS work. Because the epidemic pervades society, churches have had to look beyond HIV prevention messages to develop broader programmes in care, support, ART access, and impact mitigation. Some of the aforementioned churches, as well as Catholic and Protestant clinics, now provide treatment. In contrast to Ghana, the expansion of ART access has meant AIDS deaths in Zambia declined between 2001 and 2007 (UNAIDS 2008d).

Ghana and Zambia also differ somewhat in their religious environments, with Ghana's Christian majority being smaller than Zambia's. Since Muslims make up roughly 15 per cent of Ghana's population, there has been greater inter-religious collaboration on HIV and AIDS such as through the Compassion Campaign (US Department of State 2011; church AIDS worker, 21 October 2008, Accra). Church leaders in Ghana seemed more conscious than their Zambian counterparts about the need to reach out to Muslims (church AIDS worker, 2 December 2008, Kumasi). In contrast, Christian churches dominate the Zambian religious scene. Although there has been the development of the Zambia Interfaith Networking Group on HIV/AIDS, it appears that some of the major players on HIV and AIDS service delivery and policymaking remain the churches and increasingly, the Pentecostal churches. The dominance of Christian voices in public decision-making drove former President Chiluba to declare Zambia to be a 'Christian nation', a phrase which was then written into the country's constitution (Ranger 2008). This Christian involvement in the public sphere may have made it easier for churches to play a more prominent role in HIV/AIDS policymaking and programme development.

---

[3] Information on these churches is available at http://www.blci.info and http://www.northmeadassembly.org.

[4] There has been a slight decrease in Zambia's prevalence from 15.2 per cent in 2007 (UNAIDS 2008d). Despite this fact, the perception is that HIV/AIDS is a disease that affects many people (AIDS community worker, 19 May 2011, Kitwe).

A final contrast between the two countries is in the composition of civil society. Ghanaian civil society has a relatively high level of participation from well-educated professionals in law, academics, and the church. Ghana has significantly more of its citizens living in North America and Europe than Zambia does (UNDP 2009a 2009b), and Ghanaian civil society leaders have used these links to connect to international NGOs and UN agencies (Gifford 1998).[5] Also there tend to be strong networks between elites in civil society and state officials (Gifford 2004).

Ghana's well-organized churches with highly educated, cosmopolitan leaders could act relatively early and coherently in the Compassion Campaign. Civil society leaders' relative distance from Ghana's impoverished citizens may have caused churches to focus more on HIV/AIDS awareness and less on care, support, and treatment. Some interviewees criticized churches for not representing the voices of people living with HIV, and for avoiding the difficult issues that surround the epidemic, such as gender-based violence and poverty (pastor, 4 December 2008, Accra; AIDS NGO, 14 October 2008, Accra). Elite dominance in civil society also may have led the churches to become less concerned about HIV and AIDS over time, particularly if the disease was no longer viewed as a threat to the urban, middle class (church AIDS worker, 10 November 2008, Accra).

Unlike in Ghana, trade unions have played a large role in Zambian politics, making civil society a heterogeneous collective of working-class individuals, business professionals, church leaders, students, and lawyers. In general, Zambian civil society leaders have fewer ties to the West, academics have played a smaller role in associational life, and civil society has become increasingly divided over politics (Bartlett 2000). Zambia's three church mega-organizations are less organized and globally connected than those in Ghana (Phiri 2001). Personal networks between the churches and state officials also have changed since independence, leading to periods of church-state tension and cooperation (Freston 2001).

The relative weakness and heterogeneity of Zambian civil society meant that a high-level, coordinated church response occurred later and that churches tended to frame HIV and AIDS in terms of poverty, to develop broad efforts, and to urge ART access. More negatively, divisions in civil society led to uneven representation on the country's National AIDS Council, with Pentecostals having a larger voice than mainline Protestant leaders. As a result some church leaders complained that churches gained a seat on the National AIDS Council and access to AIDS resources because of political connections (church AIDS

---

[5] Ghana's share of total stock of emigrants in Europe is 20 percent and in North America, 22 per cent. For Zambia, these numbers are.06 per cent for Europe and.02 per cent for North America (UNDP 2009a, 2009b).

worker, 15 August 2007, Lusaka; church AIDS worker, 14 August 2007, Lusaka). The churches have been divided about how to interact with the government on a variety of socioeconomic development issues (inter-faith development worker, 30 March 2011, Lusaka; pastor, 21 May 2011, Ndola).

The implications of these societal-level findings are twofold. First, the effects of stigma in the Ghana case show how norms, beliefs, and values influence social mobilization. Despite some well-designed and well-intentioned church HIV and AIDS efforts, beliefs about spiritual causes for disease made mobilization difficult. While Ghanaian churches had high initial interest in the disease, the larger societal context made it difficult to sustain that interest. Second, African civil society is limited in its ability to urge and sustain policy changes that benefit Africa's poorest citizens. Even though civil society in each country experienced different obstacles (in Ghana, its elite dominance, in Zambia, its divisions), the outcome of civil society's weakness was that church HIV/AIDS activities were reactionary, contradictory, or short-lived. In Ghana, this led to a decline in church HIV and AIDS activities. In Zambia, this meant that HIV/AIDS responses occurred later. By 2011, it also meant that divisions among churches over church-state relations and access to donor funds led to duplication in HIV/AIDS efforts.

The State Level of Analysis

In both countries, churches have become more politically involved since they helped to facilitate the democratic transitions of the early 1990s (Ranger 2008; Gifford 1998). After 1992, church-state relations in Ghana have been relatively congenial (Gifford 1998: 68–72). Ghanaian churches have not publicly exhibited political divisions, although a few church leaders have indirectly challenged other churches' silence on corruption (*Ghanaian Times*, 23 September 2008), and the church-state relationship has become more institutionalized, through overlapping personal networks between civil society and state elites. This relationship may have led to church representation on the Ghana AIDS Commission, but it prevented churches from challenging state HIV/AIDS priorities (government official, 10 October 2008, Accra).

The long-term change in the political power and resources of the Ghana AIDS Commission also may have shaped church actions on HIV and AIDS. When it was formed in 2001, the Commission was situated in the president's office. However, by 2008, it had been placed in the relatively weak Ministry of Women and Children. The Commission's power to distribute money also changed with the establishment of the Global Fund, because the Country Coordinating Mechanism distributes Global Fund money primarily to the Ministry of Health. These changes may mean churches with representation on the Ghana AIDS Commission have less political motivation to develop HIV/AIDS efforts or to lobby for greater ART access. This dynamic may change over time, particularly since in 2010 the Ghana AIDS Commission started to receive Global Fund grants (Global Fund 2010a). While this change had the potential to urge greater church interest in the disease, it was unclear that this had occurred by 2011 (Ghanaian scholar of HIV/AIDS, personal communication, 28 September 2011, Oxford, UK).

In contrast, Zambian churches have been more politically divided on a variety of issues, particularly since 2007 when the state organized an assembly to draft a new constitution. Mainline Protestants and Catholics boycotted the constitutional assembly, while several popular Pentecostal pastors joined it (*Times of Zambia*, 12 October 2007, 25 October 2007, 29 November 2007, 8 January 2008). When the resulting constitution failed to be approved by the Zambian Parliament in March 2011, Catholic and mainline Protestant church leaders again criticized the process for wasting millions of dollars (*Church of England Newsletter*, 15 April 2011). Church-state collaboration and confrontation on these explicitly political matters may have affected church participation in HIV/AIDS policy institutions. Church representatives on the country's National AIDS Council (several of whom are Pentecostal pastors) have not publicly challenged the government. Some interviewees asserted that cooperation with the state had increased these Pentecostal pastors' power both on the National AIDS Council and within broader political circles (church development worker, 12 April 2011, Lusaka). While mainline Protestant and Catholic voices could not be ignored, their participation declined in influence (church AIDS worker, 14 August 2007, Lusaka; FBO leader, 20 August 2007, Lusaka).

Since the National AIDS Council reports to the Ministry of Health (NAC 2005), one might assume its institutional weakness would not bolster the power of churches represented on it. Yet, the Council is a crucial actor on HIV/AIDS policy making because it interfaces directly with donors. In 2003, the World Bank, Global Fund, and US government adopted the Three Ones policy, which requires countries to have one national-level HIV/AIDS coordinating authority, one country-level monitoring and evaluation system, and one national HIV/AIDS strategic framework (UNAIDS 2005). Because the National AIDS Council acts as this coordinating authority, representation on the Council heightens a church's prestige and provides opportunity to interact with bilateral and multilateral donors (bilateral donor, 15 August 2007, Lusaka). While the Ghana AIDS Commission plays a similar role in interfacing with donors, since the amount of HIV/AIDS funding Ghana receives is relatively limited, church representation on the Ghana AIDS Commission may not increase church power and interest in HIV/AIDS policy making.

The Country Coordinating Mechanisms also affected church-state dynamics in both countries. In Ghana, this institution reinforced state leadership on HIV and AIDS, since the Ministry of Health was a principal recipient of Global

Fund money and the Churches Health Association of Ghana did not get direct funding. In contrast, as a principal recipient of Global Fund money and as a key member of the Country Coordinating Mechanism, the Churches Health of Zambia had more ability to act autonomously from the state. This meant that the Churches Health Association of Zambia (and its member churches) was able to influence the state on condom advertisements, the provision of free ART, the removal of user fees, and distribution of ART in church settings.

The examination of church HIV/AIDS activities from the state level provides broader lessons on church-state relations in Africa. First, even when some church officials insist their activities are apolitical, their involvement in (or exclusion from) institutions such as the National AIDS Council affects policy decisions and resource allocation. Therefore, churches are political actors. Second, the cases show the fluidity in church-state relations. At times, churches seemed co-opted by the state; at other moments, they appeared to be autonomous. Finally, churches as institutions recognize that access to material resources (particularly for large projects such as HIV/AIDS programmes) requires that the state at least legitimate their activities. Connections to the state matter, because only the state has the 'legal command' to pass policies that address societal issues, and only the state has the international recognition to interface with donors and intergovernmental organizations (Englebert 2009, 7). Hence, while the African state is weak in capacity and political will, churches cannot fully discount it.

The International Level of Analysis

The final level examines three components – global ecumenical organizations, donor resources, and international faith-based organizations and AIDS NGOs – to explain Ghanaian and Zambian church activities on HIV and AIDS. First, although churches in both countries participate in global ecumenical organizations, these ties had more impact on Ghana than Zambia. By 2001, the World Council of Churches, the largest global ecumenical organization, developed its Plan of Action on AIDS in Africa (Kelly 2007; World Council of Churches 2009). This move led Ghanaian churches to act early and to stress awareness and compassion in HIV/AIDS messages, because of the close relations between officials at the Christian Council and the World Council of Churches (church AIDS worker, 21 October 2008, Accra; church AIDS worker, 29 August 2008, Accra). However, as Ghana's prevalence remained low, these efforts were not sufficient to sustain high-level church action or direct challenges to the state on ART access. For Zambian churches, the World Council of Churches provided ideas and technical support on HIV/AIDS mobilization, but the organization was not credited with pushing church efforts (Zambian church leader, 14 February 2008, Nairobi).

Second, the structure of donor resources in both countries affected church HIV and AIDS activities. Early money from USAID in Ghana helped push the Compassion Campaign, but as bilateral donor money decreased, church interest in AIDS declined. (Some interviewees said this correlation showed that churches were just 'on the gravy train,' while others said that churches had to have external money because they alone could not generate the funds needed for continuous AIDS efforts.) (church AIDS worker, 10 November 2008, Accra; church AIDS worker, 4 December 2008, Accra, church AIDS worker, 24 September 2008, Accra). Reliance on the Ghana AIDS Commission or the Ministry of Health for financial resources may have made churches less likely to push for ART access.

In contrast, Zambian churches tapped into increasing amounts of external funding from the Global Fund and PEPFAR. Additionally, they have benefited from international faith-based organizations such as Catholic Relief Services and World Vision, who have gotten millions of dollars from PEPFAR and who partner directly with Zambian churches (FBO worker, 15 August 2007, Lusaka). Donor funds have enabled churches to autonomously develop programmes. Moreover, PEPFAR's target to provide ART to 2 million people in its 15 focus countries by 2008 may have empowered the Churches Health Association of Zambia to advocate for free ART and the end of user fees (Patterson 2006).

Third, as a result of donor programmes, each country has different levels of exposure to the broad 'AIDS industry.' Zambia is inundated with international NGOs, AIDS experts, and AIDS organizations, many of which work closely with churches. More specifically, it has received more money for faith-based organizations from PEPFAR than most African countries; over 15 per cent of PEPFAR money for the country has gone to these groups, while the average for sub-Saharan Africa is roughly 10 per cent (Oomman et al. 2008). Two examples show this global incorporation. World Vision helped Zambian churches form the Expanded Church AIDS Trust, an organization composed primarily of evangelical churches which has received PEPFAR money (UNAIDS 2008c). And Elizabeth Mataka, the leader of the Zambia National AIDS Network (a Global Fund principal recipient), was named the UN Special Envoy on HIV/AIDS to Africa in 2007. This appointment drew attention to the positive role of Zambian civil society organizations in responding to HIV/AIDS (UNAIDS 2007). These international connections helped to sustain church interest and activity on HIV and AIDS. Similar networks are absent in Ghana, primarily because donors and international NGOs have turned their attention to other issues such as malaria eradication (FBO worker, 28 October 2008, Tamale). Even Ghana's associations of people living with HIV are less connected to the global treatment movement than similar groups in Zambia (*UN Wire*, 23 August 2002; AIDS activist, 7 March 2011, Lusaka). The outcome of these different levels of incorporation into global HIV/AIDS efforts is that Zambian churches have been able to sustain mobilization, while Ghanaian churches have become less involved with the disease with time.

Two larger conclusions emerge from these international-level findings. The first is that churches are situated within global networks which influence national- and local-level church priorities. The second is that international connections provide both opportunities and constraints for churches. Donor funds brought churches greater autonomy from the state in Zambia. But donor priorities also shape local- and national-level church activities in ways that churches may not have chosen, as was the case when donors decreased their funding for HIV and AIDS in Ghana over time.

Implications of Greater Involvement on HIV and AIDS for Zambian Churches

Because several Zambian churches have been involved with ART programmes since 2005, it is possible to analyse the effects of this involvement on the churches' role in society, their relations with donors, and their ties to the state. First, ART programmes increased the legitimacy of churches in the poor communities where these clinics were located. Clinic clients appreciated the fact that these facilities tended to be cleaner and less crowded than government clinics, and they thought that staff members were more respectful than staff at government clinics. These perceptions heightened the saliency of the churches in the lives of community members, many of whom were not church members (church clinic client, 2 March 2011, Lusaka; church clinic client, 26 May 2011, Lusaka).

Involvement with ART provision meant churches had moved beyond worship, teaching, and preaching to service provision. Encouraged by increased funding and opportunities after 2004, churches had a more visible presence in the life and health of the country's citizens. But as the number of church-related HIV/AIDS programmes grew, coordination among them remained limited (donor official, 31 March 2011, Lusaka). At times, churches seemed to duplicate what other churches were doing. At other times, there seemed to be underlying tension among churches, particularly as they competed for the finite amount of donor funds (church AIDS organizer, 20 May 2011, Kitwe; inter-faith AIDS worker, 30 March 2011, Lusaka). Thus, while churches had a growing role in the AIDS response, this role was not without controversy.

To make the transition to high levels of service provision, churches also had to become more professional. For example, the ART clinic affiliated with the Northmead Assemblies of God hired 20 staff members, who gained their positions as managers, nurses, and counsellors because of their professional qualifications. But while they were all Christians, only two were church members. Professionalization allowed the clinic to better serve the community, but it created a distance between the clinic and the congregation. Most congregation members who needed ART did not attend the clinic and few volunteered there (clinic official, 26 May 2011, Lusaka). As the clinic faced budgetary pressures in 2011, this distance made it more difficult to raise money within the congregation (clinic board member, 29 April 2011, Lusaka).

Second, greater involvement on HIV/AIDS solidified donor-church ties, as churches often became the implementers of donor projects. Playing the implementer role meant that churches had a limited influence on donors' policies (church AIDS coordinator, 14 August 2007, Lusaka). It also led to financial dependence on donors to continuously fund HIV/AIDS projects, particularly ART provision. Dependence made churches vulnerable, particularly when donor interest in the disease began to wane in 2011. And ties to donors led churches to refocus their programme attention from some of the reasons for initially becoming involved on HIV/AIDS, namely to care for the sick and dying, to meeting donor goals in treatment (Orthodox priest, 9 May 2011, Lusaka). Donors wanted efficiency and high ART adherence rates among clinic clients. In the face of declining funds and a continuous stream of HIV-positive people needing ART medications, church-based clinics began to ration services by limiting the number of new clients (ART clinic counsellor, 12 March 2011, Lusaka).[6]

Finally, the increased role of Zambian churches in ART provision influenced the dynamics in church-state relations. High levels of church involvement were a constant reminder that the state was not 'doing its job' to provide for HIV-positive citizens. Additionally, the proliferation of church-based HIV/AIDS programmes contributed to the growth of civil society, particularly as these groups gained greater donor resources.

In summary, Zambian church mobilization on HIV/AIDS met an important need in society: churches provided care, support, prevention programmes, and ART treatment. Yet as churches became more ingrained in the HIV/AIDS response, they had the potential to lose their religious fervour, to become like any other NGO, and to increasingly compete among themselves for resources and representation (Joshua 2010). The effect of such processes on the long-term development of churches themselves deserves future attention.

Conclusion

As some of the most powerful non-state actors in Africa, churches have played an important role in the HIV/AIDS response. But, as this comparative case study illustrates, their role has varied. In Ghana, churches acted early, but somewhat

6 Because government-affiliated clinics got money from the Global Fund, PEPFAR, and government revenues, they had not reached this point of rationing services in 2011.

narrowly; initial concern over HIV led to AIDS awareness campaigns in the new millennium. However, the persistence of the AIDS stigma, close relations between the state and churches, the churches' limited access to donor resources, and the country's only marginal incorporation into the global AIDS network limited the churches' long-term interest in the epidemic and particularly, ART expansion. Instead of challenging the state on HIV/AIDS and ART access, churches emphasized themes of morality and compassion.

In contrast, Zambian churches were initially slower to act on HIV/AIDS, but a decline in AIDS stigma, direct access to donor resources, increasing donor resources to faith-based organizations, church representation on the National AIDS Council and the Country Coordinating Mechanism, and the country's incorporation into global AIDS networks urged involvement over time. At times, churches bypassed state power or pushed the state to adopt more progressive HIV/AIDS policies, such as free ART. At other times, it appeared the state sought to co-opt churches, such as through selective positions on the National AIDS Council (Zambian church official, 14 February 2008, Nairobi). This involvement had the potential to affect churches, since they became professional organizations and they competed for external resources.

The Ghana and Zambia cases provide larger lessons for students of African politics and society. They show the continued limits of civil society organizations and their dependence on the state or donors, and the cases situate civil society activities in a larger context of social norms and beliefs. Additionally, the chapter illustrates the nuance and fluidity of state-church relations, ties which are situated in a global context with both religious and secular influences. Finally, the neopatrimonial nature of African politics is apparent in the ways access to material resources, personal networks, and representation on state institutions influence the timing, scope, and continuity of church activities on social issues.

This study raises two arenas of future research. First, the cross-country comparisons raise questions about the role of Pentecostal churches in social engagement. In both countries, Pentecostals participated in HIV/AIDS policy making and service delivery, and they accessed funds for HIV and AIDS. Because of their popularity, these churches have influenced HIV/AIDS programmes throughout Africa (Krakauer and Newbery 2007). Yet we know relatively little about how Pentecostals build coalitions with mainline Protestants and Catholics to lobby the state or donors.

The comparisons also raise questions about conventional notions of path dependency. In the roughly 30 years of HIV and AIDS in Africa, new actors such as Pentecostals have become more crucial in policy making and implementation and old actors such as mainline Protestants have declined in influence. Because NGOs, state AIDS institutions, and donor demands emerge, decline, and change, the issue presents continuous opportunities and constraints for churches. The levelling off of PEPFAR funding for ART in Zambia, even as the number of HIV-positive people continues to grow, presents a new scenario to which the country's churches will need to react (church ART clinic officer, 26 May 2011, Lusaka). Scholars must continually evaluate church HIV/AIDS involvement in light of the fluidity of global AIDS politics.

Acknowledgements

Research for this chapter was funded by the Fulbright Africa Scholars Program, the Calvin College Alumni Association, the Center for Social Research, the McGregor Fellowship Program, the Nagel Institute for the Study of World Christianity, the Paul Henry Institute for the Study of Christianity and Politics, and the Calvin College semester in Ghana programme. I am grateful to former Calvin student Michelle Fraser for research assistance.

References

Africa Health Dialogue 2010. *What Are the Prospects of Africa Achieving Universal Access to HIV Treatment?* [Online]. Available at: http://africahealth.wordpress.com/2010/11/22/what-are-the-prospects-of-africa-achieving-universal-access-to-hiv-treatment [accessed: 21 February 2013].

Afrobarometer 2004. *Public Opinion and HIV/AIDS: Facing Up to the Future?* Briefing Paper 12. [Online]. Available at: http://www.afrobarometer.org/publications/afrobarometer-briefing-papers/199-bp-12 [accessed: 21 February 2013].

Asamoah-Gyadu, J.K. 2005. Rethinking African Worldviews of Mystical Causality: Mission and Ecclesiology in the Era of HIV/AIDS. Paper to the World Council of Churches/Trinity Theological Seminary Consultation on Mainstreaming HIV/AIDS in Theological Education, Trinity Theological Seminary, Legon, Ghana, 12–15 June.

Bartlett, D. 2000. Civil Society and Democracy: A Zambian Case Study. *Journal of Southern African Studies*, 26(3), 429–46.

Barrett, D., Kurian, G. and Johnson T. 2001. *World Christian Encyclopedia: A Comparative Survey of Churches and Religions in the Modern World*. New York: Oxford University Press.

Boulay, M., Tweedie, I. and Fiagbey, E. 2008. The Effectiveness of a National Communication Campaign Using Religious Leaders to Reduce HIV-Related Stigma in Ghana. *African Journal of AIDS Research*, 7(1), 133–41.

Christian Health Association of Ghana (CHAG) 2005. *Annual Report*. [Online]. Available at: http://www.chagghana.org/history.htm [accessed: 21 February 2013].

Compassion Campaign 2002. *Notes from Sunyani Training*. Accra: Christian Council of Ghana.

Dilger, H. 2007. Healing the Wounds of Modernity: Salvation, Community and Care in a Neo-Pentecostal Church in Dar Es Salaam, Tanzania. *Journal of Religion in Africa*, 37(1), 59–83.

Ecumenical Pharmaceutical Network (EPN) 2004. *EPN HIV/AIDS Treatment Survey*. [Online]. Available at: http://www.epnetwork.org/index.php/hiv-and-aids-care-and-treatment [accessed: 21 February 2013].

Ecumenical Pharmaceutical Network (EPN) 2008. *Annual Report*. [Online]: Available at: http://www.epnetwork.org [accessed: 21 February 2013].

Ellis, S. and ter Haar, G. 1998. Religion and Politics in Sub-Saharan Africa. *Journal of Modern African Studies*, 36(2), 175–201.

Englebert, P. 2009. *Africa: Unity, Sovereignty, and Sorrow*. Boulder, CO: Lynne Rienner Publishers.

Fikansa, C. 2009. Reflections on the Contradictions of ARVs from a Practitioner Perspective. Paper to the conference of the International Research Network on Religion and AIDS in Africa, Lusaka, Zambia, 15–19 April.

Freedom House 2008a. *Country Report: Ghana*. [Online]. Available at: http://www.freedomhouse.org/template.cfm?page=363&year=2008&country=7400 [accessed: 21 February 2013].

Freedom House 2008b. *Country Report: Zambia*. [Online]. Available at: http://www.freedomhouse.org/template.cfm?page=22&year=2008&country=7522 [accessed: 21 February 2013].

Freston, P. 2001. *Evangelicals and Politics in Asia, Africa, and Latin America*. New York: Cambridge University Press.

Gifford, P. 1998. *African Christianity: Its Public Role*. Bloomington, IN: Indiana University Press.

Gifford, P. 2004. *Ghana's New Christianity: Pentecostalism in a Globalizing African Economy*. Bloomington, IN: Indiana University Press.

Global Fund to Fight HIV/AIDS, Tuberculosis and Malaria 2011a. *Ghana: Country Portfolio*. [Online]. Available at: http://portfolio.theglobalfund.org/en/Grant/List/GHN [accessed: 21 February 2013].

Global Fund to Fight HIV/AIDS, Tuberculosis and Malaria 2011b. *Zambia: Country Portfolio*. [Online]. Available at: http://portfolio.theglobalfund.org/en/Country/Index/ZAM [accessed: 21 February 2013].

Global Health Facts 2011. *PEPFAR Approved Funding: Fiscal Year 2010*. [Online]. Available at: http://www.globalhealthfacts.org/data/topic/map.aspx?ind=54. [accessed: 21 February 2013].

Haven, B. and Patterson, A. 2007. The Government-NGO Disconnect: AIDS Policy in Ghana, in *The Global Politics of AIDS*, edited by P. Harris and P. Siplon. Boulder, CO: Lynne Rienner Publishers, 65–86.

Jenkins, P. 2007. *The Next Christendom: The Coming of Global Christianity*. New York: Oxford University Press.

Joshua, S. 2010. A Critical Historical Analysis of the South African Catholic Church's HIV/AIDS Response between 2000 and 2005. *African Journal of AIDS Research*, 9, 437–47.

Kelly, M. 2007. The Response of the Christian Churches to HIV and AIDS in Zambia, in *Christian Ethics and HIV/AIDS in Africa*, edited by J.N. Amanze. Gaborone: Bay Publishing, 185–201.

Krakauer, M. and Newbery J. 2007. Churches' Responses to HIV/AIDS in Two South African Communities. *Journal of the International Association of Physicians in AIDS Care*, 6(1), 27–35.

Lumbe, J.M.K. 2008. Origins and Growth of Pentecostal and Neo-Pentecostal Church Movements in Zambia between 1989 and 2000. MA thesis, Department of Christian Spirituality, Church History and Missiology, University of South Africa, *Pretoria*.

Makwiza, I., Nyirenda, L., Goma, F., Hassan, F., Chingombe, I., Bongololo, G. and Theobald S. 2006. *Equity and Health System Strengthening in ART Roll Out: An Analysis from Literature Review of Experiences from East and Southern Africa*. Equinet Africa Discussion Paper Series 38. Harare: Zimbabwe.

Marshall, K. and van Saanen, M. 2007. *Development and Faith*. Washington, DC: World Bank.

Ministry of Health, National AIDS Council, and UNAIDS 2011. *Zambia Country Progress Report. UNGASS 2010 Reporting*. [Online]. Available at: http://www.unaids.org/en/dataanalysis/monitoringcountryprogress/2010progressreportssubmittedbycountries/zambia_2010_country_progress_report_en.pdf [accessed: 21 February 2013].

Moszynski, P. 2006. Zambia Scraps Healthcare Fees for Poor Rural People. *British Medical Journal*, 332(7545), 813.

Mukuka, L. and Slonim-Nevo, V. 2006. The Role of the Church in the Fight against HIV/AIDS Infection in Zambia. *International Social Work*, 49(5), 641–9.

Mwinituo, P. and Mill, J. 2006. Stigma Associated with Ghanaian Caregivers of AIDS Patients. *Western Journal of Nursing Research*, 28(4), 369–82.

National HIV/AIDS/STI/TB Council (NAC) 2005. *Zambia Country Report*. [Online]. Available at: http://data.unaids.org/pub/Report/2006/2006_country_progress_report_zambia_en.pdf?preview=true [accessed: 21 February 2013].

Ndhlovu, J. 2007. *Combating HIV: A Ministerial Strategy for Zambian Churches*. PhD thesis, Departement of *Practical Theology and Missiology*, University of Stellenbosch, South Africa.

North, D. 1990. *Institutions, Institutional Change and Economic Performance*. New York: Cambridge University Press.

Nyblade, L., Pande, R., Mathur, S., MacQuarrie, K., Kidd, R., Banteyerga, H., Kidanu, A., Kilonzo, G., Mbwambo, J. and Bond, V. 2003. *Disentangling HIV and AIDS Stigma in Ethiopia, Tanzania and Zambia*. Report for the International Center for Research on Women. [Online]. Available at: http://www.icrw.org/docs/stigmareport093003.pdf [accessed: 21 February 2013].

Oomman, N., Bernstein, M., Rosenzweig, S. and Pearson, J. 2008. *The Numbers behind the Stories*. Report for Center for Global Development. [Online]. Available at: http://www.cgdev.org/content/publications/detail/15799/ [accessed: 21 February 2013].

Patterson, A. 2006. *The Politics of AIDS in Africa*. Boulder, CO: Lynne Rienner Publishers.

Phiri, I. 2001. *Proclaiming Political Pluralism: Churches and Political Transitions in Africa*. Westport, CT: Praeger.

Ranger, T. (ed.) 2008. *Evangelical Christianity and Democracy in Africa*. New York: Oxford University Press.

Scott, J. 1998. *Seeing Like a State: How Certain Schemes to Improve the Human Condition Have Failed*. New Haven, CT: Yale University Press.

UNAIDS 2005. *The 'Three Ones' in Action: Where We Are and Where We Go From Here*. Geneva: UNAIDS.

UNAIDS 2007. *UNAIDS Welcomes Elizabeth Mataka as Special Enjoy of the UN Secretary General for HIV/AIDS in Africa*. Press release. [Online]. Available at: http://data.unaids.org/pub/PressStatement/2007/070521_liz_mataka_announcement_en.pdf [accessed: 21 February 2013].

UNAIDS 2008a. *Ghana: Epidemiological Fact Sheet on HIV and AIDS*. [Online]. Available at: www.who.int/globalatlas/predefinedReports/EFS2008/full/EFS2008_GH.pdf [accessed: 21 February 2013].

UNAIDS 2008b. *Ghana: Funding Sources*. [Online]. Available at: http://data.unaids.org/pub/report/2008/rt08_GHA.en.pdf [accessed: 21 February 2013].

UNAIDS 2008c. *Zambia Country Progress Report. Multi-sectoral AIDS Response Monitoring and Evaluation Biennial Report*. [Online]. Available at: http://data.unaids.org/pub/Report/2008/zambia_2008_country_progress_report_en.pdf [accessed: 21 February 2013].

UNAIDS 2008d. *Zambia: Epidemiological Fact Sheet on HIV and AIDS*. [Online]. Available at: www.who.int/globalatlas/predefinedReports/EFS2008/full/EFS2008_ZM.pdf [accessed: 21 February 2013].

UNAIDS 2008e. *Zambia: Funding Sources*. [Online]. Available at: http://data.unaids.org/pub/report/2008/rt08_ZAM.en.pdf [accessed: 21 February 2013].

UNAIDS 2010a. *Ghana's Progress Report on the United Nations General Assembly Special Session (UNGASS) Declaration of Commitment on AIDS*. [Online]. Available at: http://www.unaids.org/en/dataanalysis/knowyourresponse/

countryprogressreports/2010countries/ghana_2010_country_progress_report_en.pdf [accessed: 21 February 2013].
UNAIDS 2010b. *Zambia Country Report: Monitoring the Declaration on HIV and AIDS and the Universal Access*. [Online]. Available at: http://www.unaids.org/en/dataanalysis/monitoringcountryprogress/2010progressreportssubmittedbycountries/zambia_2010_country_progress_report_en.pdf [accessed: 21 February 2013].
United Nations Development Programme (UNDP) 2008a. *Human Development Report 2007/2008-Ghana*. [Online]. Available at: http://hdrstats.undp.org/countries/data_sheets/cty_ds_GHA.html [accessed: 21 February 2013].
United Nations Development Programme (UNDP) 2008b. *Human Development Report 2007/2008-Zambia*. [Online]. Available at: http://hdrstats.undp.org/countries/data_sheets/cty_ds_ZMB.html [accessed: 21 February 2013].
United Nations Development Programme (UNDP) (2009a) *Human Development Report 2009 Ghana*. [Online]. Available at: http://hdrstats.undp.org/en/countries/data_sheet/cty_ds_GHA.html [accessed: 21 February 2013].
United Nations Development Programme (UNDP) (2009b) *Human Development Report 2009 Zambia*. [Online]. Available at: http://hdrstats.undp.org/en/countries/data_sheet/cty_ds_ZMB.html [accessed: 21 February 2013].
US Agency for International Development (USAID) 2008. *Ghana: HIV/AIDS Health Profile*. [Online]. Available at: http://www.usaid.gov/missions/gh [accessed: 13 February 2013].
US Agency for International Development (USAID) 2010. *Ghana: HIV/AIDS Health Profile*. [Online]. Available at: http://www.usaid.gov/our_work/global_health/aids/Countries/africa/ghana_profile.pdf [accessed: 21 February 2013].
US Department of State 2011. *Ghana: Background Note*. [Online]. Available at: http://www.state.gov/r/pa/ei/bgn/2860.htm [accessed: 21 February 2013].
US President's Emergency Plan for AIDS Relief (PEPFAR) 2007. *2007 Country Profile: Zambia*. [Online]. Available at: http://zambia.usembassy.gov/root/pdfs/fy07country-profile2.pdf [accessed: 21 February 2013].
US President's Emergency Plan for AIDS Relief (PEPFAR) 2008. *Zambia Fiscal Year 2008 Country Allocation Plan*. [Online]. Available at: http://www.pepfar.gov/about/opplan08/102008.htm [accessed: 21 February 2013].
US President's Emergency Plan for AIDS Relief (PEPFAR) 2009a. *Partnership to Fight HIV/AIDS in Zambia*. [Online]. Available at: http://www.pepfar.gov/countries/zambia/index.htm [accessed: 21 February 2013].

US President's Emergency Plan for AIDS Relief (PEPFAR) 2009b. *Zambia-FY 2009 Approved Funding by Program Area, Agency, and Funding Source.* [Online]. Available at: http://www.pepfar.gov/about/122668.htm [accessed: 21 February 2013]

World Council of Churches 2009. *Who Are We?* [Online]. Available at: http://www.oikoumene.org/en/who-are-we.html [accessed: 21 February 2013].

World Health Organization (WHO) 2005. *Zambia: Summary Country Profile for HIV/AIDS.* [Online]. Available at: http://www.who.int/hiv/HIVCP_ZMB.pdf [accessed: 21 February 2013].

Zukoski, A. and Thorburn, S. (2009). Experiences of Stigma and Discrimination among Adults Living with HIV in a Low HIV-Prevalence Context: A Qualitative Analysis. *AIDS Patient Care and STDs*, 23 (4), 267–76.

Chapter 9

The Role of Religious Institutions in the District-Level Governance of Anti-Retroviral Treatment in Western Uganda[1]

A.M.J. Leusenkamp

Introduction

This chapter analyses how Christian development-aid organizations in Uganda, in concurrence with the Christian church, participate in the rollout and governance[2] of anti-retroviral treatment (ART) programmes for persons living with HIV/AIDS. In doing so, these faith-based organizations are becoming increasingly influential in the ART programme's initiation as well as in ART coordination. They thus engage in (re-) shaping the field of public health policy-making and service delivery.

The growing influence of Christian-based institutions in the everyday governance of ART programmes marks a significant shift from practising plain service delivery such as education and healthcare provision, activities in which Christian institutions have been engaged since the earliest missionary times. I argue that, at least at district level, in addition to having become active in ART service delivery, Christian civil-society organizations are now dominant in the governance of these services, in a role that was formally assigned to the Ugandan central government – the Uganda AIDS Commission (UAC) – and district government health departments.[3] With respect to the UAC, notably just a few years before the fieldwork leading up to this chapter was conducted, its regulatory position was acknowledged and strengthened by reinforcing the institutional structure in order to ensure its leadership for HIV/AIDS coordination and

---

[1] An earlier version of this chapter appeared in the *African Journal of AIDS Research* (AJAR) 9/4 (2010), in a special section on religion and antiretroviral therapy. Permission to reprint – in part or in whole – from that publication was kindly granted by AJAR.

[2] Governance is understood as the administration of access to and provision of rights, services and goods (Eckert, Dafinger and Behrends (2003), as quoted in Körling (2011: 30).

[3] Uganda AIDS Commission (2000: 3), Ministry of Health (2003: 13) and Republic of Uganda (1997).

policy-making[4] (Uganda AIDS Commission 2004). This chapter, however, concentrates on the latter category, the district-level health department, and its relationship with Christian institutions in processes of ART governance.

Although district ART policy is consistent with UAC guidelines, it became evident that formal public healthcare structures at this level were being superseded – both literally and figuratively – by religious actors. In addition, ART services were attuned not only to the objectives of the Ministry of Health or UAC but also to those of the Catholic bishop. What is more, ART service provision was restricted to the diocese's boundaries rather than to the district's, and the coverage and nature of ART was discussed with NGOs and donors, both within and above the district level instead of with local government institutions. Although the district's health department was formally involved as project owner, its position seems to have been marginalized due to the power and wealth of these religious actors.

Christian civil-society institutions seemed to be capable of surpassing secular NGOs both numerically as well as resource-wise (Hofer 2003). It is important to study this tendency to analyse how this process is taking shape as well as its consequences for public health management in Uganda, and possibly Africa in general. How is the increasing prevalence of religious development-aid institutions influencing ART governance and how are local ART providers affected? This chapter provides an answer to these questions by focusing on the role Christian faith-based institutions play in district-level ART governance processes in Kabarole District in western Uganda.

Institutional Challenges to ART Complexities

ART programme management offers an intriguing framework for analysing the religious institutions' agency and its effect on public healthcare administration as it marks a new and complex stage in the HIV/AIDS epidemic. ART programmes, whether in the form of prevention-of-mother-to-child transmission (PMTCT) to halt HIV infection to infants or the provision of anti-retroviral drugs (ARVs) to persons living with HIV, demand a break from earlier HIV/AIDS medical intervention practices. From an institutional point of view, the shift from a predominant focus on prevention to curb the epidemic and offering palliative treatment to persons living with HIV/AIDS to an approach that takes account of ART treatment is enormous.

---

4 This recommendation was made after a mid-term review of the National Strategic Framework for HIV/AIDS Activities in Uganda made it clear that UAC's coordinating role was structurally constrained by limited capacity and infrastructure (Uganda AIDS Commission 2004: 22–4).

The incorporation of ART practices has severe implications for every health facility involved in the process. A thorough biomedical command of the different ART regimes that presently exist and those that are continuing to be developed, along with a clear understanding of their implications for patients' well-being, is vital for ART health practitioners. Accordingly, an advanced ART curriculum for health workers needs to be compiled and mandated. And the continuous rollout of ART requires new and more proficient drug-procurement practices as well as a reconsideration of drug-storage and dispensing practices. In addition, a reconfiguration of staffing levels might be taken into account to relieve the added burden of work resulting from ART services. Correspondingly, new health facilities or new blueprints of already-existing medical constructions may be needed to accommodate all ART services and make them accessible to patients and avoid HIV/AIDS-related stigma.

It is evident that in Uganda, as elsewhere, the complexity of these relatively new ART services and their bearing on existing healthcare practices add managerial, logistic and funding challenges to often already-overstretched health systems. At the time of this research, no single healthcare facility in Kabarole District met the resources and expertise levels needed to deal with all ART concerns singlehandedly. Instead, the field of ART was being organized by an amalgam of different stakeholders, both public and private and including those of religious origin, that were cooperating with or working alongside each other.

Christian development-aid organizations in cooperation with secular institutions rose to the occasion by primarily strengthening the structures of ART-providing institutions, such as hospitals and clinics. Grants were provided to recruit and train staff and volunteers, to purchase (medical) equipment and procure ARVs. The increasing prominence of aid organizations in the management of HIV/AIDS treatment suggests a reconfiguration of the field of actors participating in ART practices, in which responsibilities are being recast. In the midst of these changes, the position of the district government, which is conventionally accredited with the legitimacy, authority and accountability of local healthcare intervention programme regulation and supervision, is being significantly affected by the interference of these (Christian) development-aid institutions.

Religions Institutions and the Public-Private Debate

For a clearer understanding of the ability of religious organizations[5] to affect public healthcare administration through the lens of ART provision in

[5] Under Ugandan law, all churches are considered as NGOs and need to register with the NGO Board of the Ministry of Internal Affairs. Notable exceptions are the Catholic Church, the Church of Uganda (Anglican) and the Uganda Muslim Supreme Council

western Uganda, an embedding of this theme into a comprehensive discussion of institutional relationships, in particular the linkages between religious organizations or the broader category of civil society and the state, is needed.

The increase of civil society in Africa is reflected in an upsurge of NGO activity that, in conjunction with a rise in the number of international donors and a withdrawal of the state, has become a major topic in academic debates on the relationship between the African state and civil society.[6] Arguments are being built on the changing position of the state in view of the global economic situation since the 1980s. In these years both the World Bank and the IMF forced structural adjustment programmes on developing countries to liberalize trade and curb public expenditure as a precondition to issuing loans and grants. These programmes activated a series of government reforms that led to a reassessment of the role of the state, resulting in schemes for economic privatization and diminishing state-led service provision in order to reduce its size. The health sector was correspondingly affected. Here too, the declining role of the state and increasing reliance on the civil and private sectors to provide and financially support healthcare practices were envisaged (World Bank 1987). Authority and governance were to be restored in more decentralized government structures, and service provision was to be placed in the hands of private and civil-society organizations. To paraphrase, states were 'rolled back' (de Torrente and Mwesigye 1999) and the private sector as well as NGOs, including religious organizations, 'jumped the gap' (Dorman 2005).

This departure of the state has in certain cases taken on such extreme forms that some question its whereabouts.[7] However, the African state has repeatedly been regarded as crumbling or failing to address the needs of its population, while at the same time being unable to control the advent of the NGO sector. Blundo (2006) comments that in many of these analyses, the state is reflected in its totality and is thus being reduced to a singular stereotype,[8] which is often imbued with a negative connotation that in comparison with the Western state model appears to be less thriving. Analyses of the African state can lead to rather static images that have negative labels such as failed, neo-patrimonial or corrupt. These opinions do not enhance our understanding. Instead of providing yet another label for the African state, it would be more appropriate to focus on

that are exempted due to their long-standing presence and activities in the country (Barr, Fafchamps and Owen 2005).

[6] See, for example, the edited collections by Igoe and Kelsall (2005), Lund (2007) and Hagmann and Péclard (2011).

[7] See Jones (2009) on Uganda and Körling (2011) on Niger as well as a range of publication describing the absence of the state in so-called failed states such as Serbia (Vivod 2011), Sierra Leone (Reno 1995) and Somalia (Menkhaus 2007; Samatar 1992).

[8] See Kawabata (2006) for an exhaustive enumeration of different types of 'the African state'.

the interrelationship between the state and non-state institutions, particularly on the subtleties of processes within and between actors in the local context, including their day-to-day encounters.[9]

Over the last few decades, religious institutions and the civil-society sector in general have grown to be a considerable social, political and economic force. They are increasingly involved in African HIV/AIDS issues and are part of HIV/AIDS policy design and implementation. Donors are contributing to these processes by claiming more prominent positions in an on-the-ground capacity and, in the process, are increasingly relocating themselves between administrative and non-state institutions (Putzel 2004). Meanwhile, the state in Uganda has embarked upon ongoing decentralization processes whereby roles and responsibilities, including the governance of public healthcare, are being reallocated (Murindwa et al. 2006; Asiimwe and Musisi 2007). In these dynamics, faith-based organizations are – although perpetually involved in the provision of healthcare and education in Africa – increasingly being acknowledged as a force for social change. According to Hofer (2003: 376), this apparent resurgence of religion within the development field can be explained by connecting the 'third wave'[10] of Christianity, the charismatic revival that is propelling the burgeoning of countless Pentecostal churches across the world, with an upswing of Christian conservatism in US politics. Both developments have catalyzed the role of faith-based organizations as development agents. Consequently, the religious institutions active in the field of HIV/AIDS (and public health-related development work in general) have rapidly grown in number, as have their financial means. The increasing visibility of religion in development arenas (Hofer 2003; Kaag and Saint-Lary 2011; Ter Haar and Ellis 2006) raises questions about how the implementation of ART affects the relationships between these actors, how perceptions and expectations among those involved are shaped, and how this in turn affects processes of ART governance.

Setting the Scene

Uganda's Kabarole District is one of many geographical areas that offer an interesting entrance point for studying ART stakeholders and understanding their interrelationships. The district is at the foot of the Rwenzori Mountains in western Uganda, close to the Congolese border. It is roughly 320 km from the nation's capital, Kampala, and has Fort Portal as its sole urban centre where

---

9 See, for example, Bierschenk and Olivier de Sardan (2003), Das and Poole (2004) and Lund (2007).

10 Based on Wagner (1980).

Kabarole's administrative offices are located. The district's first hospital was opened in Fort Portal in 1903 (Thomas and Scott 1935) and, at the time of this research, the district had 42 biomedical public and private health facilities (Kabarole District Health Department 2005a). There are currently three hospitals in Kabarole District, one public hospital, one Catholic and one affiliated to the Church of Uganda. Most of the private or NGO-run health facilities are Christian as well.

ART service provision in Kabarole District began in 2003. A process of rolling out ART to lower-level health facilities was envisaged in 2006, when level IV health centres were also accredited to provide ART services. Since then, the process has included level III health institutions too. In addition to these health facilities, the district administration unit and a number of NGOs, including some with religious origins, have been engaged in ART-related activities in Kabarole District. As elsewhere in Africa, ART is available in Kabarole District in both public and private health facilities, with the latter made up of missionary hospitals and their satellite clinics.

Delineating Methodology

A distinction is made here between those church institutions working with and for people living with HIV/AIDS but not providing ART services and church-related institutions providing (the means to facilitate) ART and PMTCT services. The analysis here is restricted to the latter category and focuses on Christian institutions involved in ART provision. Obviously many more religious groups can be found in Kabarole District, including Islamic organizations, Pentecostal churches and other independent African churches. However, since they were not engaged in ART services or involved in ART-providing health centres at the time of this research, they are not included in the analysis here.

The focus in this chapter is mainly on ART practices occurring at the district or intermediate level, excluding interactions between ART actors at the national and international level, as well as the influence of religion on global debates concerning HIV/AIDS and ART policies.[11] Nor does the article reflect on HIV/AIDS treatments other than ART or on interactions between persons working within religious or health institutions and their target audiences, namely church-going people and people living with HIV/AIDS. The chapter thus concentrates exclusively on the (behind-the-scenes) activities of district-level ART programmes and discusses interactions between ART providers (local

[11] For discussions on evangelical groups influencing global-level HIV/AIDS policies, see Kinsman (2008: chapter 4).

health facilities), district-level government authorities and NGO-sponsoring donors, including those of Christian origin.

After more than three decades,[12] the history of HIV/AIDS can be categorized as turbulent. A snapshot of the HIV epidemic in 2006, the year that most of the research discussed in this chapter was conducted, would be completely different from one taken a decade earlier. Doing research in a field as dynamic as HIV/AIDS can be challenging, especially when contrasting changes with other large-scale phenomena, such as the increasing role of civil society or, more specifically, Christian organizations. To understand these dynamics, longitudinal research was conducted to follow institutional entanglements over time. In addition, an extended research period offered the opportunity of getting acquainted with the persons working (albeit on temporary contracts) within these institutions and gaining their trust.

The data for this chapter were collected in 2006 and 2008 during multiple periods of qualitative ethnographic research on the topic of negotiation and interplay within district-level ART practices in Kabarole District. I mainly used unstructured interviews with managers at NGOs, donor institutions and hospitals, and with health workers and civil servants. In addition, I was able to read respondents' personal files and the district health department's institutional archive for reports, minutes of meetings and other relevant documentation.

Religion, the State and HIV/AIDS

Religion is omnipresent in Uganda. According to the 2002 National Population Census, more than 99 per cent of Ugandans have some religious affiliation, with the majority being Christians. This is reflected in Ugandan society, where religious buildings are a common sight, religious items feature extensively in the media, and blessings are part of everyday conversation and interaction. In Kabarole District healthcare is imbued with religious beliefs and behaviour as most Ugandans are affiliated to one of the major world religions.[13] Irrespective of the public or private nature of a healthcare facility, when walking down hospital corridors or wandering from one ward or clinic office to the next, one cannot fail to notice the numerous crucifixes on the walls, priests or nuns kneeling in

[12] For discussions on the evolution of HIV/AIDS, see Barnett and Whiteside (2002) and Iliffe (2006).

[13] According to the 2002 Uganda Population and Housing Census, 47.51 per cent of the people living in Kabarole District were Catholic; 34.12 per cent Anglican; 6.68 per cent Seventh Day Adventist; 4.96 per cent Muslim; 3.63 per cent Pentecostal; 2.66 per cent other and 0.45 per cent atheist (Uganda Bureau of Statistics 2002). The scheduled 2012 Uganda Population and Housing Census has been postponed to 2013.

prayer next to bedridden patients and health workers singing along with gospel songs on the radio.

Christianity in Uganda has always centred around the heart of political power and governance. It has a long history in the country as the first European explorers were soon followed by missionaries (Pulford 1999). The famous explorer Stanley's 'call to evangelism' prompted Christians' evangelical efforts in what is today's Uganda. Even in pre-colonial times, Christianity sought the proximity of the governing powers. When Anglican missionaries arrived in the form of the Church Missionary Society (CMS) in 1877, followed by the Catholic White Fathers in 1879 and the Mill Hill Fathers in 1895, they all chose Mengo, the capital of Buganda,[14] as their place of residence.

Kazosi (1999) describes how a ruling class of primarily Protestant families controlled the political and economic affairs in Buganda in the first half of the twentieth century, leading to a renewed rivalry with the Catholics. In this oligarchic process, religion and politics became closely interwoven. However, this changed when Milton Obote took control of the country. Religious authorities were severely curtailed in the 1960s when he abolished the kingdom's federal powers and reformed the government administration structures. Although religion was tolerated during his regime, he attempted on several occasions to influence internal religious politics, for example by interfering with the choice of head of the Anglican Church in Uganda.[15] Nonetheless, religion and politics were strictly separated.[16] Formally, this is still the case under Yoweri Museveni, although he himself is a born-again Christian and encourages the involvement of, and partnerships with, religious organizations in addressing the nation's needs.

Regarding healthcare, Christianity, with its long history of healing practices, continued to offer medical treatment following its arrival in Africa. For the early missionaries in Buganda, treating ailments was seen as an effective evangelization strategy. As Pulford (1999: 53) put it, 'care for the body was a way of winning the soul for Christ'. Initially, this slogan was adapted for practical use through what Vaughan (1991) calls sick-bed evangelization, that is missionaries making home visits to bedridden patients who then received medical treatment alongside Christian messages. Missionaries were often as much evangelists as they were doctors. And later on, when missionary posts became more established and the first clinics and hospitals were established, patients needing long-term care could

[14] Buganda is the largest of the traditional kingdoms in present-day Uganda.

[15] For this and other examples, see Kazosi (1999: chapter 4).

[16] The situation deteriorated during Idi Amin's reign and the second Obote regime. Amin favoured Muslims and expelled many missionaries, while extreme government violence against all religions was rife during Obote's second period in power.

be admitted to missionary health facilities, thus opening up 'opportunities for evangelisation afforded by longer-term care of the sick' (Vaughan 1991: 61).

Although the coexistence of public healthcare and non-state health institutions, such as missionary hospitals in East Africa, goes back to the 1870s (Iliffe 2002), the relatively rapid spread of HIV has triggered a range of non-governmental actors and new forms of state/non-state relationships. The Ugandan response to the HIV epidemic is famous, not only for its symbolic leadership and openness. Due to the political instabilities of the 1970s and 1980s, which resulted in a poor public health system, it was also characterized by its liberalism with respect to non-state actors that propagated activities aimed at reducing the further spread of AIDS. Over the last few decades, the Ugandan government has made explicit statements regarding the role of NGOs in the fight against HIV/AIDS. In addition to the religious organizations that are involved in eradicating stigma, churches and secular NGOs have been mobilized to participate in HIV/AIDS campaigns aimed at behavioural change or interventions to provide counselling, care and treatment to those infected with HIV. For example, the Antiretroviral Treatment Policy for Uganda (Ministry of Health [MoH] 2003) explicitly states that the process of developing an ART policy and guidelines should include both the public and private sectors. Christian donors, NGOs and churches (to a large extent backed by generous amounts of funding from the US President's Emergency Plan for AIDS Relief [PEPFAR]) have stepped up to provide money for ARVs and care for people living with HIV/AIDS.

Anti-Retroviral Treatment in Uganda and Kabarole District

ARV therapy became available in Uganda in 1992 through a series of clinical trials conducted at the Joint Clinical Research Centre (JCRC) in Kampala. In 1996, triple drug therapy was offered for patients who were able to pay for it, and Uganda engaged in a pilot study of four countries in 1998 that examined the provision of ART in low-resource settings (Uganda Aids Commission 2004). The government of Uganda and UNAIDS embarked on a joint pilot project called the 'HIV/AIDS Drug Access Initiative' in 1998 that was aimed at improving access to HIV/AIDS care, including ART. The project ran in five treatment centres in Kampala until March 2000. Patients were responsible for procuring their own ARVs and paying for lab tests and their physician's consulting fees, while the project covered the monitoring of patients' viral load and CD4 cell count. As of April 2000, the Ministry of Health took responsibility for managing ARV treatment access, which had been dominated by UNAIDS previously. Building on experiences gained in these pilot initiatives, the Ministry of Health, supported by the World Health Organization (WHO), developed the National Strategic Framework for Expansion of HIV/AIDS Care and Support in Uganda (2001/2–2006/7) to make ARV access part of the national health policy and the Health Sector Strategic Plan (MoH 2003; World Health Organization 2003; Richey and Haakonsson 2004). Since then, ART provision has been available at all regional referral hospitals, with a trickle-down effect ensuring ART availability at lower-level health centres too in recent years.

Coordinating ART Programmes at District Level

In 2000, the UAC developed the National Strategic Framework (NSF) for HIV/AIDS Activities in Uganda (2000/1–2005/6) (Republic of Uganda 2000) to ensure better coordination and the harmonization of the overall national HIV/AIDS programme. The NSF stated that:

> The implementation of the Strategic Framework of HIV/AIDS activities ... requires a comprehensive institutional arrangement for coordination so as to achieve effective linkages among the various tiers of organisations ... It is envisaged that the districts and sub-counties will play a pivotal role in the implementation of the Framework. (Uganda Aids Commission 2000: 70)

The role of the district administration was thus considered key in the governance of HIV/AIDS-related programmes. On the more practical point of how to do so, the NSF stated that: 'Each district shall have a committee to coordinate HIV/AIDS activities' (Republic of Uganda 2000: 72). In this regard, a new forum called the District HIV/AIDS Committee (DAC) was to be established at the district level. However, in the following years, the Ministry of Local Government acknowledged that during the implementation of the NSF, effective coordination of HIV/ AIDS programmes had not been fully realized in a number of local government structures. To fill this gap, the Ministry urged local administration to:

> invest heavily in strengthening and consolidating the capacity to deliver quality HIV/ AIDS services at all levels. The sector should primarily focus on strengthening coordination mechanisms and to ensure that, at all levels, the capacity to plan, implement and manage a wide range of interventions is built. (Ministry of Local Government 2005: 16)

Again, the crucial role of local administrative ranks in governing HIV/AIDS-related projects was underscored at the national policy level.

Kabarole District has adopted this multi-sectoral approach to HIV/AIDS control since 2002 under the Africa Multi-Country AIDS Programme (MAP) in accordance with the NSF. In compliance with recommendations previously made in the NSF, the Uganda MAP was coordinated and supervised by these propagated district HIV/AIDS committees, namely the DACs. Investments in the management and health-coordinating capacities in Kabarole District had commenced as early as 1988 when GTZ (*Gesellschaft für Technische Zusammenarbeit GmbH*), a German development organization, stepped in to help rebuild and strengthen the district's health system (GTZ 2005). As for HIV/AIDS, Kabarole District was, perhaps more than the average Ugandan district, included in long-term donor programmes due to the civil war that ended in 1986, frequent rebel/army clashes here in the late 1990s and an earthquake in February 1994.[17] In addition to restoring demolished healthcare infrastructure, improving the district's coordinating and planning capacities was considered by GTZ to contribute towards building management capacity within the team administering the district's healthcare.

The district level was considered to be key in the management and coordination of all HIV/AIDS-related intervention programmes, including ART. This policy line was not only emphasized at the national level, as stated in the NSF, but the DAC was seen as the instrument to facilitate the whole process. Specifically in Kabarole District, further strengthening of the health-coordination capacities was enabled by the support of GTZ. Altogether, conditions seemed to favour a strong district health department governance structure for ART activities in Kabarole District.

Things had changed, however, by the time my fieldwork started. GTZ, having extended its mission, had finally withdrawn from Kabarole District in 2006. Still in the process of solidifying the district's ART governance processes, GTZ's departure created a donor vacuum in Kabarole's health-development programmes that was only restored with the arrival of a small number of new development agencies two years later. The most prominent of these is the Catholic Relief Services (CRS), which is primarily focused on assisting the district with the provision of ART and PMTCT services. Since the CRS is the only international donor running health programmes on a semi-permanent basis in the district, it is an influential actor in relation to aid-receiving organizations, such as the missionary hospital and the district government. It is partly for this reason that I have chosen to highlight the relationship between the CRS and the district administration, or 'Mucwa' as the department is known by almost everybody in Kabarole District, referring to the name of the hill on which the regional administration buildings are to be found.

---

17 The epicentre of this earthquake (which measured 6.3 on the Richter Scale) was in Kisomoro village, only 40 km south of Fort Portal (GTZ 2005).

Religion, Authority and ART Governance in Kabarole District

At the district level, the District Medical Officer (DMO) is responsible for coordinating all HIV/AIDS activities within the district in addition to 'support[ing] supervision of health sub-districts, disease surveillance and mobilisation of resources for district health services' (Kabarole District Health Department 2005b: 3). The DMO is accountable to the Ministry of Health regarding healthcare in Kabarole District, including the programmes offered by non-state actors. However, with a fluctuating field of actors involved in ART and PMTCT services within the district, the question of how the DMO, or the district government for that matter, keeps track of what is happening on the ground is an important one.

To maintain an overview of the state of affairs and to regulate and coordinate when necessary, the DMO has a few options at his disposal. As for ART, the official forum for discussing relevant and emerging issues is the above-mentioned DAC, the local HIV/AIDS committee that provides technical and organizational input. The DAC is comprised of doctors from the hospitals and (public and private) health centres that offer ART, as well as representatives of other institutions involved, and the district health department's ART coordinating officer. The DAC's tasks are to monitor the progress of the different ART programmes and providers; to act as an intermediary between the hospitals and clinics and the DMO's office; and to coordinate changes affecting ARV therapy. In addition, the DAC serves as a forum for sharing experiences regarding daily practices within the ART clinics. In theory, the DAC forum, which is supposed to meet on a monthly basis, could provide the district health department with vital information regarding ART activities within the district. In turn, this information could be used to make practical adjustments or could be forwarded as management information to the Ministry of Health. However, at the time of this research, which went on until mid 2008, Kabarole's DAC had become an ineffectual governance tool and did not meet after August 2006.

Alternative means for collecting management information for the district health department in order to be able to monitor and govern ART remained weak. First of all, the health department's financial means were extremely limited during the research period. For example, the district administration did not have a regular budget to buy petrol for its vehicles or motorcycles, making supervisory or support visits to public or private health facilities a rarity. Consequently, the district was deprived of a chance to gain an overview of ART provision or to engage in constructive discussions with health workers. When asked how he kept track of the activities of non-state ART providers, the DMO referred to health statistics that all health centres are obliged to submit to the DMO's office:

> They give me the reports with all the [clinical] data. It gives me an overview of the number of patients on ART, the number of new patient enrolments, and so on.

These clinical statistics were not, however, presented uniformly. Some hospitals used an official Ministry of Health form, while others created their own. In addition, the frequency of submission of these data reports to the district health administration was not standardized at the time of this research project. Some clinics submitted on a monthly basis, others quarterly, and some did not provide any data at all.

As a result, these inverse trends between a government that seemed unable to sustain coordination, mainly due to a lack of means, and prominent donors backed by global funding agencies had profound repercussions on ART governance and the regulating authority. I illustrate this claim with a few examples involving the CRS, which was the most active and visible donor contributing to the ART and PMTCT programmes in Kabarole District.

The Case of the Catholic Relief Services

The CRS, a US-based Catholic development organization, operates in over 20 districts in Uganda and has been involved in Kabarole District since 2007. Regarding ART and PMTCT programmes, the CRS supports local project facilities, such as hospitals, as part of the AIDSRelief consortium. AIDSRelief is an institutional alliance funded by PEPFAR that makes ARVs available for patients and enables treatment and care for pregnant women. To assist PMTCT services, the CRS is funded by the United Nations Children's Fund (UNICEF), whilst the ART component is financed through PEPFAR. In Kabarole District at the time of this research, the CRS was facilitating the rollout of ARVs to 1300 patients at the Catholic mission's Virika Hospital, and to an additional 670 at Kabarole Hospital, which is affiliated to the Church of Uganda.

By doing so, the CRS is shaping the nature of ART services within the district, though it should be stressed that it is operating in Kabarole District at the request of the Ministry of Health. However, the CRS takes a more liberal approach regarding other aspects of ART and PMTCT service delivery that are not included in the government's strategic HIV/AIDS plan. One example concerns handing out mosquito nets to people who are HIV-positive. To reduce the incidences of malaria among persons living with HIV/AIDS, the staff at one of the hospitals were asked to give mosquito nets to everyone being tested for HIV. The CRS provided these nets but only on the condition that they were given solely to people who had tested HIV-positive. A hospital's medical superintendent recalled:

> We can only give mosquito nets to someone who tested HIV-positive. But then IHV positive people, that is about 10 per cent of the population. What about the other 90 per cent who would get infected with malaria? So we tell them [the CRS] that next to reducing the prevalence of HIV/AIDS, malaria as the number one disease around here should also be targeted. Then people at the CRS will say 'Okay, yes, that's the case then. We can reduce the number of times people having to go on treatment by providing them with mosquito nets'. They will buy it. But if you tell them that we want to get these nets and give them also to people who are HIV-negative, that will be disallowed. They [the CRS] will tell you to refund their money, which we spent buying these nets.

The message this medical superintendent was receiving from the CRS was that any efforts to support Kabarole's population would be sustained as long as the persons targeted are affected by HIV/AIDS. In its projects, the CRS only targets people living with HIV. However, with the decision to select people according to their HIV status and support only persons who test HIV-positive, the CRS is in fact in conflict with the Ministry of Health's non-discriminatory policy regarding medical treatment.

Another example touches on ART authority. To reduce the distance patients have to travel to obtain medical services, hospitals can open outreach posts in peripheral settlements. By doing so, access to ART is improved because people on treatment save both time and money as they no longer have to travel to Fort Portal for treatment and can receive it closer to home. Referring people on ART to outreach posts provides the opportunity to enrol additional patients eligible for ART in the hospitals. In general, the principle behind ART outreach posts is that existing lower-level health facilities – such as health centre level I or II that were at the time not accredited for ART practices but offered basic healthcare services – are visited by a delegation from an already-accredited ART service facility, like a regional referral hospital, on a regular basis. Healthcare professionals from already-accredited ART clinics can then provide ART services in an otherwise unaccredited setting.

Remarkably, the initiative to open outreach posts in Kabarole District came from the CRS and not from the hospitals concerned, nor from the district government that was not even consulted about the decision to open new ART posts. A respondent working for the CRS office in Fort Portal explained:

> Under PMTCT [practices], what was lacking was that you are testing these people, the pregnant women and also their families, as it is a family approach. You encourage these people to come in for a test. But the question then was: if they are eligible for ART, where do you take them? So that was already an issue, which we are trying to link to AIDSRelief. So it's our initiative that AIDSRelief should open up outreaches. Because when you look at AIDSRelief, its partners

> [the Christian ART providing hospitals and clinics] are in Kabarole. But now, we're encouraging them [these health facilities] to open up outreaches within their catchment area. Now when you talk about their catchment area, you see, it is the diocesan catchment area. So when you talk about Virika Hospital, you ask – What is their catchment area? – it is not district-ruled, but it is diocesan. So when you talk about the diocese of Virika – or the Fort Portal diocese – it covers Kamwenge, Kyenjojo and Bundibugyo [that is adjacent districts bordering Kabarole District]. Thus that is the Catholic diocese. Now when we go to the Church of Uganda [to which Kabarole Hospital is affiliated], it's also the diocesan catchment which covers all these potential ART clients. So that is the development we are taking ... then when we talk about the catchment area we are able to cross to the other districts ... So there will be one outreach in Kyenjojo District by Kabarole [Hospital], then there will also be one outreach by Virika [Hospital] in Kyakatara, which is also in Kyenjojo District. So there will be two new ART outreaches in Kyenjojo District. Then there will be only one big outreach by Virika Hospital in Kamwenge District. And then there is another second outreach because they are going to take two outreaches each; the second outreach for Kabarole [Hospital] is in Urahura, which is in Kabarole District. But it's far from Fort Portal, which is good for us. Now the other target, the outreach in Bundibugyo District. But Bundibugyo, you know, EGPAF [Elizabeth Glaser Pediatric AIDS Foundation] has [done] a lot, so we are not worried about that.

This passage reveals several interesting points. The first is the establishment of outreach ART posts based on the CRS's initiative. The district health department, though not against the decision to introduce ART services in remote areas since this would also enable the enrolment of new ART clients in Fort Portal's hospitals, was not consulted on this decision but was only 'informed' of it. Consultation was not deemed necessary by either the CRS or the hospitals because, as one doctor explained, 'by nature of being a hospital you are allowed to have outreaches'.

Secondly, the decision as to which geographical areas ought to be selected for ART and PMTCT was taken in negotiations between the CRS and the other development organizations involved in ART and PMTCT programmes, such as the Elizabeth Glaser Pediatric AIDS Foundation (EGPAF). At the time of this research, CRS staff members were frequently communicating with staff from EGPAF, the World Harvest Mission or other NGOs regarding programme practicalities. Achieving more efficient service provision was at stake here. However, bearing in mind the role of the district government (that is the coordination of all HIV/AIDS activities), questions about the degree and level of the involvement of the Ministry of Health's representative arise. In addition, the fact that remote places are being favoured in outreach planning suggests that locations are being selected where already-accredited ART services are lacking.

In practice though, remote and rural areas that have only the most basic medical care facility are being targeted in outreach planning.

A third observation is about extending the CRS's operational area to a territory that respects the diocesan boundaries, instead of the district border. Neither Virika Hospital nor Kabarole Hospital is a regional referral hospital but both are general hospitals, although this does not mean that they are restricted to serving a clearly demarcated population. Nonetheless, the broadening of the CRS's area of operations derives from its ties with clerical structures (that is the Catholic diocese). The same CRS representative explained:

> When we come to Uganda, or any other country, it's under the auspices of the Catholic secretariat. We have our affiliation to the church. So that when we are working here, you find the bishop monitoring things. The bishop can tell the CRS directors at the US headquarters that they don't need me here, and if that is the case, the CRS will fire me. So the church is also involved. The diocese monitors our activities. So they are powerful. Whenever they want something from us, we'll listen to them.

The expansion of the CRS's activities to areas outside those assigned by the Ministry of Health came at the request of the bishop's office. He was aiming to secure an equal level of service delivery across the entire diocese, instead of service provision to solely that part of the diocese population living in Kabarole District.

The above example shows how religious actors are capable of shaping the nature of ART services. However this is not to say that secular institutions engaged in similar ART activities would not be equally influential. The CRS was clearly pressed into territory by the local diocese that it would perhaps not have engaged in if it had been a secular NGO. By encouraging the CRS to cover the entire diocesan catchment area, the Catholic Church provided itself with an opportunity to expand its reach and influence, albeit not in the biomedical sense of ART provision but at a moral level. The question of how this affects the NGO/state/donor relationship is intriguing. The example above describes a situation where NGOs rely heavily on their donors. Clearly public authority is at stake and one might wonder whether the district health department is able to supervise and coordinate all ART services within their district. When asked about how ART activities in Kabarole District should be controlled, the DMO stressed that 'it is just collaboration, mutual collaboration. Not control as such.'

Similarly, when I asked representatives of the donors and NGOs whether the district government still figured in their ART plans and activities, it was emphasized that the district government is and should be the only stakeholder in charge of ART coordination and that it should decide what activities ought to be carried out. This contradicts the earlier statements that Mucwa does not need to be informed about opening up new outreach posts. Returning to the CRS case, a similar explanation was given by a representative:

> It is for the district to say. It is up to the district directors to tell us where we should go ... EGPAF has a signed agreement with the district government. We [the CRS], have also a signed agreement with the district government. When we discuss ART topics, like in our coordination meetings, I think that's where we realize that when we are having our coordination meetings all shareholders should be present – the EGPAF should be there, the CRS and the local government, and the district – so that we talk the same language ... So when we invite all of them, we can always strike a balanced blow.

This quote suggests that according to the CRS it should be the district health department to coordinate ART matters. And when asked about the role of the DMO in these meetings:

> Yes, he is there. When we go to meetings, they [the district health department] are supposed to chair the meeting. They have to open and close [the meeting]. You see ... we're a bit strategic here. We don't want to chair meetings. Even if it concerns the meeting's opening remarks, it shouldn't be us. It should be the district. Because it is *their* programme [emphasis added] ... So we are also telling the DMO that he should provide us with an office, so that when we are at Mucwa we are always able to reach them. And then we also say that all these coordination meetings should take place in their building [Mucwa]. We don't want to rent hotel space [for meetings] here in Fort Portal. We are partners and they [the district health department] are the owners of this. So we encourage these meetings to take place there at Mucwa.

The district government is thus pushed forward as the institution responsible for ART coordinative processes. But although the district health department is formally involved as the project owner, their position seems marginalized. The statements made above are in line with the theoretical idea of de-politicizing development interventions and the way they intersect with the refashioning of the state, as described by Ferguson (1994) in his widely acclaimed book *The Anti-Politics Machine*. According to him, by needing to construe their role as 'apolitical', development-aid institutions continue to see the government as a 'neutral' machine for delivering services. Although he does not mention religious institutions or distinguish between these and secular development-aid institutions, this theoretical principle holds true for the case described above.

When the CRS opts to initiate ART activities in institutions and areas other than those accredited by the Ministry of Health, this has consequences for the target population, as well as the care providers and local politicians. People outside Kabarole's administrative border who are medically eligible for ART might be lucky enough to live within the catchment area of the diocese and be treated at one of these newly established ART outreach posts. The satellite ART clinics are under the direct supervision of Fort Portal hospital staff and these doctors and nurses make frequent visits to the new ART posts.

The outreach posts, however, surpass the conventional patient/health-worker relationship, as even local politicians are recruited to lobby for the outreach posts. The direct mobilization of political support by the CRS when stepping into unknown territory is in line with Ferguson's (1994) conceptual idea. A staff member at the CRS explained it as follows:

> When we are going to local communities for project sensitization, we need political support. We can go there [to the community] because the district people [from the district administration's health department], they are civil servants. And therefore the population doesn't know them [the civil servants]. But they do know the local politicians. So that's why we ask these politicians to come with us.

To gain access to local communities, the CRS seeks the support of political persons who are well known to the communities. In the process, political authority is endorsed and their efforts are legitimized for the local public at the same time.

Conclusion

Religious institutions, whether churches or civil-society organizations driven by spiritual inspiration, do not exist in isolation. They engage in both short-lived and enduring partnerships and interactions within and outside the religious realm. In Africa, as elsewhere, these spiritual organizations have complemented their religiously inspired practices with more mundane services, most notably in the fields of education and healthcare. Testimony to these accomplishments are the countless Christian schools and health facilities that were set up by missionary associations in pre-colonial times, many of which still exist today.

Conditions have changed in Africa over the years. States have been founded and formed; governments have waxed and waned; and societies have been caught up in processes of amalgamation and diversification. In the midst of all these dynamics, religion has remained an important presence. It continues to be a vital aspect of many people's lives[18] and still has a significant influence on societal developments. The vitality of religion is testimony to both the strength

18 See Kaba (2005) for a discussion on the number of religious people in Africa.

of people's faith as well as the capacity of faith-based institutions to thrive under shifting circumstances.

The above has explained how formal public structures at ground level may be superseded – both literally and figuratively – by religious actors if ART-related services are attuned not only to the needs of the Ministry of Health but also to those of the Catholic bishop. This occurs if, for example, service provision is restricted to diocese boundaries rather than to those of the district, and if the coverage and nature of ART is discussed with NGOs and donors, both at and above the district level, instead of with the local government.

Though the district health department is formally involved as the project owner, its position in ART governance has been marginalized over the last few years. Notably, however, although the CRS's activities in and outside Kabarole District are shaped by its affiliation to the diocese and its geographical boundaries, the ways in which the CRS affects district-level ART programme coordination do not derive from the ideological nature of its relationship with the diocese but rather from its organizational independence from existing district structures. In this respect, this chapter has provided cases highlighting the power struggles taking place within the context of ART, and discussed how influence is being established by Christian actors, not because they are religious per se but because they belong to a configuration of religiously inspired institutions that exceed state and secular stakeholders in both ART coverage and resources. Since these were not present within a comparable, more secularized cluster of ART institutions in Kabarole at the time of this research, the CRS was able to shape Kabarole's ART practices in the ways described above.

Although ART-related authority and coordination capacities seem to have shifted from the district government to civil-society actors (for example the CRS), Kabarole District's health department does not need to be classified as having failed or crumbled, as many authors have suggested with respect to the African state. Regarding this issue, I agree with Cohen (2006) who, building on the ideas of Ferguson (1994), questions the idea that NGOs have caused the state to retreat. He feels that it is far from the norm to bypass the state and that NGOs instead have good reason to work together with the state, for example as subcontractors. NGOs usually have no wish to be a substitute for the state in the management of public affairs or to weaken it. In other words, these NGOs want to exercise influence, not power. In doing so, they may frantically position themselves as neutral, as shown in the quotes above. Most NGOs are engaged in solving local problems – the 'technical fix-it stance' – but do not have the capacity or the desire to deal with the underlying structural causes of underdevelopment. The position of the Catholic Church in this case seems even more ambiguous. As already mentioned, the Catholic diocese is used as a matrix in which the Catholic CRS is compelled to operate. This not only displays the power relations in which both organizations are confined in comparison to the local government, but it also accentuates how legitimacy and authority fluctuate with respect to different matters of ART governance.

The concept of accountability seems to gain importance as it closely relates to issues of responsibility and liability and refers to the answerability of persons or institutions to their supporting (or superior) members. In terms of HIV/AIDS-related governance, accounts regarding drafted policy plans and all derived activities are given to both the public and the corresponding legislative institutions. So when the local government in Kabarole District, the district health department, was positioned as formal project owner, and subsequently presented to all as being in charge of coordinating ART activities, the question of who holds accountability is then answered. This also explains why the CRS insisted on the district health department's approval. Private organizations like the CRS have no desire for a position that claims 'ultimate responsibility',[19] and are likely to present themselves as working for, under or together with the district government. In the case of the CRS, the contrast with reality was apparent, as the NGO produced formal documents delineating each actor's responsibilities. These memorandums of understanding were subsequently given to the DMO for their stamp of approval. This serves once again as an illustration of how the CRS decides how, and sometimes where, to operate in Kabarole District, while the DMO is placed in a situation where he is ultimately accountable for HIV/AIDS-related activities, although he lacks the means to monitor them properly.

Kabarole's health department, or Kabarole local government, seems weaker regarding issues of authority and coordination now than it was a few years ago. There are several possible reasons for this situation, with the most likely being a lack of resources in contrast to the relative wealth of some of the (religious) actors involved in expanding accessibility to ART. However, this does not explain whether an NGO's influence on the ART landscape is structural or generally ad hoc. To answer this question, more comparative case studies both within[20] and outside Uganda and involving a more longitudinal dimension are required to explain whether it is the rising power of non-state actors that is leading to state decline or rather the absence or capability of the state that is enabling NGOs to proliferate in the field of HIV/AIDS interventions.

The CRS was the primary NGO/Christian actor 'on the ground' regarding HIV/AIDS in Kabarole District. But there are similar faith-based development agencies working in other parts of Uganda and across Africa too. After decades in which secularist discourses inattentive to religious-based development institutions have dominated instrumentalist academic debates on development work, this

---

[19] One could argue whether ultimate responsibility exists at all and, if so, to what extent it resides in the upper echelons of the Roman Catholic Church.

[20] See Christiansen (2009).

situation has changed only recently,[21] although more academic attention to the interconnectivity of religion and development is still needed. The context of the HIV/AIDS epidemic, and specifically ART, is suitable for studying these relationships. As an intervention, ART is both unique and complex in nature: it extends beyond the field of medical procedures and its availability is creating high demands in the social, political and economic sphere, thus challenging both regulating and operational institutions. Studying this dynamic field of actors contributes not only to a better understanding of ART practices but also uncovers the underlying forces that are shaping these developments.

References

Asiimwe, D. and Musisi, N.B. (eds) 2007. *Decentralisation and Transformation of Governance in Uganda.* Kampala: Fountain Publishers.

Barnett, T. and Whiteside, A. 2002. *AIDS in the Twenty-First Century: Disease and Globalization.* New York: Palgrave Macmillan.

Barr, A., Fafchamps, M. and Owens, T. 2005. The governance of non-governmental organizations in Uganda. *World Development*, 33(4), 657–79.

Bierschenk, T. and Olivier de Sardan, J.-P. 2003. Powers in the village: Rural Benin between democratisation and decentralisation. *Africa*, 73(2), 145–73.

Blundo, G. 2006. Dealing with the local state: The informal privatization of street-level bureaucracies in Senegal. *Development and Change*, 37(4), 799–918.

Bornstein, E. 2005. *The Spirit of Development: Protestant NGOs, Morality, and Economics in Zimbabwe.* Stanford, CA: University Press.

Christiansen, C. 2009. Conditional certainty: Ugandan charismatic Christians striving for health and harmony, in *Dealing with Uncertainty in Contemporary African Lives,* edited by L. Haram and C.B. Yamba. Uppsala: Nordiska Afrika Institutet, 48–71.

Cohen, S. 2006. *The Resilience of the State: Democracy and the Challenge of Globalisation.* London: Hurst & Co.

Das, V. and Poole, D. 2004. *Anthropology in the Margins of the State.* New Delhi: Oxford University Press.

Dorman, S.R. 2005. Studying democratization in Africa: A case study of human rights NGOs in Zimbabwe, in *Between a Rock and a Hard Place: African NGOs, Donors and the State*, edited by J. Igoe and T. Kelsall. Durham, NC: Carolina Academic Press, 35–62.

21 See for example Bornstein's (2005) analysis of two Protestant NGOs in Zimbabwe: World Vision International and Christian Care.

Eckert, J., Dafinger, A. and Behrends, D. 2003. Towards an anthropology of governance. *Reports 2003*. Halle: Max Planck Institute for Social Anthropology, 19–30.

Ferguson, J. 1994. *The Anti-Politics Machine: 'Development', Depoliticization, and Bureaucratic Power in Lesotho*. Minneapolis, MN: University of Minnesota Press.

GTZ 2005. *Building a Healthy Population: Seventeen Years of Basic Health Services in Western Uganda*. Eschborn: Deutsche Gesellschaft für Technische Zusammenarbeit (GTZ) GmbH.

Hagmann, T. and Péclard, D. (eds) 2011. *Negotiating Statehood: Dynamics of Power and Domination in Africa*. Chichester: Wiley-Blackwell.

Hofer, K. 2003. The role of Evangelical NGOs in international development: A comparative case study of Kenya and Uganda. *Afrika Spectrum*, 38(3), 376–98.

Igoe, J. and Kelsall, T. (eds) 2005. *Between a Rock and a Hard Place: African NGOs, Donors and the State*. Durham, NC: Carolina Academic Press.

Iliffe, J. 2002. *East African Doctors: A History of the Modern Profession*. Kampala: Fountain Publishers.

Iliffe, J. 2006. *The African AIDS Epidemic: A History*. Oxford: James Currey.

Jones, B. 2009. *Beyond the State in Rural Uganda*. Edinburgh: Edinburgh University Press.

Kaag, M. and Saint-Lary, M. 2011. The new visibility of religion in the development arena. *Bulletin de l'APAD* 33.

Kaba, A.J. 2005. The spread of Christianity and Islam in Africa: A survey and analysis of the numbers and percentages of Christians, Muslims and those who practice indigenous religions. *The Western Journal of Black Studies*, 29(2), 553–70.

Kabarole District Health Department 2005a. *Kabarole District HIV/AIDS Strategic Plan 2005/6–2010/11*. Fort Portal: Kabarole District Health Department.

Kabarole District Health Department 2005b. *Quarterly Report on HIV/AIDS Activities Implemented in Kabarole District*. Fort Portal: Kabarole District Health Department.

Kawabata, M. 2006. *An Overview of the Debate on the African State. Afrasian Centre for Peace and Development Studies*. Shiga: Ryukoku University. Working Paper Series No. 15.

Kazosi, A.B.K. 1999. *The Social Origins of Violence in Uganda, 1964–85*. Kampala: Fountain Publishers.

Kinsman, J.F. 2008. Pragmatic Choices: Research, Politics and AIDS Control in Uganda. PhD thesis, Amsterdam Institute for Social Science Research, University of Amsterdam.

Körling, G. 2011. *In Search of the State: An Ethnography of Public Service Provision in Urban Niger*. Uppsala Studies in Cultural Anthropology 51. Uppsala: Acta Universitatis Upsaliensis.

Leusenkamp, A.M.J. 2010. Religion, authority and their interplay in the shaping of antiretroviral treatment in western Uganda. *African Journal of AIDS Research*, 9(4), 419–27.

Lund, C. 2007. *Twilight Institutions: Public Authority and Local Politics in Africa*. Oxford: Blackwell Publishing.

Menkhaus, K. 2007. Governance without government in Somalia: Spoilers, state building and the politics of coping. *International Security*, 31(3), 74–106.

Ministry of Health 2003. *Antiretroviral Treatment Policy for Uganda*. Kampala: MoH.

Ministry of Local Government 2005. *The Revised HIV/AIDS-Sector Strategic Plan (2005–10)*. Kampala: AIDS Control Programme Desk, Ministry of Local Government.

Murindwa, G., Tashobya, C.K., Kyabuggu, J.H., Rutebemberwa, E. and Nabyonga, J. 2006. Meeting the challenges of decentralised health service delivery in Uganda as a component of broader health-sector reforms, in *Health Systems Reforms in Uganda: Processes and Outputs,* edited by C.K. Tashobya, F. Ssengooba and V.O. Cruz. London: London School of Hygiene and Tropical Medicine, Health Systems Development Programme, 97–107.

Pulford, C. 1999. *Eating Uganda: From Christianity to Conquest.* Banbury: Ituri Publications.

Putzel, J. 2004. The politics of action on AIDS: A case study of Uganda. *Public Administration and Development*, 24(1), 19–30.

Reno, W. 1995. *Corruption and State-Politics in Sierra Leone*. Cambridge: Cambridge University Press.

Republic of Uganda. 1997. *Local Government Act.* Kampala: Government Printer.

Richey, L.A. and Haakonsson, S.J. 2004. *Access to ARV Treatment: Aid, Trade and Governance in Uganda*. Copenhagen: Danish Institute for International Studies (DIIS) Working Paper 2004/19.

Samatar, A.I. 1992. Destruction of state and society in Somalia: beyond the tribal convention. *The Journal of Modern African Studies*, 30, 625–41.

Ter Haar, G. and Ellis, S. 2006. The role of religion in development: Towards a new relationship between the European Union and Africa. *The European Journal of Development Research*, 18(3), 351–67.

Thomas, H.B. and Scott, R. 1935. *Uganda*. London: Oxford University Press.

de Torrente, N. and Mwesigye, F. 1999. *The Evolving Roles of the State, Donors and NGOs Providing Health Services in a Liberal Environment: Some Insights from Uganda*. Kampala: Centre for Basic Research. CBR Occasional Paper No. 2.

Uganda AIDS Commission 2000. *The National Strategic Framework for HIV/AIDS Activities in Uganda: 2000/1–2005/6*. Kampala: Uganda AIDS Commission (UAC).

Uganda AIDS Commission 2004. *The Revised National Strategic Framework for HIV/AIDS Activities in Uganda: 2003/4–2005/6*. Kampala: Uganda AIDS Commission (UAC).

Uganda Bureau of Statistics 2002. *2002 Uganda Population and Housing Census: Main Report*. Kampala: Uganda Bureau of Statistics.

Vaughan, M. 1991. *Curing their Ills: Colonial Power and African Illness*. Stanford, CA: Sanford University Press.

Vivod, M. 2011. Stronger than the state? *Etnofoor*, 23(2), 99–114.

Wagner, C.P. 1980. *The Third Wave of the Holy Spirit: Encountering the Power of Signs and Wonders Today*. Ann Arbor, MI: Vine Books.

World Bank 1987. *Financing Health Services in Developing Countries: An Agenda for Reform*. Washington, DC: World Bank.

World Health Organization 2003. *Scaling Up Antiretroviral Therapy: Experiences in Uganda: Case Study*. Geneva: WHO.

World Health Organization 2006. *Progress on Global Access to HIV Antiretroviral Therapy: A Report on '3 by 5' and Beyond*. Geneva: WHO.

Chapter 10

Negotiating Holistic Care with the 'Rules' of ARV Treatment in a Catholic Community-Based Organization in Kampala

Louise Mubanda Rasmussen

Introduction

Based on a case study of a Catholic community-based NGO in an impoverished area of Kampala, this chapter illustrates how involvement in the scale-up of antiretroviral treatment (ARV/ART) may pose new questions for religious organizations concerning the social and spiritual aspects of suffering and healing. It is argued that the highly medicalized and individualized transnational governmentality surrounding ARV treatment provision in Uganda is contributing to a reconfiguration of Catholic ideals of holistic HIV/AIDS care.

The Roman Catholic Church was one of the religious organizations that engaged early on with a comprehensive response to HIV/AIDS across Africa (Patterson 2011: 54–7). Despite this, most discussions surrounding the Catholic Church have focused solely on its contentious condom policies and only recently have studies discussed the relationship between religious and institutional Catholic practices and HIV/AIDS more broadly (Behrend 2007; Joshua 2010; Leusenkamp 2010). As the largest denomination in Uganda, the Catholic Church has been an important player in the country's successful AIDS response since it started in 1986 (Parkhurst 2001).

This chapter focuses on a community-based organization in Kampala called the Kamwokya Christian Caring Community (KCCC), which grew out of Catholic lay mobilization in the late 1980s. It is one of the three Catholic organizations involved in providing treatment, care and support to people living with HIV/AIDS that I studied for my PhD thesis. I have selected this organization here to illustrate that, when it comes to Catholic community-based action, it is not only moralistic standpoints regarding HIV-prevention that have dominated but that there have also been attempts to reach out to AIDS patients with compassion as a Christian obligation.

Alongside similar Catholic initiatives in Eastern and Southern in Africa that started in the late 1980s (Blinkhoff et al. 1999; Czerny 2007; Nsambya Home Care 2007; Fikansa 2009), the KCCC initially formulated care for people living with HIV/AIDS as a holistic endeavour. Material, medical and spiritual forms of assistance were meant to restore AIDS patients' dignity and mitigate the social impacts of AIDS. KCCC received PEPFAR funding for ARV treatment provision in 2004. Its involvement in the ART scale-up reinforced an unfolding process of institutional growth and professionalization that had already contributed to redefining the terms of holistic care with a more secular and neoliberal focus.

This chapter illustrates how the KCCC's involvement in global AIDS treatment has resulted in it becoming involved in a particular bio-political project. As part of this, counsellors and community workers concentrate on counselling and disciplining clients[1] so that they 'learn' that, in order to benefit from their ARV treatment, they have to take responsibility for addressing any social, economic or emotional barriers they may face in adhering to the medicine and its social 'rules'. In this context, the terms of holistic care are being dramatically redefined and spiritual assistance is now seen as a form of psycho-social support.

I do not suggest that such a form of bio-power produces a unified cohort of responsible individuals or 'therapeutic citizens' (Mattes 2011; Nguyen 2005). Rather, in the context of prevailing social inequalities, the organization's disciplining techniques help create significant divides in people's abilities to benefit from treatment. Dissident voices within the KCCC are challenging the dominant rules of ARV treatment, with some counsellors and clients stressing the continued relevance of spiritual assistance in order to come to terms with the disease and the relevance of material assistance as a form of enactment of divine presence.

A Foucault-Inspired Ethnography

The analysis presented here of Catholic AIDS treatment practices and care rests on a Foucault-inspired framework combined with ethnographic studies. Foucault's concept of bio-politics has become popular in the study of medical anthropology (Lock and Nguyen 2010) as well as in the study of HIV/AIDS (Nguyen 2009; Biehl 2007). The term bio-politics is useful when analysing the ways in which life itself can become the object of political interventions.

---

[1] 'Client' is the term widely used for people living with HIV in Uganda. It is connected to the initial opposition to the term 'patient' and to the importance of counselling in HIV-related programmes (Hampton 1992).

Bio-politics is characterized by intervening at the mass level of the population (Foucault 2009) and making use of forms of knowledge, such as statistics and forecasts, to determine and describe specific populations (Foucault 2004: 246–9). With regard to the AIDS epidemic, we can point to how the epidemic has been made known and intervened in terms of HIV prevalence rates, mortality rates and now 'lives saved' as a result of ARV treatment. However, it is vital to bear in mind that the politicization of certain health problems may not necessarily only reflect a bio-political ambition to optimize life but also a concern with how subjects govern themselves (Larsen 2011: 202–203). In other words, bio-political ambitions sometimes have to be combined with concerns of 'governmentality'.

The term 'governmentality' denotes a way of studying government as 'the conduct of conduct' along two lines of inquiry (Bröckling et al. 2011: 2). First, governmentality indicates an interest in 'the contact between technologies of domination of others and those of the self' (Foucault 1988: 19) because if government is to govern how others conduct themselves, forms of political government have to resort to 'processes by which the individual acts upon himself' (Foucault 1993: 203). Secondly, with governmentality, Foucault (2009: 311) also points to the way the problematic of how to govern was increasingly rationalized, i.e. worked out according to calculations of force, relations, strength and wealth.

The discussion here focuses on these two sides of governmentality and analyses how counsellors and community workers in the KCCC have attempted to govern how people with HIV/AIDS govern themselves, thus emphasizing the neoliberal rationalities of government that have been dominating development assistance in recent decades. With neoliberal development rationalities, I am not referring here to an economic ideology but more to technologies of government that work through the creation of responsiblized citizen-subjects (Ferguson 2010: 172). I refer also to the problematic reflected in discussions of sustainable development: how to ensure that development assistance does not create passive recipients but self-activating individuals and communities that can take responsibility for their own development (Kelsall and Mercer 2003; Swidler and Watkins 2009).

The analysis focuses on how bio-political ambitions, neoliberal development rationalities and Catholic notions of healing are negotiated in the KCCC in debates on the provision of HIV/AIDS treatment and care. Regarding Catholic notions of healing, the chapter considers how counsellors and community workers are employing Catholic notions of healthcare as an imitation of Christ's mission and as a practice aiming to restore wholeness (Cochran 1999: 28–9). I am also concerned with the continuities between Catholic approaches to AIDS treatment and care and practices of Christian medical missionaries who attempted to achieve not merely physical transformations of the body but also new subjectivities through evangelization (Vaughan 1991: 73–4).

Methodologically, the discussion is based on an ethnographic study that focused on practices of counselling and home visiting. With participant observation of counselling sessions, home visits and broader everyday organizational practices, my aim was to highlight how counsellors and community workers take up, transform and negotiate central rationalities and technologies of government. Additionally, I conducted qualitative interviews with programme managers, counsellors, community workers and clients and held two focus-group discussions with staff members to discover the role of Christianity in the work of the KCCC.

The names of all the informants featuring in this chapter are fictitious, with the exception of that of the KCCC's founder, Sr Miriam Duggan. The KCCC represents a particular Kampala phenomenon among Catholic AIDS projects in Uganda. A number of such organizations in Kampala started with voluntary activities among the laity and have gradually developed into professional NGOs. In contrast, Catholic AIDS projects outside Kampala are usually positioned within existing health institutions or are coordinated by the diocese. The case of the KCCC is interesting as its trajectory as a self-proclaimed pioneer in holistic HIV/AIDS care illustrates how becoming involved in the ART scale-up can pose questions for religious organizations concerning the social and spiritual aspects of suffering and healing.

The KCCC's Beginnings and the Development of Holistic Care

This section considers how KCCC informants narrated the organization's beginnings as being rooted in a unique Christian community-based approach to holistic HIV/AIDS care. These narratives should not be read as objective histories but as collective-building narratives that have come to produce an ideal of holistic care that managers, counsellors and community workers in the KCCC adopt today in debates on how to provide treatment, care and support to people with HIV/AIDS. Before turning to these narratives, some general points about holistic care are considered first.

The notion of a holistic approach to health and healing has a long history in Catholic healthcare practice (Cochran 1999) and it is part of the mission of Catholic health services in Uganda (UCMB 1999). More generally, faith-based organizations in African countries today often frame their contributions to development as holistic approaches that bridge material and spiritual transformations (Bornstein 2005; Dilger 2009).

In the field of HIV/AIDS, the idea of a holistic approach is tied to the notion that AIDS is not merely a medical issue but a multi-sectoral challenge that also involves social, economic and cultural facets. In the 1990s, holistic HIV/AIDS care was in line with the general international discourse on the need for multi-sectoral approaches (O'Manique 2004). Consequently, a number of Catholic NGOs in Kampala, including the KCCC, were able to grow in the 1990s and 2000s by accessing international funding to run programmes targeting the medical, social, spiritual, emotional and economic needs of people living with and families affected by HIV/AIDS. Today the term holistic HIV/AIDS care is used by a variety of organizations in Uganda and other parts of Africa. With its widespread use, it is fair to ask whether holistic care is merely an empty catch phrase.

The notion of holistic care does, however, illustrate a central feature about how healing can be framed from a Christian perspective in a way that links medical healing with spiritual and material transformations. As such, holistic HIV/AIDS care has historical parallels with the way Christian missionaries in East Africa envisioned medical healing to be part of a larger project to tackle ignorance and poverty (Vaughan 1991).

The Beginnings of the Kamwokya Christian Caring Community

The KCCC is situated in Kamwokya, one of Kampala's oldest and more 'attractive' slum areas. Kamwokya is centrally located to the northeast of the city centre and has a vibrant informal economy that has attracted an ethnic mix of people from all over the country who are looking for economic opportunities.

On my first visits and during the initial interviews with programme coordinators, the story of how the KCCC began was repeated over and over again. Details of the story varied but the emphasis was always on its origins in Kamwokya's small Christian communities and the pivotal role played by Sr Dr Miriam Duggan, a Franciscan missionary from Ireland who had previously been the medical superintendent at Nsambya Hospital.[2]

Establishing Small Christian Communities (SCCs) was a strategy that was begun in the 1970s by Catholic Church leaders across Africa who had been inspired by the base communities in Latin America. Catholics were supposed to organize themselves in small, neighbourhood communities (SCCs) where they could engage in Bible reading, prayers and self-help projects. Their purpose was to encourage church members to take more responsibility for their own Christian formation and socialization. It was hoped that this form of 'spiritual empowerment' would help mobilize the laity into wider social and political action (Kassimir 1998: 69–70). SCCs in Uganda were never, however, established as voluntary organizations but as the lowest unit of the Church's territorial administrative system (ibid.: 70–71; Christiansen 2010).

Prior to 1987, the SCCs in Kamwokya functioned primarily as administrative units. In 1987, the newly arrived Fr Tony Darragh introduced his parishioners

2 A Catholic hospital in Kampala that opened in 1903.

to the idea of SCCs as forums of everyday Christian action. The response was slow at first but soon the number of church members that were active in their respective *kabondo* (the Luganda term for SCCs) started growing (Williams and Tamale 1991: 20).

The *bubondo* (pl: *kabondo*) in Kamwokya became connected to the mobile team from Nsambya Hospital's AIDS programme in 1988, which led to their efforts regarding caring for neighbours in need being gradually redirected towards HIV/AIDS care (ibid.: 20–22). In 1990, three Franciscan missionary sisters, including Sr Duggan, moved to Kamwokya. According to KCCC informants, they provided medical resources that were central in transforming the practices into a fully-fledged HIV/AIDS intervention. With the help of Sr Duggan, a small clinic was opened by the church and clinic staff could then refer patients to Nsambya Hospital. Additionally, a group of volunteers would meet at the church every day after morning mass and split up into groups and go to visit the sick (interview with Damian, a pastoral worker, 28 April 2008).

The volunteers provided a combination of practical assistance and spiritual support. Informants mentioned help such as washing clothes, bathing the sick, doing housework and fetching water. There was also a monthly collection in church to buy basic food items for the poor that were then distributed by *kabondo* members (Williams and Tamale 1991: 11). In terms of spiritual support, volunteers would lead prayers, read Bible passages or sing hymns (interview with Christine, a community coordinator, 21 April 2008). A number of informants stressed how the mere presence of these carers had a spiritual significance for the sick. This included the pastoral workers/counsellors, Damian, Anthony and Charles. Damian and Anthony spoke about the 'sacrament of presence' that had a particular significance when people with HIV/AIDS were left to die alone:

> There is what we call a sacrament of presence, for you being there is very meaningful to a patient who has been in a room for a week without a visitor. When you visit someone at home, you have consoled, you have healed, you have changed that person's mind and feelings. They say oh thank you for coming, since last week, I never got a visitor. Nobody pays a visit to me, nobody! (Interview with Damian, 28 April 2008)

Charles described this act of presence as a matter of 'journeying' with people living with HIV/AIDS. It implies being with them and supporting them in whatever they are going through, including helping them to die with dignity (focus-group discussion, 16 June 2008). Informants described how they helped those with AIDS to die in peace in the knowledge of God's love with a community of volunteers praying and singing at the time of death (focus-group discussions, 12 and 16 June 2008).

Several informants described these initial care practices as stemming from the resolve of the *bubondo* to 'put the Gospel into reality'. As Damian argued, they were trying to find a way of practically enacting the Christian obligation to love one's neighbour in their day-to-day lives in Kamwokya:

> It was just the values we had in Christianity that motivated us to reach out to our people ... there was that love, that drive, that love of Christ, you know, love one another as I have loved you ... We would read a scripture, after reading it, then we'd apply it in our day-to-day life. God is to help people, let's go and help. It was practical, what we share is what we do. (Interview with Damian, 28 April 2008)

In such discussions, informants often referred to a particular biblical passage: 'For I was hungry and you gave me food, I was thirsty and you gave me drink, a stranger and you welcomed me, naked and you clothed me, ill and you cared for me, in prison and you visited me' (Matthew 25:35–36, *The African Bible*). This passage invokes a centrality of material help and mere presence in caring for the suffering and lonely as a reflection of one's love of Christ. What informants described as their unique Christian community-based approach to AIDS treatment and care is thus defined by a holistic commitment to combine medical assistance with spiritual and material support.

The Development and Expansion of Holistic Care

The initial treatment and care practices discussed above have developed into an encompassing practice of holistic care, as the volunteers were 'journeying' with people with HIV/AIDS and were realizing the wide-ranging social problems they faced. Community coordinator Christine explained:

> This was chronic illness which didn't have even a treatment so many of them couldn't work ... many of them they do petty trade, and if they don't work, they don't have anything to eat, their children will not go to school, they will not pay their rent, and the moment you don't pay rent, they send you out of the house ... So many of them used to be in a no-hope situation and very sick ... also we found it very difficult that you cannot even give treatment because when somebody has not eaten, even the treatment will not ... will weaken ... So all the programmes you see here ... they have been lessons learnt ... on the long road we are moving on with these HIV/AIDS patients. (Interview with Christine, 21 April 2008)

This exemplifies the model of holistic care that is central to how the KCCC identifies itself as a unique Christian community-based initiative. In this model, social, medical, spiritual and familial support has to be combined to provide AIDS patients with a comprehensive form of healing.

The KCCC expanded its services in Kamwokya in the 1990s and 2000s with a wide portfolio of programmes that aimed to provide holistic care to people with HIV/AIDS. Many of these started as impromptu initiatives but, with the help of donor funding, gradually turned into more formal programmes. These include, among others, a Child Welfare Department, a primary school, a vocational training centre, a micro-credit programme, a youth HIV-prevention and sports centre, a post-test club, a community mental health programme, a clinic for both HIV-positive clients and the general public, and various food support programmes.

In the process of expanding and mobilizing donor funds for all these programmes, the KCCC was transformed from being a Catholic lay initiative into an NGO. It was registered as an NGO at the Ministry of Internal Affairs in 1994, officially taking the name of Kamwokya Christian Caring Community. Its transformation into an NGO entailed a shift from working with volunteers to employing paid staff. After 1993, volunteers started to receive a salary and the KCCC's work was divided into different areas of expertise with more employees being gradually hired. At the time of this research in 2008 and 2009, most of the 140 full-time employees were Catholics but there were also a number of Anglicans and a few Muslim and Pentecostal employees too.

The notion of being a Christian community committed to holistic care was still actively evoked in the organization at this time. For example, each working day started with morning prayers for all employees and volunteers, which included praise songs, hymns, prayers and official announcements. In the focus-group discussions old and new employees presented holistic care as the essence of their Christian community-based approach. For example, the pastoral counsellor Anthony, who started as a volunteer during the KCCC's first years, explained:

> When we are reaching out to the sick ... we look at the person we are caring for in a holistic way ... there are a lot of needs, there is social need, there is spiritual need, there are psychological needs and there are physical needs. So the approach we use on this person has to be holistic. (Focus-group discussion, 16 June 2008)

Rose, a Catholic counsellor who started working for the KCCC in 2004, explained it similarly:

> As a Christian you need to treat him wholly, holistic care, that's what one should approach, you treat the psycho part, the body ... the social, the mental part, and the economic comes afterwards, at least when the mind is set, he will even appreciate the medicine. (Focus-group discussion, 16 June 2008)

Despite the prominence of holistic care rationalities in such normative discourses, my experience when observing counselling and home visits was that these ideals of holistic care were under pressure from the bio-political concerns associated with the expansion of ARV treatment in Uganda and the dominance of neoliberal rationalities in international development. The following sections discuss how counsellors and community workers in the KCCC negotiated the ideals of holistic care in this changing context. The discussion begins with an introduction to ART as a global bio-political project and then analyse how counselling and home visiting have been redefined as governmental technologies in the context of ART and, finally, how the introduction of ART in the KCCC has coincided with an intensified importance of neoliberal development rationalities that have contributed to a redefinition of holistic care.

A Global Bio-political Project to Save Lives in Africa

The issue of ART in Africa has undergone a dramatic shift in the past decade. From a situation where treatment was deemed beyond the reach of most Africans and donors viewed ART provision in Africa as an unfeasible solution to the AIDS crisis (Jones 2004; Ngoasong 2009), expanding access to ARV treatment has now come to be seen as a humanitarian necessity (Nguyen 2009). It was estimated that about 10,000 people were receiving ARV treatment in Uganda in 2003 (Richey and Haakonsson 2004). By the end of 2010, this figure had risen to 248,200, which constitutes a coverage of 47 per cent (UNAIDS 2012). One of the major donors to ART programmes in Uganda has been the US President's Emergency Plan for AIDS Relief (PEPFAR), which has channelled funding to a number of faith-based organizations as well as to government institutions.

Access to ART was constituted a humanitarian emergency in the wake of a global treatment activist movement. Activists helped push for a dramatic reduction in the price of generic first-line ARV medicines (Hein 2007) and, more importantly, argued that access to ARV treatment constituted a right to life and one that should not be denied to the poorest people in the world (Smith and Siplon 2006).

In the context of framing 'treatment as a right to life', the large-scale funding initiatives that were meant to expand ARV treatment in Africa were, in turn, framed as compassionate projects that would 'save lives'. PEPFAR was, for example, introduced in this way:

> [T]onight I propose the Emergency Plan for AIDS Relief, a work of mercy beyond all current international efforts to help the people of Africa. (US President George W. Bush, State of the Union Address, 28 January 2003)

For the transnational consortia of NGOs, FBOs, foreign donor governments, private philanthropists and Northern universities involved in the ART scale-up, providing ART has thus come to constitute a way of literally saving lives in Africa. Their success is demonstrated by figures illustrating how many lives or years have been saved by the individual programmes (Nguyen 2009: 209). In a Foucauldian sense, this network is tied together in a bio-political project that aims to optimize life through the deployment of technologies targeting, describing and aiming to regulate specific populations (ibid.: 199).

This bio-political project is characterized by specific rationalities and technologies of government that are related to how ARV treatment works as a medical technology and to the challenges of under-funded health sectors, poverty and food insecurity that were initially seen as a barrier to ART provision in Africa (Jones 2004). As a medical technology, ARV treatment is premised on a strict treatment regime: medication must be taken every day at the same time for the rest of one's life in order to delay drug resistance and suppress the virus permanently. For the individual patient and the global project of achieving successful treatment outcomes, stringent adherence to the medicine is critical. Due to initial fears among Northern donors that expansion of the treatment in Africa would lead to 'antiretroviral anarchy' (Whyte et al. 2004: 17), ART provision in Africa has been characterized by a strict emphasis on treatment adherence (Mattes 2011; Meinert et al. 2009; Richey 2012; Kalofonos 2008).

To ensure treatment adherence, clinics employ a number of monitoring and disciplining techniques and combine the medical criteria for ART eligibility with social criteria. In addition, the expected challenges of ensuring treatment adherence in contexts of poverty and high food insecurity have been resolved in many programmes by complementing the treatment with food support programmes, micro-credit schemes and other forms of social support (Kalofonos 2008; Whyte et al. 2010). However, my experience in Uganda suggests that, as access to ARV treatment has expanded and the number of patients on life-long treatment has increased, programmes like these are now facing questions concerning sustainability.

New Technologies of Counselling and Home Visiting

When the KCCC began to provide ARV treatment in 2004, counselling and home visiting became central technologies of government to ensure the proper government of ARV clients. Prior to the start of the new ART programme, five new counsellors (to complement the original four) and 33 community health workers were recruited and trained to deal with the new counselling and follow-up procedures.

These counsellors and community workers counsel, educate and discipline their clients to follow a set of rules that are defined as central to achieving good treatment outcomes and preventing the spread of HIV. 'The rules' stipulate that clients on ARV treatment have to take their medicine every day at the same time, be punctual for clinical appointments, eat a balanced diet, avoid smoking, drinking, unprotected sex and overwork, disclose their HIV status and maintain a positive attitude. These rules illustrate how Ugandan ART providers are attempting to overcome the above-mentioned challenges of providing treatment amid widespread poverty by shifting a large part of the responsibility for ensuring that the treatment works as effectively as possible onto the individual patient (Meinert et al. 2009; Richey 2012).

Counselling

Clients are introduced to the rules prior to beginning their ARV therapy. When their CD4 count indicates that it is time to start treatment, their counsellor takes them through the rules and the implications of starting therapy. They are then referred to an ART enrolment group counselling session handled by a counsellor called 'Jagwe' In these sessions, the clients are taught that this is a treatment that comes with rules and that if they want the treatment to work well, they will have to abide by them.

A central technique used in the sessions is to educate clients about 'the enemies of the CD4'. A CD4 cell count indicates the level of immune deficiency caused by HIV. This has become a central indicator for when to start ART and how to assess the efficacy of treatment. In Luganda, Jagwe calls the CD4 cells *aba silikale* (our soldiers) and asks clients during sessions who the enemies of their CD4 cells are. After getting their suggestions, he then summarizes the five main enemies: poor nutrition, worry, overwork, illness and childbirth. Educating clients about what they themselves can do to increase 'the soldiers' in their blood is a way of encouraging and enabling them to achieve treatment success by taking responsibility for managing their CD4 cells.

In addition to such educational techniques that focus on enabling the clients' responsible self-government, more disciplining techniques are also used by counsellors and medical doctors. The disciplining of clients is centred on appointments. It is a general feature in ART programmes that the medicine is only provided in limited doses. At the KCCC, the first batch of ARV medicine lasts for two weeks and if the client does well during this period, the amount prescribed can be increased to last for a month and later to two or three months. When clients receive their ARV medication, they are given an appointment for a check-up when they will receive a new batch. Appointments and regular check-ups serve a medical function, since close monitoring is especially critical in the first month. However, they also serve to discipline clients to 'keep to time' and not to interrupt the treatment, as well as to offer doctors and counsellors an opportunity to assess whether clients are sticking to the rules. When a client comes for his/her appointment, the doctor usually asks the client how s/he is taking the pills. The counsellor may explore any social, emotional or economic problems the client is facing. When asking such questions, the counsellors and doctors do not know for sure if the client is telling the truth but the appointments offer the opportunity to continuously remind clients about the rules. The disciplining aspects of appointments are also reflected in the fact that clients who successfully honour their appointments and generally demonstrate a good adherence record are rewarded by having their supply of medication increased to cover two or three months, while clients who fail to keep appointments and/or have a poor adherence record will usually be kept on monthly dosages. Clients are also warned that if they demonstrate extremely poor adherence, they may be taken off the programme.

Home Visiting

Community workers involve 'the home' as a way of encouraging the family to assist in clients' responsible self-government. At the KCCC, home visiting was part and parcel of their initial efforts to offer a combination of material, practical and spiritual support. Prior to starting their ART programme, a new home-based care programme was initiated with the aim of ensuring effective adherence to the ARV treatment and the support of families and communities (Byansi 2006: 2).

Part of the home-based care programme includes assessing the client's home situation prior to starting treatment. A feasibility study has to be undertaken by the client's designated community worker to determine where the client lives and who will be responsible as a 'caretaker'. Though this policy is not always followed to the letter, it reflects how community workers attempt to render the home responsible for the client's adherence to the rules. Sometimes community workers also try to address complicated family relations that may impact upon a client's ability to follow the rules.

Apart from this emphasis on producing responsible families, the community workers' home visits are first and foremost focused on ART follow-up. After greeting the client, the community workers usually begins the visit by asking how the client is taking the medicine. They ask questions like 'Have you missed any medicine this month?' or 'Are you taking the drugs regularly?' A community worker may also check their client's pill jar and adherence card, which is a form clients have to tick every time they swallow a pill on time. Apart from checking the adherence card, the community workers often count the remaining pills to check whether the number matches the date of the next appointment.

The practice of pill-counting illustrates the 'ART surveillance' responsibility with which community workers are charged. This is reflected in the way their performance is evaluated in direct correlation with the ART programme indicators, such as levels of adherence, mortality rates and the percentage of clients 'lost to follow-up' – in short, the community workers' ability to effectively 'save lives' through ARV treatment. For example, at one of the daily morning praise sessions at the KCCC, the Executive Director used such programme indicators to single out the allegedly poor performance of the community workers (here called CBVs, which is short for community-based volunteers).[3] He said:

> You CBVs have a very big challenge, your patients and your performance have gone down according to the indicators we have put down: (a) many of them have disappeared. Why? That means it's either the follow-up or the recruitment. And (b) so many ART patients have died, these people are not supposed to die. Those people who gave us the money are now saying, what is the use of these people, when people are dying? How do we justify the existence of these people? One of our roles as CBVs is to ensure life continuation, isn't it so Mr Bisase? (Field notes, 27 January 2009)

This interaction reveals how counsellors and community workers are themselves disciplined and governed with the help of the statistics that the KCCC produces for their donors. These are the statistics that are, in turn, used in PEPFAR's accumulated account of how many 'lives' they have saved.

The above analysis illustrates how counsellors and community workers are preoccupied with encouraging and disciplining their clients to follow the rules as a matter of individual and familial responsibility. This raises questions about what space there is left for the provision of the kind of spiritual, material and social support that characterized the KCCC's beginnings.

Negotiating Holistic Care with Neoliberal Development Rationalities

In the context of the introduction of ART at the KCCC, the ideals of holistic care have come under pressure. KCCC informants still consider social, material and spiritual support to be important for the treatment and care of people living with HIV/AIDS. But with regards to social and material support new questions have emerged in Uganda about whose responsibility it is to provide such care, as access to ARV treatment has dramatically expanded. At the same

---

[3] The community workers have a status somewhere between volunteer and employee and receive a stipend, not a salary.

time, the KCCC had ambiguous experiences with their social services in the 1990s. Tracing the historical transformations in their social services and pastoral care approaches over the years illustrates the increasing importance of neoliberal development rationalities and how these have gained new significance in the context of the ART scale-up.

When the KCCC expanded its social services in the 1990s, it faced dilemmas related to the challenges of being a small NGO grappling with the wider structural inequalities underlying the AIDS epidemic in Uganda. In a slum area like Kamwokya and in a general context of persistent inequalities and limited social services, providing services such as free schooling, lenient micro-credit and food support raises questions about whether it is justifiable to offer such services only to people with HIV/AIDS. A number of the programmes that addressed the needs of people living with HIV/AIDS were therefore opened up to the general community in Kamwokya. This was the case with child-welfare services, which changed from initially helping their clients' children to generally helping a wider group of orphans and vulnerable children. When the services were expanded in this way, the number of people trying to access child-welfare support grew substantially. At present, 5 to 10 people are coming into the office every day asking for help, many from outside Kamwokya, according to the child-welfare coordinator. The department's core intervention is now support with school fees but because the waiting list to access such support is very long, there appeared to be very few instances where school fees came to function as a form of support for the KCCC's impoverished clients.

Expanding social services, often with the help of funding from small European and American faith-based organizations, raised questions about the sustainability of programmes. The KCCC's micro-finance programme was restructured in 2004 in response to donor concerns that it had become unsustainable. Previously, it had provided grants and interest-free loans to people living with HIV to help them start income-generating activities. According to my informants, this practice created the attitude that this was 'church money' and that clients did not need to pay it back. The programme therefore suffered from poor repayment rates and yet was facing increasing demand. The programme's donors subsequently gave the KCCC a final grant and asked it to propose a new programme that could continue without any more funding (interview with Anthony, 2 February 2009). The micro-credit programme was thus transformed into an independent Savings and Credit Cooperative (SACCO), which now functions as a revolving fund and has been expanded to include anyone living in Kampala District, and not just people with HIV. The SACCO requires a person to open a savings account first and s/he can then apply for a loan after two months but, to do so, has to provide security and have one or two guarantors. Most of the clients found these new loan requirements either unattainable or frightening. According to the SACCO director, 25 per cent of their members are people living with HIV/AIDS. However, in my experience and according to the KCCC, these loans have become largely inaccessible to their poorest clients (Ntale and Cunningham 2008: 45).

Another major change in the KCCC was the discontinuation of the USAID-supported food programme in 2006. This change was part of a general development in Uganda whereby food support to people with HIV/AIDS was discontinued in many programmes between 2006 and 2008, and abandoned as a priority within World Food Programme Uganda (WFP 2009). While food support was previously considered a therapeutic measure complementing ARV treatment, general food support to ARV clients began to be viewed by donors and many implementing organizations as an unsustainable measure.[4] This change can be placed in the context of the ART scale-up. Donors and implementing organizations are now providing treatment and care to a growing number of clients who are living longer and in better health, so providing food support to all has become questionable.

A number of counsellors and community workers in the KCCC regretted these developments, especially the discontinuation of food support. They saw many clients who were struggling to follow the rules because they did not have enough to eat, were worried about their children's future because they could not afford school fees, and had limited opportunities to generate an income to help themselves. However, there was also a general perception, especially among programme coordinators, that many of these social services had produced passive, demanding clients and that it was time for them to take responsibility for their own social situation. Counsellor and pastoral worker Damian, who has worked in the KCCC since it started, explained how, as much as they thought holistic care was essential, they had learnt that many forms of social and material support were unsustainable:

> HIV and AIDS, it is multi-sectoral, it is holistic, you have to deal with the total personality, and you are not going to give drugs only and think that the person will improve. There is food, there is rent, but the question is: are they sustainable? Like we used to pay for house rent, but we couldn't sustain it. And years went by and we started refraining from paying house rent. Because now after getting ARVs, our patients are getting better. And why do we want them to get better? It is so that they can look after themselves. They have to sustain themselves. (Interview with Damian, 28 April 2008)

Damian not only outlines how the KCCC has come to question the sustainability of interventions like rent and food support but also how the introduction of

[4] However, emergency food support for the most malnourished clients has remained a feature of most programmes.

ART has changed the terms of such support. Unlike in the early years of the epidemic, their clients now have the opportunity to improve in a way that might allow them to return to providing for themselves. The way the KCCC provides care and support had thus to change from helping 'helpless' clients to assisting them in 'helping themselves'.

Despite the opportunity that ART has given people to return to productive lives, the counsellors and community workers have experienced situations where their counselling has not worked because their clients had social needs that they could not address. Nevertheless, many of them maintained that all they could provide was information and counselling because social support, especially food support, was not sustainable in the long run. The coordinator of the home-based care programme, Mr Bisase, explained:

> There is also that dependency syndrome, waiting to be given. We tell them: 'It's high time, you start supporting yourself, you have been given the medicine for free, so the least you can do is work for yourself'. You see we found that food support was not sustainable. (Informal conversation, 19 December 2008)

The premise outlined by Mr Bisase exemplifies the dominance of neoliberal development rationalities in the KCCC today: when clients access the right to free ARV treatment, they are in turn obliged to take responsibility for addressing any social and economic barriers to treatment success they may encounter.

Such barriers were often referred to as 'psycho-social problems' and could include issues like 'lack of rent, no school fees and domestic violence', as Mr Bisase explained (field notes, 5 January 2009). Defining problems as psycho-social reflects the transformation of the rationalities around holistic care. Whereas the KCCC earlier attempted to help clients by paying their school fees or providing food or capital to start a small business, they now counsel clients on how to overcome such problems. Counselling involves addressing problems in the psychological and emotional realm rather than those of a socioeconomic nature. Clients now have to work on how they relate to problems like having no income and not being able to pay their children's school fees.

With this understanding of psycho-social support, a certain kind of pastoral care still has relevance. In a few post-test counselling sessions, pastoral care techniques were central in the counselling of clients who were finding it hard to come to terms with having tested HIV-positive. Pastoral care techniques were also relevant in community workers' attempts to offer the client hope and consolation in the face of a desperate social situation. Visiting a couple who were both taking ARV treatment, struggling to get by and felt they had been abandoned by everyone, the HIV-positive community worker Beatrice shared her own story of how the KCCC had helped her, assuring them that 'God will make a way for you' (field notes, 9 January 2009). Anthony explained that when clients come to him with social problems, he prayed with them, encouraging them to 'lift these problems up to God, and we believe that God will provide' (focus-group discussion, 16 June 2008).

A shift can thus be noted in terms of the Christian rationalities in the KCCC's work. In the late 1980s and early 1990s, they were 'feeding the hungry, giving drinks to the thirsty and visiting the sick'. They were *giving* material things and their time in an attempt to embody the presence of God. Today, they can offer 'only' prayers, consolation and counselling to help clients have faith and the determination to find ways of overcoming their struggles.

I therefore argue that we can characterize the change in how the KCCC conceives the treatment and care of people living with HIV/AIDS as having moved from an approach of helping to ensure their dignity in the face of serious illness to enabling them to 'follow the rules' in order to benefit from the life-prolonging potentials of a biomedical therapy. In other words, the KCCC is now focusing on how to produce responsible individuals who can govern themselves according to specific health-prolonging advice.

Living by the Rules Is Not Always Easy

Dilger, Burchardt and Van Dijk (2010: 379) have observed that the new era of ART has not produced 'the medicalised, disciplined or responsible patients that a project of this size anticipated' and point to how religious ideas, moralities and practices continue to play an important role in the way patients, families and health personnel ascribe meaning to life, death and healing. Apart from the continued importance of religion, the crucial material aspects of the 'incomplete reach' of the bio-political project of saving lives with ART need to be highlighted.

As organizations like the KCCC place the burden of addressing any social or economic barriers to the success of ARV treatment on individual clients and their families, most clients are coming to rely on the kind of material support they can access through kinship relations. Though a few clients found other avenues for support in post-test clubs, in Pentecostal churches or by gaining employment as 'Ambassadors of Positive Living',[5] most clients were attempting to follow the rules in the context of family and kinship relations. Following the rules is also contingent upon aspects such as stigma, denial and difficulties with disclosure. Such challenges were, however, often closely intertwined with social and economic factors so, for clients whose options for material support from kin were limited or unreliable, taking ARV treatment has come to constitute a

[5] Some people with HIV/AIDS are employed in AIDS clinics, home-based care programmes and HIV sensitization projects where they function as examples and support for their peers on how to live positively.

remarkably uncertain path to survival. I therefore argue that ART programmes are contributing to significant social divides between those who can manage to follow 'the rules' and those who struggle to do so. In this way, ART programmes interact with and are reinforcing existing social and economic inequalities in Uganda.

In the context of many clients' continued material challenges to benefiting from ARV treatment, some KCCC counsellors and community workers have questioned the premise of producing economically responsible clients. Anthony, for example, argued that, as a Christian, he sometimes felt obliged to help impoverished clients with a small contribution:

> Counsellors are not supposed to give hand-outs but in some situations when someone shares something with you and you find you have tears in your eyes, you may be forced to go into your own pocket and say, if I have 2000, let me at least offer 1000, but practically in training, they don't encourage us to give ... but in some situations because you believe in God, you go an extra mile ... God has given me, let me also give ... in counselling training, they told us not to give, but what does God say? If I really have 5000, why don't I offer 1000? (Interview, 2 February 2009)

For some of the original KCCC volunteers, there still appeared to be a close connection between embodying the presence of God and providing material support. During a home visit with Anthony and Damian, Damian emphasized how they were failing to encourage clients to see God as the provider. As he was explaining the situation of the woman we were visiting, he said:

> One of the daughters is on our child sponsorship programme. When her fees are paid, she feels OK, if not, it will stress her. If there are basic needs not addressed, you can keep counselling without it helping. Sometimes you need to have other practical interventions like rent and food but it's not sustainable, which donor will fund that? That is when we as counsellors also get affected ... If we say God is the provider, but there's no provision today, tomorrow, so why don't I leave God? (Field notes, 2 February 2009)

Damian thus emphasized the close connection between the provision of material support, enacting the presence of God and the client's sense of hope for the future. More generally, Damian, Anthony and Charles regretted that pastoral care had been sidelined in the KCCC's treatment and care efforts. Damian and Anthony blamed the neglect of pastoral care on the KCCC's professionalization and the fact that since the introduction of ART, home visiting has been left almost entirely to community workers who, as mentioned above, were first and foremost focused on ART follow-up and have not necessarily prioritized pastoral care.

A home visit to a client called David, who was a member of and preacher at a local Pentecostal church, exemplified how some clients felt a continued need for spiritual support and how this form of support also had material aspects. David lived in a slum area adjacent to Kamwokya with his ageing mother and a number of children. Community worker Doris (a devout Anglican) had come to visit him to discuss the fact that he had begun to preach on the street again. David was taking both ARV medication and mental health drugs, and had previously been admitted to the national mental hospital three times. According to Doris, the doctors at the KCCC were concerned about the effects on his mental and general health of standing in the sun all day preaching on the street. However, as the visit unfolded, it was clear that Doris's concerns were broader and involved Pentecostal churches having a negative influence on clients' commitment to the rules of ART, as the rumours of Pentecostal pastors discouraging members of their congregation from taking their ARV medicine abounded in the KCCC.

Doris discouraged David from spending so much time at his church, especially 'all the shouting' and the overnight prayers. She cautioned him that 'you cannot treat with the word of God alone'. But David insisted that going to church and praying on the street was crucial for his physical and mental well-being. He explained that he had attempted to return to his job as a school teacher but, given his mental problems, he found it too stressful:

> I tried to go back to teaching, but it's straining. But in church, you can just sit, not participate and you pass the day, like on Fridays we start at 3 pm and go to 6 in the morning. The problem is staying alone in the house with nothing to do. It is not the church that makes me sick, it's being idle. If I stay home, idle, my body will feel sick, even if I have a fever or flu, when I go to church, I'll come back when I'm delivered.

His mother then intervened and said that the church looked after him well and showed him love. David explained that the KCCC used to provide porridge and oil. 'So now we're badly off. In my church, there is always food and they give USh 700 to women to buy milk' (field notes, 12 December 2008). David thus claims to have found a sense of community and belonging in the church that delivered him from worries and minor illnesses. This would seem to be a form of community and a 'Positive Living' practice that the KCCC could not offer him. And in contrast to the KCCC, the church provided him with some food. Thus to David, the way the KCCC insisted he followed the rules was an incomplete strategy towards living positively. He therefore tried to insist that he needed to combine his ARV medicine with another form of spiritual and community-based support.

Conclusion

This chapter has shown that when the KCCC became involved in the ART scale-up, it also became part of a particular bio-political project. As a result, counsellors and community workers at the KCCC are now concentrating on counselling and disciplining their clients to follow the rules of ARV treatment and to take responsibility for any social, economic or spiritual barriers they face in adhering to them. In this context, the terms of holistic care have been dramatically redefined: material assistance has been gradually reduced and spiritual assistance is now defined as a form of psycho-social support. Though access to ARV treatment means that the KCCC are no longer confined to helping people die with dignity but can help their clients live longer, involvement in this particular bio-political project has raised a number of dilemmas in terms of how they should approach the social and spiritual aspects of suffering and healing.

The analysis above resonates with those who argue that global HIV treatment regime offers only a degraded form of belonging to people with HIV/AIDS in African countries through their highly medicalized and individualized approach to addressing suffering related to HIV/AIDS (Kalofonos 2008; Seckinelgin 2008). Large-scale ART programmes not only help to obscure the political and economic conditions of suffering (Kalofonos 2008) but also potentially sideline pastoral care approaches to suffering. For Catholic organizations, it is remarkable how involvement in the ART scale-up has contributed to a process whereby an approach to healing that focuses on ensuring dignity through spiritual and material assistance has been replaced by an emphasis on promoting individual self-government. However, this bio-political project does not resolve the uncertainties of living with HIV/AIDS but instead creates new concerns over how to follow the rules and may lead to inequalities between those who can and those who fail to follow them. Practices of pastoral care and material support as enactments of divine presence thus continue to have relevance for some counsellors and community workers and for many people living with HIV/AIDS.

References

The African Bible. Nairobi: Pauline Publications.

Behrend, H. 2007. The rise of occult power, AIDS and the Roman Catholic Church in western Uganda. *Journal of Religion in Africa*, 37(1), 41–58.

Biehl, J.G. 2007. *Will to Live: AIDS Therapies and the Politics of Survival*. Princeton, NJ: Princeton University Press.

Blinkhoff, P., Bukanga, E., Syamalevwe, B. and Williams, G. 1999. *Under the Mupundu Tree: Volunteers in Home Care for People with HIV/AIDS and TB in Zambia's Copperbelt*. Strategies for Hope No. 14. Oxford: Strategies for Hope Trust.

Bornstein, E. 2005. *The Spirit of Development: Protestant NGOs, Morality, and Economics in Zimbabwe*. Stanford, CA: Stanford University Press.

Bröckling, U., Krasmann, S. and Lemke, T. 2011. From Foucault's lectures at the Collège de France to studies of governmentality: An introduction, in *Governmentality: Current Issues and Future Challenges*, edited by U. Bröckling, S. Krasmann and T. Lemke. New York and London: Routledge, 1–33.

Byansi, P.K. 2006. Working towards accountability: The experience of Kamwokya Christian Caring Community in Uganda. *Learning about Community-Based Worker Systems Newsletter* 5 [Online]. Available at: http://www.khanya-aicdd.org [accessed 21 February 2013].

Christiansen, C. 2010. Development by churches, development of churches: Institutional trajectories in rural Uganda. PhD thesis, Department of Anthropology, University of Copenhagen.

Cochran, C.E. 1999. Institutional identity; sacramental potential: Catholic healthcare at century's end. *Christian Bioethics*, 5(1), 26–43.

Czerny, M.F. 2007. ARVs when possible, in *AIDS in Africa: Theological reflections*, edited by B. Bujo and M.F. Czerny. Nairobi: Pauline Publications, 97–103.

Dilger, H. 2009. Doing better? Religion, the virtue ethics of development, and the fragmentation of health politics in Tanzania. *Africa Today*, 56(1), 89–110.

Dilger, H., Burchardt, M. and van Dijk, R. 2010. Introduction – The redemptive moment: HIV treatments and the production of new religious spaces. *African Journal of AIDS Research*, 9(4), 373–83.

Ferguson, J. 2010. The uses of neoliberalism. *Antipode*, 41(S1), 166–84.

Fikansa, C. 2009. Reflections on the contradictions of ARVs from a practitioner perspective. Paper to the Prolonging Life, Challenging Religion Conference, Lusaka, 15–17 April.

Foucault, M. 1988. Technologies of the self, in *Technologies of the Self: A Seminar with Michel Foucault*, edited by M.H. Luther. Amherst, MA: University of Massachusetts Press, 6–49.

Foucault, M. 1993. About the beginning of the hermeneutics of the self. *Political Theory*, 21(2), 198–227.

Foucault, M. 2004 [1976]. Society must be defended, in *Lectures at the Collège de France 1975–76*, edited by M. Bertani and A. Fontana, translated by D. Macey. London: Penguin Books.

Foucault, M. 2009 [1979]. The birth of biopolitics, in *Lectures at Collège de France 1978–79*, edited by M. Senellart, translated by G. Burchell. Basingstoke: Palgrave Macmillan.

Hampton, J. 1992. *Living positively with AIDS: The AIDS Support Organisation (TASO), Uganda*. Strategies of Hope No. 2. London and Nairobi: ActionAid, CAFOD and AMREF.

Hein, W. 2007. Global health governance and WTO/TRIPS: Conflicts between 'Global Market-Creation' and 'Global Social Rights', in *Global Health Governance and the Fight against HIV/AIDS*, edited by W. Hein, S. Bartsch and L. Kohlmorgen. Basingstoke: Palgrave Macmillan, 38–66.

Jones, P.S. 2004. When 'development' devastates: Donor discourses, access to HIV/AIDS treatment in Africa and rethinking the landscape of development. *Third World Quarterly*, 25(2), 385–404.

Joshua, S.M. 2010. A critical historical analysis of the South African Catholic Church's HIV/AIDS response between 2000 and 2005. *African Journal of AIDS Research*, 9(4), 437–47.

Kalofonos, I. 2008. 'All I eat is ARVs': Living with HIV/AIDS at the dawn of the treatment era in Central Mozambique. PhD thesis, Department of Anthropology, University of California.

Kassimir, R. 1998. The social power of religious organisation and civil society: The Catholic Church in Uganda, in *Civil Society and Democracy in Africa: Critical Perspectives*, edited by N. Kasfir. London: Frank Cass and Co, 54–83.

Kelsall, T. and Mercer, C. 2003. Empowering people? World Vision and 'Transformatory Development' in Tanzania. *Review of African Political Economy*, 30(96), 293–304.

Larsen, L.T. 2011. The birth of lifestyle politics: The biopolitical management of lifestyle disease in the United States and Denmark, in *Governmentality: Current Issues and Future Challenges*, edited by U. Bröckling, S. Krasman and T. Lemke. New York: Routledge, 201–24.

Leusenkamp, A.M. 2010. Religion, authority and their interplay in the shaping of antiretroviral treatment in western Uganda. *African Journal of* AIDS *Research*, 9(4), 419–27.

Lock, M. and Nguyen, V-K. 2010. *An anthropology of medicine*. Chichester: Wiley-Blackwell.

Mattes, D. 2011. 'We are just supposed to be quiet': The production of adherence to antiretroviral treatment in urban Tanzania. *Medical Anthropology*, 30(2), 158–82.

Meinert, L., Mogensen, H. and Twebaze, J. 2009. Tests for life chances: CD4 miracles and obstacles in Uganda. *Anthropology and Medicine*, 16(2), 195–209.

Ngoasong, M.Z. 2009. The emergence of global health partnerships as facilitators of access to medication in Africa: A narrative policy analysis. *Social Science and Medicine*, 68, 949–56.

Nguyen, V-K. 2005. Antiretroviral globalism, biopolitics, and therapeutic citizenship, in *Global Assembalges: Technology, Politics and Ethics as*

Anthropological Problems, edted by O. Aihwa and S.J. Collier. Malden, MA: Blackwell Publishing, 124–44.

Nguyen, V-K. 2009. Government-by-exception: Enrolment and experimentality in mass HIV treatment programmes in Africa. *Social Theory and Health*, 7(3), 196–217.

Nsambya Home Care 2007. *Nsambya Home Care 1987–2007*. Kampala: St Raphael of St Francis Nsambya Hospital.

Ntale, C.L. and Cunningham, A. 2008. *Independent Evaluation Report: Kamwokya Christian Caring Community, Uganda. January 2004–December 2007*. Development Research and Training, Uganda and Kairos Consultancy, UK.

O'Manique, C. 2004. *Neoliberalism and AIDS Crisis in Sub-Saharan Africa: Globalization's Pandemic*. Basingstoke: Palgrave Macmillan.

Parkhurst, J.O. 2001. The crisis of AIDS and the politics of response: The case of Uganda. *International Relations*, 15(6), 69–87.

Patterson, A.S. 2011. *The Church and AIDS in Africa: The Politics of Ambiguity*. Boulder, CO: Lynne Rienner Publishers.

Rasmussen, L.M. 2011. From dying with dignity to living with rules: AIDS treatment and 'Holistic Care' in Catholic organisations in Uganda. PhD thesis, Centre of African Studies, University of Copenhagen.

Richey, L.A. 2012. Counselling citizens and producing patronage: AIDS treatment in South African and Ugandan clinics. *Development and Change*, 43(4), 823–45.

Richey, L.A. and Haakonsson, S.J. 2004. *Access to ARV Treatment: Aid, Trade and Governance in Uganda*. Copenhagen: Danish Institute for International Studies.

Seckinelgin, H. 2008. *International Politics of HIV/AIDS: Global Disease – Local Pain*. New York: Routledge.

Smith, R.A. and Siplon, P.D. 2006. *Drugs into Bodies: Global AIDS Treatment Activism*. Westport, CT: Praeger.

Swidler, A. and Watkins, S.C. 2009. 'Teach a man to fish': The sustainability doctrine and its social consequences. *World Development*, 37(7), 1182–96.

Uganda Catholic Medical Bureau 1999. *Mission Statement and Policy of Catholic Health Services in Uganda*. Kampala: Uganda Episcopal Conference.

UNAIDS 2012. *AIDS Info Country Fact Sheets – Uganda* [Online]. Available at: http://www.unaids.org/en/dataanalysis/tools/aidsinfo/countryfactsheets/ [acessed: 29 June 2012].

Vaughan, M. 1991. *Curing their Ills: Colonial Power and African Illness*. Palo Alto, CA: Stanford University Press.

Whyte, S.R., Whyte, M. and Kyaddondo, D. 2010. Health workers entangled: Confidentiality and certification, in *Morality, Hope and Grief: Anthropologies of AIDS in Africa*, edited by H. Dilger and U. Luig. New York and Oxford: Berghahn Books, 80–101.

Whyte, S.R., Whyte, M., Meinert, L. and Kyaddondo, B. 2004. Treating AIDS: Dilemmas of unequal access in Uganda. *Journal of Social Aspects of HIV/AIDS Research Alliance*, 1(1), 14–26.

Williams, G. and Tamale, N. 1991. *The caring community: Coping with AIDS in urban Uganda*. Strategies of Hope No. 6. London and Nairobi: ActionAid, CAFOD and AMREF.

World Food Programme 2009. *Country strategy for WFP in Uganda (2009–14)* [Online]. Available at: http://www.wfp.org/sites/default/files/Draft%20-%20Uganda%20Country%20Strategy%202009-2014.pdf [accessed: 22 June 2010].

Chapter 11

Notions of Efficacy around a Chinese Medicinal Plant: Artemisia annua – an Innovative AIDS therapy in Tanzania

Caroline Meier zu Biesen

> In the first decade of the AIDS epidemic there was no effective treatment for HIV/AIDS and patients were faced with nearly certain premature death. At that time, there were regular hypes offering hope for life. But with the introduction of ART, alternative treatments are now marked for many additional purposes too ... Biomedical practitioners generally discourage the use of alternative medicines, fearing interactions with ART and also through the concern that patients may stop using ART.
>
> (Hardon et al. 2008: 2)

Introduction

In the face of the underrepresentation of government-provided healthcare services in Tanzania and the resulting grave lack of treatment for AIDS patients – antiretroviral medications (ARVs) were only introduced in 2005 (The United Republic of Tanzania 2009: 1) – medical-technical and/or psycho-social care is often provided by NGOs, HIV self-help groups or (new) religious movements (Dilger 2005). Under the catchword of 'empowerment' many of these organizations have tried to develop and implement strategic concepts that help affected individuals to represent their own interests in a self-determined way. The 'empowerment approach' is based on the assumption that people living with HIV/AIDS can develop strategies of action and ways of designing their lives ('technologies of the self' cf. Foucault 1988), which allow them to approach their illness in a self-determined way and actively participate in the development of their therapy (cf. Seidel 1993; Schoepf 2001: 350; Dilger 2012: 68ff.).

In the context of anthropological research on the interaction between notions of 'health' and 'identity' (cf. Petryna 2002; Rose and Novas 2004: 440f.; Whyte 2009: 7), the concept of 'therapeutic citizenship' (Nguyen 2004: 126) was developed. It theorizes the (social, cultural) conditions necessary for active engagement with one's own state of health. This explicitly comprises the ability to indicate as well as demand medical care requirements (ibid.: 142). One of the central expectations – through which the concept's explicit relationship to daily practice is addressed – is that by claiming or enabling positive patient identities, access to medicines will be facilitated (cf. Comaroff 2010: 27). This focus on access to pharmaceuticals as the most important means to overcome therapeutic marginality has, however, been criticized by Nichter (1998) and Ecks (2005: 241f.) as part of a process of 'pharmaceuticalization' of healthcare provision. Pharmaceuticals provide more autonomy in healthcare, yet (new) dependencies on markets and health politics regimes are simultaneously created. Furthermore, the model of therapeutic citizenship does not adequately address the question of the balance between therapeutic and economic autonomy, as well as the question of patients' options for agency outside of treatment with biomedical medication – for example, through the consumption of 'traditional medicine'.

In Tanzania's government-run healthcare institutions, access to ARVs is tied to certain rules and regulations. Individuals desiring antiretroviral therapy (ART), for instance, have to prove that they are 'adherent patients' (Whyte, Van der Geest and Hardon 2002: 68). The regulations that patients are subjected to show that the central requirement of therapeutic citizenship's conceptual framework of healthcare improvement, based on largely unrestricted access to therapeutic resources, has hardly been achieved. The notion that access to ARVs is equivalent to a form of patient empowerment has to be at least partially revised in the face of extensive (medical) controls and disciplinary mechanisms, which can be seen as a disempowering measure (Mattes 2011: 160ff.).

The difficulties that AIDS patients in Tanzania encounter are not limited to restricted access to medicinal treatment. Even where medicines are available – and in the best case quality of life is positively influenced – patients still face new challenges. ARVs must be taken for an entire lifetime and this 'lifelong contract' (Swahili: *mkataba wa kudumu*) is experienced by many as a burden (cf. Dilger 2012: 74). The schedule for taking the tablets is not only complicated, but the therapy can have either no effect or unwelcome side effects (Liu 2007: 295). There is, moreover, no guarantee that ARVs will be continually available.

This multitude of uncertainties correlates with the large number of treatment options, especially in the extensive spectrum of traditional medicines. The market for medical-therapeutic substances for the treatment of HIV/AIDS could be described as prosperous and highly dynamic – innumerable new remedies have appeared in the therapeutic realm in the last 15 years (Hardon et al. 2008: 1). These remedies are heterogeneous, both with regard to their efficacy and their geographical origin. In Tanzania, the HIV epidemic has reinforced the need to integrate traditional medicines for the (symptomatic) treatment of HIV/AIDS within the (bio-) medical treatment sector (Kayombo et al. 2007; Stangeland, Dhillion and Reksten 2008: 290). The appeal of traditional treatment concepts is partially explained by the fact that in the framework of biomedical therapy, while an HIV infection is 'controllable' through biomedicine, the drugs do not lead to a cure and therefore do not offer a 'solution' (Bruchhausen 2010: 252). Another reason is that patients want to delay beginning a lifelong dependency on the drugs for as long as possible. Others have experienced the effective treatment of opportunistic infections through traditional medicines, or they have experienced that taking ARVs is only manageable when combined with herbal medicines (Hardon et al. 2007: 662). Government hospital control programs nevertheless often discourage patients from consuming supplementary substances, fearing that these substances will interact negatively with or endanger the continual consumption of ARVs (Hardon et al. 2008: 5).

This chapter explores the controversial tendency of Tanzanian patients to turn to medicinal plants in the case of an AIDS illness. At the center of this exploration is the Chinese medicinal plant *Artemisia annua* L., which has played a decisive role in the therapy management of an HIV self-help group in Musoma (Mara region) since 2003. The clinical utility of a component from the Chinese plant ('*Artemisinin*') has stimulated global interest in medicinal plants as potential sources of new antimalarial drugs (cf. Hsu 2006; Meier zu Biesen 2010, 2013). A series of pharmacological and medical studies – conducted by research institutions, European universities, as well as the international NGO Anamed ('Action for Natural Medicine') – suggest that the plant ingredients also have a palliative effect on AIDS-associated illnesses. It has been observed, for instance, that *Artemisia* – consumed in regular doses as tea – can lead to a stabilization of the immune system's T4 helper cells (Hirt, Lindsey and Balagizi 2004: 21; Efferth et al. 2008; Lubbe et al. 2012).

In the following I outline the influence that *Artemisia* has had on the medical care of HIV patients in Musoma and will elucidate that the adoption of the medicinal plant is based on complex negotiations about and attributions of its efficacy. Since *Artemisia* continues to be an important component in the treatment repertoire among HIV patients and is subsequently often combined with ARVs, this chapter makes a contribution to a field which has received little attention to date:

> The efficacy claims of alternative medicines often reinforce a biomedical paradigm for HIV/AIDS, and fit with a healthy living ideology promoted by AIDS care programs and support groups ... More interdisciplinary research is needed on the experience of people living with HIV/AIDS with these alternative medicines, and on the ways in which these products interact (or not) with anti-retroviral therapy at pharmacological as well as psychosocial levels. (Hardon et al. 2008: 5)

The available possibility in Musoma to bolster biomedical treatment for HIV/AIDS sicknesses with *Artemisia* is closely linked to the religious organization of the society. In 2003, the faith-based NGO Anamed – which works in collaboration with churches and missionary institutions – introduced the *Artemisia* plant to Musoma. Upon the initiation of Anamed, knowledge of the cultivation and utilization techniques were imparted, particularly to the members and medical experts of the largest and most influential church in the area, the 'African Inland Church of Tanzania' (AICT). The AICT plays an important role with regard to the health and social safeguarding of HIV/AIDS patients in the region and has expanded access to medical care through its healthcare service 'HUYAMU' (*Huduma ya Afya Mara/Ukerewe*) as well as its own church-led dispensary. One of HUYAMU's HIV/AIDS self-help groups ('*Kaza Roho*') has taken up the therapeutic use of *Artemisia*. The self-empowerment process initiated by this group enables patients to determine their therapeutic approaches and medical resources through the use of *Artemisia*.

This article examines the processes of the construction of *Artemisia*'s efficacy by focusing on the role of the AICT, HUYAMU and particularly its HIV self-help group *Kaza Roho*. The Christian beliefs in this group decisively influence the therapeutic concept and religious messages that are instrumentalized in the acceptance of *Artemisia*. In the *Kaza Roho* group, an environment of adherence and trust has been established, and empowerment has been institutionalized, all of which have an influence on the (perceptions of) efficacy of this plant-based therapy. Particular attention will be paid to the extent to which access to innovative therapeutic resources, such as *Artemisia*, is achieved through the group's activities. The construction of efficacy in this context encompasses forms of legitimization as well as the instrumentalization of (medical) knowledge. The appropriation of *Artemisia*, as observed in the *Kaza Roho* group, represents a new case in terms of access to therapeutic care. Special attention is directed to the economic independence of patients and the strengthening of the community. The question is whether an improvement in healthcare can be achieved primarily through access to ARVs – a question implied in the critique of the pharmaceuticalization of healthcare provision – or if other factors – for example, the dynamics of belonging or mutual support group forums for HIV affected individuals – are also significant for the expansion of patients' power to act.

***Kaza Roho* and *Artemisia annua*: the incorporation of a new remedy**[1]

The living conditions of people suffering from HIV/AIDS (*ukimwi*) in Musoma were precarious for a long time. Throughout the 1990s, a growing number of infected persons – recent estimates place the prevalence rate for the Mara region

[1] The chapter is based on the results of field research between 2006 and 2008 (Meier zu Biesen 2013). Through qualitative interviews with *Kaza Roho* members (aged 27–73) as

at 3.5 per cent (The United Republic of Tanzania 2007: 9) – could not receive sufficient care. In 2003, the HUYAMU healthcare service of the AICT began to respond to this shortage. Within their own dispensary, HIV/AIDS patients were offered services free of charge. Additionally, the group *Kaza Roho* (the Swahili verb *kukaza* means 'to fortify', *roho* means 'psyche, soul' and/or 'spirit') was formed especially for HIV/AIDS patients, and today claims 120 members in Musoma. The group's name reflects its constitutive formula 'be brave and strong': members not only receive access to medical care but also psycho-social support (*shauri nasaha*) to 'strengthen their souls'.

Kaza Roho adopted Anamed's medicinal *Artemisia* plant therapy concept as well as the idea of self-sufficiency and trust in personal strength (*siasa ya kujitegemea*), the latter of which was initially a politically motivated idea in Tanzania, though one which is transferable to the realm of healthcare. The use of *Artemisia*, a therapeutic source available at cost price and through personal production, is the focus of the group's activities. *Kaza Roho* dedicated a plot of land on which *Artemisia* is cultivated by all group members. The *Artemisia* tea is then processed and dispensed to members by the group leaders. Since *Kaza Roho* cooperates with the AICT dispensary, the *Artemisia* tea is also dispensed from there.

In order to guarantee long-term membership to *Kaza Roho* and thus access to its therapeutic resources, members must actively engage in the production of the *Artemisia* tea.[2] The personal cultivation of *Artemisia* demonstrates that patients can have a direct influence on their therapies. This type of therapeutic self-help is also relevant in relation to the socioeconomic profiles of the group's members, the majority of whom are widowed with little schooling. Most of them bear the sole responsibility for their children (cf. Dilger 2005: 189ff.).

In Tanzania, the AIDS epidemic has strongly affected the economically productive segment of the population between the ages of 20 and 50. At highest risk of infection are young women (The United Republic of Tanzania 2007: 8). The economic consequences for those affected are often dramatic: in addition to loss of work and lack of income they are often faced with high costs for medical treatment. According to the reflections shared with me by patients in Musoma, upon receiving a seropositive diagnosis for HIV, the women often experienced potent fear for their economic survival. Since the majority of the *Kaza Roho* members stem from economically impoverished backgrounds, the fact that participation in the *Artemisia* therapy was free made it economically advantageous.

---

well as my regular participation in the group meetings, I was able to document their specific orientation.

2 The group is funded exclusively through AICT donations. The space for action is thus limited and the programme can only function through the support of all participants.

Discussions of *Artemisia*'s efficacy among *Kaza Roho* members demonstrated that the low cost of the treatment, achieved through self-planting, constitutes an important factor influencing the preference for this remedy. Therapy with *Artemisia* is also associated with a form of 'natural healing' (*matibabu asilia*), as the tea represents a notion of 'harmlessness' in contrast to pharmaceuticals, since it is said to be 'free from side effects' (*haina madhara*). Interpretations of its efficacy contain further somatic idioms connoting strength: the tea's treatment effectiveness is described as vitalizing (*unapata nguvu*).

The following extracts taken from the biographical illness narratives of two women in Musoma are examples of the search for a suitable therapy that many HIV positive people undertake:

> I was informed in the hospital [in 2002, before ARVs were rolled out] that I am HIV positive. I was given Septrin tablets,[3] but I didn't feel better ... One day a relative told me about *Kaza Roho* ... I went there and they gave me *Artemisia*. After I drank the *Artemisia* tea I still had diarrhea but I wasn't as weak. The wounds (*vidonda*) and abrasions (*magonjwa ya ngozi*) began to heal ... I remember that at the beginning I didn't trust the tea, because I had taken traditional medicines (*dawa ya kienyeji*) before and paid a lot for them but they didn't help. But the *Kaza Roho* group encouraged me to drink the tea ... After my relatives and neighbors saw that I was doing better they wanted to know what happened. I had to explain *Artemisia* to them. (Angavu,[4] f., 41)

> In 1999 I tested positive for tuberculosis. I took the medication I was given at the hospital but my condition did not improve. The doctors advised my relatives to have an HIV test done. And I tested positive ... My family didn't want to believe it, they thought I had been bewitched (*kulogwa*) and they took me to several healers (*waganga*) ... but they couldn't help me ... My family took me to the hospital but there was no medicine. I then decided to join *Kaza Roho* ... My family began to isolate (*kutengwa*) me and I reported it to *Kaza Roho*. In response, they [group counselors] went to talk to my family ... I've had AIDS for ten years now, but I don't take ARVs. At the moment my CD4 count is so high[5] that it's not necessary. I only ever wanted to take herbal medicine and told them that in the hospital ... Because you suffer side effects (*madhara*) from modern medicine (*dawa ya hospitali*). (Sarah, f., 40)

---

[3] This antibiotic combination was by then the only care provided to HIV patients.

[4] All names have been anonymized.

[5] The CD4 helper cell in a HIV negative adult is usually between 600 and 1,200 CD4 cells/ml. The value which defines illness for AIDS patients is a CD4 count of less than 200 cells/ml (The United Republic of Tanzania 2008).

As Angavu and Sarah report, an HIV test was not only difficult to accept, but was also considered essentially useless by the *Kaza Roho* members since before 2006 there was no access to ART in Musoma. When positive HIV results were confirmed, members sought out various institutions offering therapies. Traditional healers were generally the first to be consulted, followed by hospital stays. According to the experiences of my interview partners, the therapies offered by healers or in hospitals frequently delivered no palliation for their medical condition. Since at this point financial resources were often exhausted, patients were finally 'ready' to try the herbal therapy offered by *Kaza Roho*. This therapy is described as a 'technique for health maintenance': in many cases, the tea contributed to a quick physical recovery, which enabled the consumers to improve their economic situation through the resumption of work or to reduce their care dependency on those closest to them. *Kaza Roho* members who receive the *Artemisia* tea at no cost experience, at least to a limited degree, alleviation from their financial burdens.

'You have to believe in this medicine. It only helps if you believe in it': Faith and Notions on *Artemisia*'s Efficacy

Approximately two-thirds of the *Kaza Roho* members are also members of the AICT. They receive support from the congregation and regularly participate in church services. The group's main meetings are also held in a building made available by the church. Integration into church activities makes membership in *Kaza Roho* more appealing to some individuals. The following statements make this clear, as well as the fact that Christian beliefs decisively influence the therapeutic conceptualization of *Artemisia*:

> It is my faith that keeps me alive ... Since I joined *Kaza Roho* I have promoted it everywhere, heralded the Gospel and have spoken about *Artemisia* ... after I saw that many people are suffering from HIV/AIDS and that it is a [emphasized] *normal* illness (*ugonjwa wa kawaida*) ... *Artemisia* gives us hope. We tell the patients that *Artemisia* increases the CD4 count (*Artemisia inaongeza afya mwilini*). I thank God that not a single person has complained that it didn't work. (Nabhani, m., 43)

> If this AIDS illness comes, you have to believe in God, deep in your heart. And then when you take herbal medicine, you have to believe in this medicine. It only helps if you believe in it. (Charles, m., 73)

The fact that influential church representatives propagandized in favour of *Artemisia* in Musoma established the basis of trust for some later members.

The affirmative line of the AICT towards *Artemisia* is rooted in biblical passages, which express high regard for herbal medicine.[6] However, the church's attempt to classify the *Artemisia* plant in a particular way can also be seen as an effort to conform to local expectations. With regard to the relationship between religion and medicine in Tanzania, Bruchhausen (2004) refers in his work on (traditional) medicine to assimilation processes, which are shaped by intercultural contacts. According to this theory, healthcare in Tanzania has changed continually due to the influence of various forms of medical practice – stemming from African, European, Islamic and Christian origins. Providing documentation from a medical history perspective, Bruchhausen has shown that the classification of processes related to illness and healing are significantly influenced by the interests of those who make the classifications. In the case of the AICT, the endeavour to classify the treatment with *Artemisia* in a particular way can be seen as an attempt to strategically correlate it in line with local expectations.

On the one hand, the appropriation of *Artemisia* by the AICT occurred in close connection with existing treatment options from traditional medicines that are trusted among the local population of Musoma. On the other hand, in light of the historical legacy and ongoing reservations that many contemporary churches hold toward traditional medicine (cf. Illife 1998: 29; Bruchhausen 2010: 249; Marsland 2007: 757), it is comprehendible that the AICT has simultaneously made attempts to redefine the treatment approach with medicinal plants and to disassociate themselves from certain traditions. The AICT's programmatic orientation – described as a middle way between Western and traditional medicine, conveyed through transparency and scientificity (Hirt and M'Pia 2000: 18) – enables them to take up a strategically convenient position in the Tanzanian medical landscape: in contrast to customary local 'traditional' medicine (here: *dawa ya kienyeji*), the classification of *Artemisia* tea as 'natural' medicine (here: *dawa ya asili*) provides a distance from spirit cults and witchcraft that is both politically and religiously motivated.

In church circles in particular, the definition of *Artemisia* tea as 'natural medicine' presents the possibility of legitimizing it for medical-therapeutic use. This strategic classification enables church leaders to avoid the transfer of their critical beliefs regarding occult practices – which they associate with the (polemical) category of 'traditional medicine' – to *Artemisia*:

---

6 AICT members often cite biblical passages referring to natural healing. Moreover, Christ's way of life – marked by his emphasis on practical action, which among others was manifested as healing – serves as a model for the AICT's work.

> Many people say traditional medicine (*dawa ya kienyeji*) is a sin. But I recommend *Artemisia* to my parish because I want to go back to the roots of our tradition (*mila*). (Mjeya, Bishop Anglican Church)

> The church says that only modern medicine (*dawa ya kisasa*) is allowed but not traditional medicine (*dawa ya kienyeji*) ... We try to help explain the difference between natural medicine (*dawa ya asili*) and witchcraft (*uchawi*). They are convinced by the truth of the Christians. (Mayari, AICT)

> People thought we were going against the *Lord*. They prayed for us because they thought we had become atheists. They scorned us when we carried *Artemisia* plants from the field ... It took almost a year until we could sell *Artemisia* in the dispensary. (Hara, *Kaza Roho* Group Leader)

The church's consecrations of *Artemisia* have had a major influence to the extent that the plant is currently used by a growing portion of *Kaza Roho* members for the symptomatic treatment of malaria as well as HIV/AIDS. In addition to the theological legitimization of the plant and the conveyance of its treatment potential,[7] *Artemisia*'s provenance has also influenced its acceptance and use by group members. Many anthropological studies show that the 'power of healing' is based on the transcending of boundaries, geographic as well as metaphoric. When viewed historically, the cross-pollination of natural healing practices, substances or (healing) knowledge across socio-cultural boundaries has always existed (cf. Luedke and West 2006: 4, Langwick 2006: 151), and the appropriation of the *Artemisia* plant in Musoma from another socio-cultural context (China) is an example of this mobility.

With regard to the acceptance of Chinese medicine in Tanzania – which has particular relevance from a historical perspective – we might turn to Hsu's (2007: 22) reference to 'social efficacy,' an efficacy that results when patients consciously turn to a specific therapeutic service that is regarded as effective in the context of social relations (cf. Whyte, Van der Geest and Hardon 2002: 23ff.).[8] The *Artemisia* plant is exemplary of this phenomenon, whereby medical goods 'from the outside' (can) assume a special potency in people's consciousness or expectations (cf. Evans-Pritchard 1937; Whyte 1988; Van Dijk 2006). Since Chinese medicine has a good reputation in Tanzania, the plant's association with China has a positive influence on its acceptance:

---

7 The potential as well as the limits of *Artemisia* therapy – immune strengthening, palliative care, alleviation of AIDS–associated illnesses, but *no* elimination of the HIV virus – are firmly conveyed to the members.

8 For a critical examination of how efficacy has been conceived of in medical anthropology, see Etkin (1988: 300f.) and Waldram (2000: 603ff.).

> *Artemisia* is really effective (*inafaa*). Since the plant comes from far away many people believe it is good medicine (*dawa nzuri*) ... And when you tell them that *Artemisia* is something foreign (*ni kitu kigeni*) that comes from China, it helps them to accept the plant because Chinese medicine (*dawa ya Kichina*) is well-known in Tanzania. (Kito, Anamed employee)

That *Artemisia* 'comes from far away' (*inatoka mbali kwenu*) is decisive for many patients, church wardens or medical experts. Furthermore, similar to medications that are associated with the technological advancement of their countries of origin, *Artemisia*'s acceptance has been positively influenced by the fact that European members of the NGO Anamed shaped *Artemisia*'s introduction through scientific directives for its indication from the Western context. The fact that the WHO's current recommendation for antimalarial medication is made from an active ingredient from the plant ('*Artemisinin*') has promoted further trust – among those people aware of this connection – of the efficacy of *Artemisia*.

Dynamics of Belonging and Trust: Accepting a New Therapy

According to my observations, the decision to pursue therapy with *Artemisia* requires a whole series of conditions. Firstly, such a decision is not solely dependent on the patient's personal preferences but is also influenced by family networks, which are activated when it comes to health-related issues. Some patients occasionally defied the directives of their social milieus; however, the decision (positive or negative) regarding *Artemisia* therapy coincided for the most part with an intersubjective consensus. One example of how important a role the private network plays in the decision is provided by the *Kaza Roho* initiators. They propagate the consumption of *Artemisia* in family settings – and thus integrate family members from the outset in the therapy programme:

> We teach patients and their families about *Artemisia* and tell them they should believe in God ... Many people come who don't even know they are HIV positive. We encourage them to get tested ... and we start the *Artemisia* therapy (Pauli, *Kaza Roho* Group Counselor)

> When I received my [HIV positive] result, I cried a lot. But I thought that maybe it is God's plan ... I decided to join *Kaza Roho*. The counselors asked me if I was ready to deal with my illness [emphasis] *openly*. They told me I should tell my relatives the truth and follow the motto 'Living with hope' (*kuishi kwa matumaini*) ... That was really encouraging. (Ruth, f., 36)

> My relatives were annoyed because I didn't want to take the traditional medicine (*dawa ya kienyeji*) from the healer (*mganga*) anymore. They even put me out. I wanted to take the natural medicine (here: *Artemisia*) because it is scientifically tested ... It was God who helped me. (Jonasi, m., 43)

The rituals of collective production and consumption of *Artemisia* seem to be only two of a number of activities that promote community spirit among *Kaza Roho* group members. The activities are also accompanied by the singing of self-composed, often religiously influenced songs. The songs address life with HIV/AIDS and the hope that many have (newly) achieved through *Artemisia*. That this hope is borne largely by the *Artemisia* plant is epitomized by a famous song called 'We live with hope' (*tunaishi kwa matumaini*) and the integration of *Artemisia* branches into dance performances. Statements by *Kaza Roho* members about their health condition usually follow these performances.

Lyrics of other songs like 'let's talk of *anamed* and natural medicine to overcome the suffering nation [in Ghana, Kongo, Kenya, Tanzania]', or 'wake up, let's focus far and welcome *anamed* to have a healthy nation tomorrow'[9] reflect that Anamed is (trans-) nationally active, and that its concept of the medical-therapeutic use of *Artemisia* has expanded to become a worldwide project. Other phrases such as 'let us unite and get *Artemisia* to overcome the wilds of malaria' and 'let's have a new start and face HIV' demonstrate the composers' conviction of overcoming (bodily) suffering through natural medicine. Moreover, it becomes evident that through the forming *of* and belonging *to* groups ('let us unite'), claims for *Artemisia* can be made and therapeutic improvements achieved. The forming of new, self-aware patient identities – as postulated in the *Kaza Roho* group, in which patients are emboldened to have an 'affirmative' self-perception and deal openly with their seropositive status – can be interpreted as the central requirement for access to medical resources.

The form of patient identity fostered by *Kaza Roho* and exemplified well by those songs is supported by the experience of (and belief in) the possibility of self-transformation on the basis of taking a proactive approach to one's HIV status (cf. Nguyen 2004: 126; Whyte, Whyte and Kyadondo 2010: 83). One of *Kaza Roho*'s special characteristics, for instance, is its implementation of a specific form of the concept of a symbolically hopeful 'positHIVe' life (cf. Dilger 2001). The group takes on this concept as an awareness raising measure and ties it to the collective empowerment associated with *Artemisia*.

Individual psychological aspects – such as patients' expectations – as well as (emotional) connections to remedies also play an important role in the acceptance of their efficacy (cf. Van der Geest 1997: 909; Luedke and West 2006: 9). Discussing the context of Tanzanian healers and their relation to healing

9 See: http://www.anamed.net/Report_Kenya_2009_English.pdf.

substances, Steven Feierman argues that the efficacy of substances is based on what he calls 'relational efficacy.'[10] According to Feierman, the prerequisite for the perception of or belief in the efficacy of a substance is the development of a relationship between the therapy provider and the therapeutic substance to be used. A medical doctor or healer can claim to be 'in agreement' (*kubaliana*) with the substance and this relationship of trust is carried over to the patient, which results in the patient experiencing the substance as effectual. This means that in addition to the medical effects, other factors such as relationality and trust in the substance play a role in its efficacy (cf. Feierman 1981: 357; Bruchhausen 2004: 133; Langwick 2011: 79).

In particular, for those people in Musoma who have been living with HIV for many years, who started to consume *Artemisia* while in a despairing state, and who still rely exclusively on the plant for strengthening their body's immune system, they perceive and communicate *Artemisia* as a bearer of hope. They thoroughly 'identify' with both the therapeutic concept and the medicinal plant itself. Here the previously mentioned relationship between health, trust and identity, as referred to by Whyte (2009: 7), should be taken up. To emphasize the process-related character of identity, Whyte suggests that an adjectival expression such as 'to identify with something' is preferable to the substantive ('identity') because of its emphasis on the process-related and transformative character of human identities. While 'identity' is an indicator of passive characteristics, pride about or the confession of belonging to a certain therapy is a proper act of 'medicinal cultural politics': a person who expresses loyalty to a specific therapy as part of an opinion-building process takes a stand and positions him- or herself in opposition to other possibilities. Furthermore, it is not only loyalty to but also trust in a therapy that can influence patients' therapy seeking choices (as well as the therapy's success). Thus, in addition to the perceived medical efficacy of *Artemisia*, numerous other factors play a role in determining its popularity and efficacy. Along with (self-) staging in the *Kaza Roho* group – and the associated (re-) activation of self-confidence – the fact that *Artemisia* has been declared a trustworthy medicine by the church has also influenced the therapy's acceptance.

I would like to examine another characteristic more closely in the following section: *Kaza Roho* practices a form of medical care oriented to individual needs. By now, many patients combine ARVs with the *Artemisia* therapy offered by *Kaza Roho*. In the following passages, I describe the consequences of the introduction of ARVs for HIV patients in Musoma and examine whether conflicts have resulted from simultaneous use.

---

[10] 'Relational efficacy': lecture delivered by Steven Feierman at the workshop 'Trust and intimacy in relationships of health and healing: Perspectives from Africa, past and present' on 11 February 2011 at the Freie Universität Berlin.

Establishing Proof? Chinese Medicine and its Interaction with ARVs

In 2006, the 'Care and Treatment Clinic' (CTC) for HIV/AIDS in the government hospital in Musoma was built and equipped with the latest technology. Today, the clinic is visited daily by up to 200 patients. Considering the high patient numbers and relatively small staff, the regional HIV/AIDS coordinator speaks of excessive structural demands. With the introduction of ARVs (*dawa ya kurefusha maisha*), a set of new control technologies, medical terms and treatment protocols have been established. As part of a three-day standard training that all HIV positive patients must undergo, patients are taught about possible opportunistic infections (*magonjwa nyemelezi*), the necessity of conducting regular CD4 counts (*kinga ya mwili*) and the correct way to take ARVs. Through interviews and observations, I noted that the measurement of CD4 counts was taken very seriously by many patients. The majority of the patients I interviewed not only shared their CD4 counts with me, but also carried their patient identification cards (*kadi ya utambulisho*) with them at all times. This open sharing of their viral load correlates to the process of 'personal identification' with diagnostic values described by Comaroff (2010: 27) or De Bruijn and Van Dijk (2012: 8).

The possibility of measuring the progress of an HIV infection through CD4 counts allows for the 'monitoring' of one's personal contribution to one's health improvement. Above all, for those patients who relied exclusively on the *Artemisia* tea – and who visited the hospital only for examinations but not for ART – the CD4 count provided a means of 'proving' their subjectively experienced improved state of health. The CD4 tests provided diagnostic evidence (cf. Adams 2002: 203) by demonstrating whether the CD4 count rose or stabilized as a result of the *Artemisia* therapy.

Two-thirds of *Kaza Roho*'s members were also taking ARVs in addition to the *Artemisia* therapy. In most cases, they were explicitly advised to do so by biomedical doctors. At the start of the ART programme, patients are instructed on how to maintain the rigid rules established by the medical staff (cf. Mattes 2011: 167). In addition to the requirement for healthy nutrition, they must avoid alcohol and integrate their medication in a disciplined manner into their daily routines. They are also instructed not to take any (supplementary) traditional medicine. This rule is justified on the grounds that cross-reactions can occur due to the intake of medications from various sources. Patients recounted to me that they were threatened with exclusion from the ART programe for non-compliance with this rule.

A consequence of this threat of sanctions is that patients often defy the rule regarding use of supplementary substances, though they conceal this from the biomedical personnel. *Kaza Roho* members justified their decision to me by pointing out that they experienced benefits through the *Artemisia* plant that they did not want to be denied. A decisive factor for the majority was that ARVs were only tolerable in combination with the plant. Through treatment with *Artemisia*, many patients experienced not only a stimulation of their immune system, but that the side effects of the ARVs, which are worsened by malnutrition, were reduced.

In some cases, the 'unofficial' *Artemisia* therapy functioned almost as a prerequisite for ART. In order for a patient to be eligible for ART a whole series of conditions needs to be met; the result of a CD4 test is the most important indicator. Officially, all patients with a CD4 count below 200 cells/ml are eligible to receive ARVs (The United Republic of Tanzania 2008: 30). However, patients with CD4 counts over 200 cells/ml are still provided with medication as long as they are already suffering from AIDS-specific symptoms, while patients whose CD4 counts are under 50 cells/ml are at a higher risk of their opportunistic infections worsening through the intake of ARVs (ibid.: 158), and thus are often not initiated onto ART. In this respect, my initial assumption that supplementary (and successful) *Artemisia* therapy resulting in CD4 counts exceeding the limit would mean that patients are denied ART was invalid. Actually the opposite occurred. According to the interviewed patients, it was an intensive *Artemisia* 'cure' that allowed them to stabilize their CD4 counts and achieve a bodily condition that finally enabled them to begin ART.

The interview segments presented below address some of the previously discussed aspects (such as the hospital prohibition against taking traditional medicine) and demonstrate how *Artemisia* and ART can be integrated from the patients' point of view.[11] The interviews also show how the attempt is often made – not only by hospitals but also by families or healers – to dictate which therapy HIV positive persons should use, and how these dictates sometimes constitute a form of test aimed at gaining experimental knowledge on the efficacy of a certain therapy:

> At *Kaza Roho* I took the *Artemisia* tea ... At the hospital they treated me with Septrin. Then I secretly combined *Artemisia* with Septrin, because the hospital does not allow mixing (*kuchanganya*) traditional (*dawa ya kienyeji*) with hospital medicine (*dawa za hospitali*). But since we have seen that *Artemisia* helps our health condition (*hali ya afya*) to improve we combine it anyway. Dr. [*] explained to me in the hospital that I would be very tired (*kuchoka sana*), if I only took medicinal plants ... We told him about *Artemisia* and *Moringa*[12]

[11] It should be noted that there is some methodological bias here, since the interview partners already belonged to the *Kaza Roho* group and had been using the *Artemisia* therapy for several years.

[12] Many *Kaza Roho* members add *Moringa* (*oleifera*) powder to their food as a nutritional supplement. The ingredients of *Moringa* are well-balanced (cf. Hirt and M'Pia 2000: 100f.).

> and he confirmed that anyone taking ARVs is not permitted to combine these with plants ... I remember a healer who said that his medicine would heal us. He said he wanted to test his medicine on a group of persons. I took his medicine for a year and I got better ... Then I got medicine from another doctor, who said we would be healed. But after I took his powder for two months, I was still HIV positive ... Then I tried *Artemisia* and started with ARVs. I can't attest that *Artemisia* cures (*kupona*) AIDS ... but if I didn't have *Artemisia* and hope, I would have died. (Nyanglo, f., 30)

> I was shocked [after I was diagnosed with HIV] ... At the hospital, they suggested I register for *Kaza Roho*. When I got there, I was really weak. I had a CD4 count of 300. At the beginning, I didn't get ARVs, but now I take ARVs because the doctors insisted (*walishikilia*). I still take *Artemisia* and *Moringa* as well. And that is good for my body. In the morning, I drink the tea and in the evening I take the ARVs. My last CD4 test was 437 ... I wasn't afraid to try *Artemisia*, because I was familiar with traditional medicine ... In my church congregation [Mennonite Church] they know that I am ill and that I use natural medicine (*dawa ya asili*, here: *Artemisia*) but they don't say anything because they're all familiar with it ... Without *Kaza Roho* I might already be dead, but now I live in peace, I see the future and there is hope. (Karoli, f., 47)

> The first time I took ARVs, I was nauseous (*kichefuchefu*) but I feel good now. When you use natural medicine, you get your appetite back (*inaongeza hamu ya kula*) ... In the [Catholic] church they know that I am living with AIDS and take *Artemisia*. They asked me if it is dangerous to combine ARVs with natural medicine ... In the hospital, they knew that I took both because they heard from the church and from *Kaza Roho*. We were instructed by the hospital to take the ARVs in the morning so we had to take the natural medicine in the afternoon. This way the ARVs could take effect (Jauhar, f., 36)

Patients and medical personnel from the AICT dispensary recounted to me in hindsight that the activities of *Kaza Roho* initially met with strong opposition from the personnel of the CTC Center, especially with regard to the introduction of ARVs. In particular, the criticism was made that treatment with *Artemisia* was not sufficiently controllable, and subsequently the safety of the medicine could not be guaranteed. This reservation is understandable since 'improper' consumption (i.e. contra to the indications of the *Kaza Roho* leaders) could not be ruled out. I observed, for example, that in spite of the guidance given by *Kaza Roho* or Anamed, patients did not always consume the tea (whether quantitatively or qualitatively) according to the guidelines.

Conflicts between *Kaza Roho* and hospital representatives resulted not only from their differing views on the efficacy of the *Artemisia* therapy. Significantly more straining on the relationship were the long-standing rumors that *Kaza Roho* discouraged its members from taking ARVs:

> In our district health committee there is a pharmacist, who accused us of forbidding patients to take ARVs and that some patients died because of this. But we do not forbid patients to take ARVs ... One day I met up with one of the members from the hospital and he told me that he heard many patients come to us [AICT dispensary]. They [personnel from the regional hospital] believe that we convince (*kushawishi*) patients to take plant medicine [emphasized] *instead* of ARVs. I think it was just jealousy because we have more patients than any other dispensary. This leads to competition (*ushindani*) among the [healthcare] institutions and envy (*wivu*). Sometimes patients are not treated successfully in the hospital and then they decide to come here of their own accord. (Dr. Rahema, Clinical Officer AICT dispensary)

In addition to medically based criticism, reservations concerning the *Artemisia* therapy were thus also reputedly the result of jealousy regarding the high client numbers of *Kaza Roho*, working in cooperation with the AICT dispensary. This makes clear how competitive HIV therapy management can become. Many patients perceived hospital consultations as a form of emergency care, and since, according to *Kaza Roho* members, the hospitals do not have enough capacity to respond to individual needs, it is understandable that patients look for an alternative. According to my observations, the choice offered to *Kaza Roho* members of either taking the plant medicine or combining it with ARVs made it an attractive option.

Over time, there developed a gradual cooperation between the CTC and the AICT health service HUYAMU regarding HIV positive patients' medical care. Those who initially hid their concurrent use of *Artemisia* and ARVs, or who started at a later point in time, benefited from the work of the 'pioneers' who introduced the *Artemisia* therapy to the hospital personnel. Furthermore, by visiting *Kaza Roho*, the biomedical hospital staff was able to overcome their concern that patients would stop using ARVs if they took them concurrently with *Artemisia* as they realized that the group leaders encouraged their members to continue with ART. The most commonly expressed reservation – that *Artemisia* can negatively impact the efficacy of the ARVs – was ultimately refuted by the evident improvements to patients' health. The appropriation of the *Artemisia* plant moreover initiated innovation processes, resulting in the patients' active participation in therapy procedures. The dynamics of the phenomenon of assuming personal responsibility as an ill person for medical-therapeutic care and actively participating in health betterment will be discussed in the concluding section.

Conclusions: Participation and Empowerment – the Shaping of a New Therapeutic Solution

In Tanzania, *Artemisia* therapy – originally developed in Asia for the treatment of feverish infections – has been integrated into a new socio-cultural context and modified for new therapeutic applications, namely HIV/AIDS. The therapeutic use of the plant demonstrates in an exemplary manner a medical landscape being transformed through dynamic interactions (cf. Luedke and West 2006: 6). The emphasis on the dynamic character of therapeutic practices is extremely relevant for my research context. If the *Artemisia* therapy appears upon initial examination to be a peripheral (and increasingly marginalized) practice in the otherwise institutionalized context and 'legal framework' of prescribed ART, the therapeutic landscape has proven in actual social praxis to be characterized less by a coexistence of techniques or therapeutic substances as by their interrelatedness.

To begin with, the appropriation of new medical practices must be construed against the background of (continual) resource scarcity; i.e. innovations may come about as a reaction to a deficiency. Pioneers of the *Artemisia* therapy were responding to the fact that ARVs in Musoma were available only in limited quantities. As the patients recalled, *Kaza Roho* compensated for these deficiencies – at least partially – through *Artemisia*. The motivation for patients to utilize the *Artemisia* therapy at *Kaza Roho* is in turn closely related to the given facts of the health institutions of Musoma. The fact that patients experience treatment in the overcrowded CTC as compromising leads to the situation that many use this institution solely for diagnostic purposes, and rather decide in favour of medical-therapeutic treatment with *Kaza Roho*. The CTC also ties access to ARVs to certain requirements that extend beyond medical control values, prescribing both therapy guidelines and a (partially) 'normalized' lifestyle. Likewise, however, patients can only become members of *Kaza Roho* under certain circumstances, making access to *Artemisia* regimented as well. The actions of the *Kaza Roho* members are strongly oriented to the rules of their respective social milieus, and the AICT and its religious messages are instrumentalized in acceptance of the plant.

A further aspect of the dynamic interaction between various medical fields is demonstrated by the increasing significance of modern technology-based diagnostic procedures for traditional healing practices (cf. West 2006: 24). This is exemplified by this case study in Musoma, since following the introduction of the technology for measuring CD4 counts, patients have the option to monitor their subjectively experienced changes brought about by *Artemisia* therapy. In addition, through this process the *Artemisia* therapy, which was at first regarded with strong scepticism by the hospital personnel, has become acceptable to them, as they can objectively verify its therapeutic value. Furthermore, over time the hospital employees realized that there were no harmful interactions, and they got to know the activities of the *Kaza Roho* members better. Subsequently, patients were actually referred by the hospital staff to *Kaza Roho*, and the two institutions have slowly developed a cooperative relationship out of an initially conflictual one.

Through the case study of *Kaza Roho* and *Artemisia* therapy, it also becomes clear that an understanding of (therapeutic) efficacy based on apparently universal factors has little meaning. Therapeutic efficacy can only be meaningfully defined against the background of respective culturally specific expectations in which both biological as well as social and cultural behavioral dimensions play a role (Van der Geest and Hardon 2006: 1). While the hospital personnel now see the curative efficacy of *Artemisia* tea as having been proven through the above described 'experimental' processes – the result of a change in perspective that took place over several years – other factors play a much more significant role for HIV patients in the construction of efficacy. Social and relational efficacy, trust, as well as the fact that the religious group *Kaza Roho* created space for this innovative therapy and institutionalized collective empowerment have all influenced the perception of efficacy and consequent acceptance of the therapy.

The rhetoric of participation and empowerment is widespread among many HIV/AIDS groups in Tanzania (cf. Mercer 1998: 250). However, while many groups simply use the call for empowered action as a slogan (cf. Schoepf 2001: 347), *Kaza Roho* puts it into practice as members are entrusted with a high degree of personal responsibility for their situation. The consistency of the group's approach makes this an innovative and exemplary element for the praxis of NGOs in Tanzania. The offer of a medical treatment with a medicinal plant, achieved through participatory action, presents a strategy for helping to improve the health condition of HIV positive persons through personal empowerment.

The strategies for action and 'technologies of the self' developed through the confrontation with illness are symbolically presented through the *Artemisia* plant, which is applied through personal initiative. Empowerment appears in this context to be the result of self-determined medical praxis. Knowledge of and access to medication are understood as an opportunity to reduce dependency on healthcare institutions. *Kaza Roho* promotes inclusion and the creation of new social ties, and attempts to counter to the greatest extent possible familial and societal exclusion. In this sense, the group possesses strategies of empowerment and is involved in the production of specific (self-determined) values and subjects.

Medical practices are established within the areas of tension between local, national and international economic and political interests (Lock and Scheper-Hughes 1990; Farmer 2001; Biehl 2007). Religiously influenced initiatives and institutions have a special position that enables them to create new social spaces. As represented by *Kaza Roho*, this unique role is characterized firstly by a deep cultural rootedness, and secondly through political and economic independence. Both aspects were of major significance in the case of the introduction of *Artemisia* and with regard to its legitimization among the population of Musoma. Firstly, the internationally operating organization Anamed, who first introduced the *Artemisia* plant to Musoma, brought Western scientific standards to bear on the efficacy of the herbal therapy. Furthermore, through newly negotiated relationships between biomedicine and traditional healing practice (brought about by the differentiation between 'good' and 'bad' traditional processes, between 'natural' and 'traditional' healing practices), a connection was made between *Artemisia* and pre-existing widespread local practices, which had a strongly integrative impact. In this way, the main advantage of the *Artemisia* therapy – namely the possibility of self-sufficiency supported through self-production – could take effect on the basis of a broad cultural consensus. The church-based *Kaza Roho* organization represents a unique junction in a network of diverse traditions, forces and interests. This position alone made it possible to achieve such a strong influence over the introduction and acceptance of *Artemisia*.

The significance of local individuals' ability to act and their creative potential in dealing with globally circulating ideas are frequently emphasized in theoretical works. The activities of the *Kaza Roho* group show that 'persistent processes and new arrangements' (Hörbst and Krause 2004: 50) are created through the local confrontation with biomedical offers and their limitations. The initial critique presented in this article argued that through treatment with ARVs, patients are medically cared for and can 'operate' socially, but are simultaneously excluded from participation in social and political life (cf. Biehl 2007). With regard to the integration of the *Artemisia* plant into the therapeutic lives of patients in Musoma, it has been shown that innovative approaches to (unauthorized) medicinal products and to social participation can prove to have a positive effect on the therapeutic process.

Kaza Roho members have overcome territorial and categorical demarcations through the self-aware utilization of a medicinal plant by – especially at the beginning – resisting the strict official guidelines for HIV/AIDS treatment. This 'disobedience' towards prescribed rules of behavior seems at the same time to be a defence of personal preferences in the configuration of the therapy. Patients – even those 'without means' in global relations – can either advance or inhibit developments in the healthcare field. The *Kaza Roho* group provides an exemplarily demonstration of this.

References

Adams, V. 2002. Establishing proof: Translating 'science' and the state in Tibetan medicine, in *New Horizons in Medical Anthropology: Essays in Honour of Charles Leslie*, edited by M. Nichter and M. Lock. London: Bergin and Garvey, 200–20.

Biehl, J. 2007. *Will to Live: AIDS Therapies and the Politics of Survival*. Princeton, NJ, and Oxford: Princeton University Press.

Bruchhausen, W. 2004. *Medizin zwischen den Welten. Geschichte und Gegenwart des medizinischen Pluralismus im südöstlichen Tansania*. Bonn: University Press.

Bruchhausen, W. 2010. Heiltraditionen oder 'traditionelle Medizin'? Von Förderung und Verweigerung des biomedizinischen Paradigmas in Tansania, in *Medizin im Kontext. Krankheit und Gesundheit in einer vernetzten Welt*, edited by H. Dilger and B. Hadolt. Frankfurt am Main, Berlin, Bern, Brussels, New York, Oxford and Vienna: Peter Lang Verlag, 245–66.

Comaroff, J. 2010. Beyond bare life: AIDS, (bio) politics, and the neoliberal order, in *Morality, Hope and Grief: Anthropologies of AIDS in Africa*, edited by H. Dilger and U. Luig. New York and Oxford: Berghahn Books, 21–42.

De Bruijn, M. and Van Dijk, R. 2012. Connecting and change in African societies: Examples of 'ethnographies of linking' in anthropology. *Anthropologica*, 54(1), 45–60.

Dilger, H. 2001. 'Living positHIVely in Tanzania'. The global dynamics of AIDS and the meaning of religion for international and local AIDS work. *Afrika spectrum*, 36(1), 73–90.

Dilger, H. 2005. *Leben mit AIDS. Krankheit, Tod und soziale Beziehungen in Afrika. Eine Ethnographie*. Frankfurt: Campus-Verlag.

Dilger, H. 2012. Targeting the Empowered Individual: Transnational Policy-Making, the Global Economy of Aid and the Limitation of 'Biopower' in the Neoliberal Era, in *Medicine, Mobility, and Power in Global Africa: Transnational Health and Healing*, edited by H. Dilger, A. Kane and S. Langwick. Bloomington, IN: Indiana University Press, 60–91.

Ecks, S. 2005. Pharmaceutical citizenship: Antidepressant marketing and the promise of demarginalization in India. *Anthropology and Medicine*, 12(3), 239–54.

Efferth, T., Romero, M.R., Wolf, D.G., Stamminger, T., Main, J.J.G. and Marschall, M. 2008. The antiviral activities of artemisinin and artesunate. *Clinical Infectious Diseases*, 47, 804–11.

Etkin, N.L. 1988. Cultural constructions of efficacy, in *The Context of Medicines in Developing Countries: Studies in Pharmaceutical Anthropology (Culture, Illness and Healing)*, edited by S.R. Whyte and S. van der Geest. Amsterdam: Het Spinhuis, 299–326.

Evans-Pritchard, E.E. 1978 [1937]. *Witchcraft, Oracles and Magic among the Azande*. New York: Oxford University Press.

Farmer, P. 2001. *Infections and Inequalities: The Modern Plagues*. Berkeley, CA: University of California Press.

Feierman, S. 1981. Therapy as a system-in-action in northeastern Tanzania. *Social Science and Medicine*, 15(B), 353–60.

Foucault, M. 1988. Technologies of the self: A seminar with Michel Foucault, in *Technologies of the Self*, edited by H.M. Luther, H. Gutman and P.H. Hutton. Amherst, MA: University of Massachusetts Press, 16–50.

Hardon, A, Akurut, D., Comoro, C., Ekezie, C., Irunde, H.F. and Gerrits, T. 2007. Hunger, waiting time and transport costs: Time to confront challenges to ART adherence in Africa. *AIDS Care*, 19(5), 658–65.

Hardon, A., Desclaux, A., Ergot, M., Simon, E., Micollier, E. and Kyakuwa, M. 2008. Alternative medicines for AIDS in resource-poor settings: Insights from Exploratory Anthropological Studies in Asia and Africa. *Journal of Ethnobiology and Ethnomedicine*, 4, 1–6.

Hirt, H.M. and M'Pia, B. 2000. *Natürliche Medizin in den Tropen*. Winnenden: Anamed – Aktion Natürliche Medizin.

Hirt, H.-M., Lindsey, K. and Balagizi, I. 2004. *Natural Medicine in the Tropics: AIDS and Natural Medicine*. Winnenden: Anamed – Aktion Natürliche Medizin.

Hörbst, V. and Krause, K. 2004. 'On the Move' – Die Globalisierungsdebatte in der Medizinethnologie. *Curare*, 27(1 and 2), 41–60.

Hsu, E. 2006. Reflections on the 'discovery' of the antimalarial Qinghao. *British Journal of Clinical Pharmacology*, 61(6), 666–70.

Hsu, E. 2007. Chinese medicine in East Africa and its effectiveness. *IIAS Newsletter*, 45(Autumn), 22.

Illife, J. 1998. *East African Doctors: A History of the Modern Profession*. Cambridge: Cambridge University Press.

Kayombo, E.J., Uiso, F.C., Mbwambo, Z.H., Mahunnah, R.L., Moshi, M.J. and Mgonda, J.H. 2007. Experience of initiating collaboration of traditional healers in managing HIV and AIDS in Tanzania. *Journal of Ethnobiology and Ethnomedicine*, 3(6), 1–9.

Langwick, S. 2006. Geographies of medicine: Integrating the boundary between 'traditional' and 'modern' medicine in Tanganyika, in *Borders and Healers: Brokering Therapeutic Resources in Southeast Africa*, edited by T.J. Luedke and H.G. West. Bloomington, IN: Indiana University Press, 143–66.

Langwick, S. 2011. *Bodies, Politics, and African Healing: The Matter of Maladies in Tanzania*. Bloomington, IN: Indiana University Press.

Liu, J. 2007. An overview of clinical studies on complementary and alternative medicine in HIV infection and AIDS, in *Traditional, Complementary and Alternative Medicine: Policy and Public Health Perspectives*, edited by G. Bodeker and G. Burford. London: Imperial College Press, 295–308.

Lock, M. and Scheper-Hughes, N. 1990. A critical-interpretive approach in medical anthropology: Rituals and routines of discipline and dissent, in *Medical Anthropology: Contemporary Theory and Method*, edited by T. Johnson and C. Sargent. New York: Praeger, 47–72.

Lubbe, A., Seibert, I., Klimkait, T. and Van der Kooy, F. 2012. Ethnopharmacology in overdrive: The remarkable anti-HIV activity of *Artemisia annua*. *Journal of Ethnopharmacology*, 141(3), 854–9.

Luedke, T.J. and West, H.G. (eds) 2006. *Borders and Healers: Brokering Therapeutic Resources in Southeast Africa*. Bloomington, IN: Indiana University Press.

Marsland, R. 2007. The modern traditional healer: locating 'hybridity' in modern traditional medicine, Southern Tanzania. *Journal of Southern African Studies*, 33(4), 751–65.

Mattes, D. 2011. 'We are just supposed to be quiet': The production of adherence to antiretroviral treatment in urban Tanzania. *Medical Anthropology*, 30(2), 158–82.

Meier zu Biesen, C. 2010. The rise to prominence of *Artemisia annua L.* – The transformation of a Chinese plant to a global pharmaceutical. *African Sociological Review. Revue Africaine de Sociologie*, 14(2), 24–46.

Meier zu Biesen, C. 2013. *Globale Epidemien – lokale Antworten. Eine Ethnographie der Heilpflanze Artemisia annua in Tansania*. Frankfurt: Campus-Verlag.

Mercer, C. 1998. Reconceptualising state-society relations in Tanzania: Are NGOs making a difference? *Royal Geographical Society*, 31(3), 247–58.

Nguyen, V.-K. 2004. Antiretroviral globalism, biopolitics, and therapeutic citizenship, in *Global Assemblages: Technologies, Politics, and Ethics as Anthropological Problems*, edited by A. Ong and S.J. Collier. Malden, MA, and Oxford: Blackwell Publishing, 124–44.

Nichter, M. 1998. The mission within the madness: Self-initiated medicalization as expression of agency, in *Pragmatic Women and Body Politics*, edited by M. Lock and P.A. Kaufert. Cambridge Studies in Medical Anthropology. New York: Cambridge University Press 327–53.

Petryna, A. 2002. *Life Exposed: Biological Citizens after Chernobyl*. Princeton, NJ: Princeton University Press.

Rose, N. and Novas, C. 2004. Biological citizenship, in *Global Assemblages: Technologies, Politics, and Ethics as Anthropological Problems*, edited by A. Ong and S.J. Collier. Malden, MA, and Oxford: Blackwell Publishing, 439–63.

Schoepf, B.G. 2001. International AIDS research in anthropology: Taking a critical perspective on the crisis. *Annual Review of Anthropology*, 30, 335–61.

Seidel, G. 1993. The competing discourses of HIV/AIDS in sub-Saharan Africa: Discourses of rights and empowerment vs. discourses of control and exclusion. *Social Science and Medicine*, 36(3), 175–94.

Stangeland, T., Dhillion, S.S. and Reksten, H. 2008. Recognition and development of traditional medicine in Tanzania. *Journal of Ethnopharmacology*, 117(2), 290–99.

The United Republic of Tanzania 2007. *Health Sector HIV and AIDS Strategy Plan (HSSP) 2008–12*. Zero Draft, 25th May 2007.

The United Republic of Tanzania 2008. *National Aids Control Programme: National Guidelines for the Management of HIV and AIDS*. Ministry of Health Tanzania, Dar es Salaam.

The United Republic of Tanzania 2009. *Progress Report on the Implementation of the National Care and Treatment Programme*. Dar es Salaam: National AIDS Control Programme.

Van der Geest, S. 1997. Is there a role for traditional medicine in basic health services in Africa? A plea for a community perspective. *Tropical Medicine and International Health*, 2(9), 903–11.

Van der Geest, S. and Hardon, A. 2006. Social and cultural efficacies of medicines: Complications for antiretroviral therapy. *Journal of Ethnobiology and Ethnomedicine*, 2(48), 1–5.

Van Dijk, R. 2006. Transnational images of Pentecostal healing: comparative examples from Malawi and Botswana, in *Borders and Healers: Brokering Therapeutic Resources in Southeast Africa*, edited by T.J. Luedke and H.G. West. Bloomington, IN: Indiana University Press, 101–24.

Waldram, J.B. 2000. The efficacy of traditional medicine: Current theoretical and methodological issues. *Medical Anthropology Quarterly*, 14(4), 603–25.

West, H.G. 2006. Working the borders to beneficial effect: The not-so-indigenous knowledge of not-so-traditional healers in northern Mozambique, in *Borders and Healers: Brokering Therapeutic Resources in Southeast Africa*, edited by T.J. Luedke and H.G. West. Bloomington, IN: Indiana University Press, 21–42.

Whyte, S.R. 1988. The power of medicines in east Africa, in *The Context of Medicines in Developing Countries: Studies in Pharmaceutical Anthropology (Culture, Illness and Healing*, edited by S.R. Whyte and S. van der Geest. Amsterdam: Het Spinhuis, 217–35.

Whyte, S.R. 2009. Health identities and subjectivities: The ethnographic challenge. *Medical Anthropology Quarterly*, 23(1), 6–15.

Whyte, S.R., Van der Geest, S. and Hardon, A. (eds) 2002. *Social Lives of Medicines*. New York: Cambridge University Press.

Whyte, S.R., Whyte, M.A. and Kyadondo, D. 2010. Health workers entangled: Confidentiality and certification?, in *Morality, Hope and Grief: Anthropologies of AIDS in Africa*, edited by H. Dilger and U. Luig. New York and Oxford: Berghahn Books, 80–101.

Willcox, M.L., Burton, S., Oyweka, R., Namyalo, R., Challand, S. and Lindsey, K. 2011. Evaluation and pharmacovigilance of projects promoting cultivation and local use of Artemisia annua for Malaria. *Malaria Journal*, 10(84), 1–24.

Index